Plexus Anesthesia

Volume I

Perivascular Techniques of Brachial Plexus Block

D1327648

ALON P. WINNIE, M. D.

Professor and Chairman
of the Department of Anesthesiology,
University of Illinois
Chicago, USA

LENNART HÅKANSSON

Editor

POUL BUCKHÖJ

Medical artist

KARSTEN HJERTHOLM

Photo

POUL BUCKHÖJ

Layout

CHURCHILL LIVINGSTONE
EDINBURGH LONDON MELBOURNE
AND NEW YORK 1984

CHURCHILL LIVINGSTONE
Medical Division of Longman Group Limited

Distributed in all areas except USA and Scandinavia by
Churchill Livingstone, Robert Stevenson House, 1-3 Baxter's
Place, Leith Walk, Edinburgh EH1 3AF.

Distributed in the USA by
W. B. Saunders, West Washington Square, Philadelphia,
Pa 19105, USA.

Distributed in Scandinavia by
Schultz Medical Information ApS, 21, Møntergade,
DK-1116 Copenhagen K

First published 1983

ISBN 0 7216 1172 9 (Saunders)
      87 569 1106 8 (Schultz)
      0 443 03222 X (Churchill Livingstone)

British Library Cataloguing in Publication Data
Plexus Anesthesia
vol 1: Perivascular techniques of Brachial
Plexus Block
1. Choroid Plexus 2. Anasthesia
i Winnie, Alon P.
617'.967481 rd594

Printed in Denmark by
J. H. Schultz A/S

Plexus Anesthesia

Volume I

Contents

Foreword

A hundred years ago, Koller introduced the first local anesthetic agent into surgical practice, and the impact was enormous. A couple of hours in the medical library of the University of Oxford reveal that within a short period many dozens of doctoral theses were written on different methods of producing local and regional analgesia, some of them quaint to a degree. These hail from medical schools on the mainland of Europe where the art and science of general anesthesia had been strangely disregarded. The price for this neglect in terms of mortality and morbidity was great, and the remedy seems to have been local analgesia for pain relief. For decades afterwards in these parts of the globe local analglesia was commonplace in the operating theatre, general anesthesia exceptional.

But research into general anesthetics continued in the English-speaking countries, and here these were used almost to the exclusion of locals. The pendulum now is swinging backwards, and we find regional analgesia increasingly in use. Two factors have contributed to this: there is a much greater variety of agents to choose from, so that the effects can be tailored to any particular surgical procedure; pain relief can be assured throughout the actual operation, and if required well into the post-operative period. Of equal importance, a more detailed knowledge of the anatomy involved has led to the development of more precise techniques to deposit the local anesthetic solution for optimum effect.

Over the past few years, I have seen the production of a new and greatly improved breed of books on these important subjects which reflect an ever increasing interest in regional analgesia and a greater understanding of the problems involved and how these can be overcome. And now to these contributions is added this splendid masterpiece by Alon Winnie. For the twenty years I have known him the disposition of the fascia surrounding muscles, nerves and vessels has been one of his main interests in his professional life, and many are the hours he has spent in the post-mortom room to confirm the impressions formed in the operating theatrè.

This book will be of great practical help to every anesthetist, junior and senior. Moreover, it makes a fascinating story of research and discovery. If medical eponyms are still in vogue, surely "Winnie's fascia" should find its way into our nomenclature.

Robert Macintosh

Dedication

Authors often acknowledge persons "without whom this work would not have been possible," an obvious exaggeration but one that is indicative of gratitude and a certain degree of indebtedness to secretaries, artists, proofreaders, editors, and even to wives, sweethearts, and mistresses, depending upon the nature of the author's literary product. Clearly, the work *could* have been completed without the specific individual or individuals being acknowledged, though the product might have taken longer to produce or, perhaps, might even have taken on a different character or format, depending on the degree of participation of the individual or individuals to whom the author is expressing gratitude.

It is my privilege, as author of this book, which is the product of a major part of my professional life, to acknowledge a group of individuals without whom this work *really* would not have been possible, for without them I would not have survived to undertake the present work. So I acknowledge and dedicate this book to those physicians to whom I am indebted for life itself, my fellow interns and residents of Cook County Hospital who, exhausted from their own demanding call schedules, took an additional call to protect me from the possible malfunction of the ventilator upon which my life depended while I was totally paralyzed from acute poliomyelitis. Repeatedly, when my ventilator malfunctioned or failed, these vigilant young physician friends succeeded in keeping me alive until the ventilator could be repaired. Clearly, without them this work would *not* have been possible.

Plexus Anesthesia to me represents the epitome of the science of anesthesiology, the application of fundamental anatomic principles to form a clinical concept which, carried out with sufficient technical skill and clinical judgment, results in enhanced safety for the surgical patient. If this book can provide an understanding of the principles upon which the concept of plexus anesthesia is based and make available this safe and effective form of anesthesia to patients in whom it might be appropriate, then my efforts will not be in vain. And if, in just one instance, the resultant ability of an anesthetist to provide this safer alternative to general anesthesia proves to be life-saving, then I feel that those colleagues who saved my life repeatedly and made this book possible will finally see a rewarding return on their investment in me. For this work is the result of their friendship and dedication.

Preface

Both the axillary and supraclavicular approaches to percutaneous brachial plexus block anesthesia, introduced in 1911, were received enthusiastically as much safer alternatives to general anesthesia and all its dreaded complications. This enthusiasm increased over the next decade, giving rise to a multitude of reports of the advantages and disadvantages of this new form of anesthesia, which was given an even greater impetus by the first World War because of the many upper extremity injuries that invariably result from war. However, in the two decades following World War I, as technical and pharmacological advances rendered general anesthesia safer and as anesthesiology began to evolve as a medical discipline, regional anesthesia was utilized less and less and general anesthesia was utilized more and more for upper extremity surgery. Surgeons no longer had to be proficient in regional anesthesia in order to avoid general anesthesia, and new physician-anesthetists, not being surgeons, were certainly less familiar with the anatomical knowledge necessary for regional anesthesia than their surgeon-anesthetist predecessors. In those parts of the world where nurses were recruited to become anesthetists, their training was almost exclusively in the techniques of general anesthesia.

As stated succinctly by Macintosh, "to the advantages of local anesthesia, both to patient and surgeon, there is common assent. Among its disadvantages is the uncertainty of bringing the local anesthetic into contact with the nerves carrying sensory impulses from the field of operation." In 1940 Patrick described a technique of supraclavicular brachial plexus block that went a long way toward "the removal of this uncertainty" by obviating need to actually locate the brachial plexus with the needle. Rather than having the anesthetist probe repeatedly in an attempt to identify the precise location of the plexus, this technique called for the anesthetist to deposit a "wall of local anesthetic" on top of the first rib extensive enough to ensure that the brachial plexus would be blocked.

Medical educators are well aware that the simple publication of a new technique in no way guarantees its acceptance. This is particularly true when that publication reports a regional anesthetic procedure to a population of anesthetists absorbed in the rapidly evolving technology of general anesthesia. Thus it fell to Sir Robert Macintosh and William Mushin, two of the greatest educators of all time in anesthesiology, to popularize this "solution" to the problem of brachial plexus anesthesia by the publication of their excellent monograph entitled "Local Anesthesia: Brachial Plexus". Giving full credit to Patrick for the development of the technique, "which for the first time enabled the procedure to be undertaken with assurance that anesthesia would result", they presented a classic monograph "in which the main instruction is conveyed by pictures instead of by the written word". The pictorial format was a result of their observation that "it has sometimes been difficult to learn a particular technique from textbooks," especially when compared with "the comparative ease with which a considerable amount can be learned from *watching* masters of the art"; and since not everyone has the opportunity to learn by watching the masters, they "can be given many of the advantages of the eye-witness if they are taught by a pictorial method". The success of their efforts is attested to by the fact that the monograph came out in four editions, the first in 1944 and the last in 1967, a span of almost a quarter of a century!

Nonetheless, in 1946 John Lundy stated, "I know of no one who can describe a technique which is certain in all cases. However, I expect that sooner or later someone will make a sufficiently close examination of the anatomy involved... that an exact technique will be developed." Certainly Patrick's technique, as effective as it is, is not "an exact technique"; in fact, it was designed to obviate the need for an exact technique. However, the present author feels that the "plexus block" concept does provide the anatomical basis for Lundy's "exact technique". That concept results from the fact that all of the plexuses, at some point in their formation and/or distribution, pass between two muscles, and hence may be considered to be "invested" by the fascia of those muscles. At this point the plexus lies in a potential "interfascial compartment", so if this compartment can be identified and entered by a needle, then the plexus can be blocked by a single injection rather than by the multiple injections required to lay down the "wall of anesthetic" called for by Patrick's technique. Injection of an appropriate volume of anesthetic into such an "interfascial compartment" allows the solution, rather than the needle, "to seek out the nerves of the plexus."

This interfascial concept was first introduced by this author in 1964, as the "perivascular concept of brachial plexus block" since both the vessels and the nerves occupy the "interfascial compartment" in the case of the upper extremity. Since that time continuing efforts to popularize this simple approach to brachial plexus anesthesia have included scientific exhibits, lectures, and publications. However, the production of a pictorial monograph similar to that of Macintosh and Mushin awaited the discovery of the right artist and a publisher willing to include illustrations in color. As stated in the preface to the first edition of Macintosh and Mushin, "a venture of this sort must necessarily come to naught unless supported by an artist whose main aim is to convey clearly the details of the author's practice to the eye of the reader." The moment I saw the work of Poul Buckhöj I knew I had found the appropriate artist, a man with the unique artistic talent necessary to portray the anatomy in a manner meaningful to the student of regional anesthesia. But to obtain his services and to find a publisher that was willing to produce Poul's work in full color, so important in the delineation of fine anatomical detail, to a limited market at a time when the cost of full color is prohibitive, appeared to be impossible, and my plans for this monograph similarly appeared to be an impossible dream. The impossible became possible and, indeed, a reality through the efforts of Mr. Lennart Håkansson of Information Consulting Medical, who brought together the unlikely combination of an American author, a Swedish artist, and a Danish publisher, and coordinated the activities of all three to produce the present work. It is my earnest hope that this unique, international cooperative effort of author, artist, and publisher will present information that enables the anesthetist not only to learn the perivascular techniques of brachial plexus anesthesia but also to comprehend completely the anatomical principles upon which the techniques are based.

In addition, as a firm believer that "those who do not remember the past are condemned to relive it," I have provided an unusually extensive historical review of brachial block techniques, utilizing a format that I hope will achieve two objectives: while the text deals with the role of each of the major contributions of brachial plexus anesthesia in the evolution of current techniques, the accompanying figures present each author's original description and illustration of his technique, so that the devotee of regional anesthesia, if he so desires, can actually learn each of the various techniques from the original description and also understand their advantages and disadvantages from the discussion in the text. It is hoped that this section will serve to place the role of the perivascular techniques in the proper perspective.

Finally, I would like to acknowledge the assistance of Miss Haidi Mayer, who translated many of the original German articles into English for me, and the tierless efforts of Mrs Lourdes Magpali, who typed and retyped the many revisions of the original manuscript.

I. Anatomical Considerations

"Regional anesthesia is simply an exercise in applied anatomy."

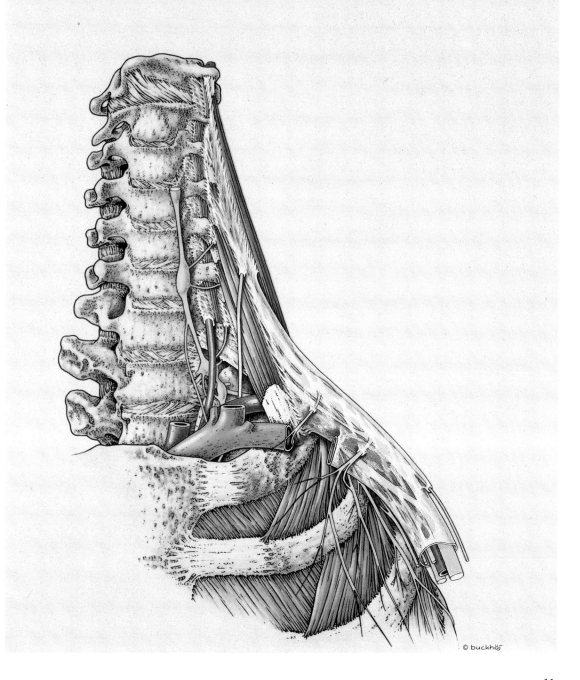

© buckhöj

Introduction

Knowledge of the formation of the brachial plexus and of its ultimate cutaneous and muscular distribution is absolutely essential to the intelligent and effective use of brachial plexus anesthesia for surgery of the upper extremity. For any anticipated surgical procedure or manipulation, it is the neuroanatomical considerations that will indicate the most suitable technique and the appropriate volume of anesthetic solution to achieve the desired level of anesthesia. In addition, close familiarity with the vascular, muscular, and fascial relationships of the plexus throughout its formation and distribution is equally essential to mastery of the various techniques of brachial plexus anesthesia, for it is these perineural structures which serve as the landmarks by which the needle may accurately locate the plexus percutaneously.

Formation of Brachial Plexus

vical nerves and the first thoracic nerve, with frequent contributions from the fourth cervical nerve above and the second thoracic nerve below.

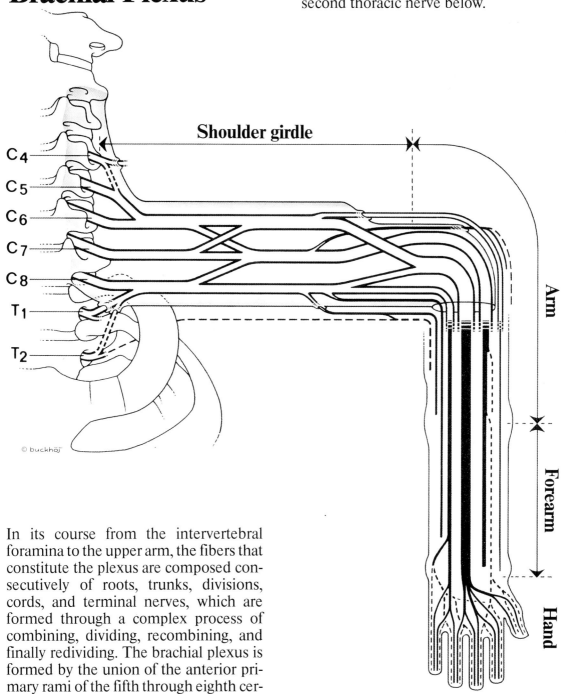

Shoulder girdle

C₄
C₅
C₆
C₇
C₈
T₁
T₂

Arm

Forearm

Hand

© buckhöj

In its course from the intervertebral foramina to the upper arm, the fibers that constitute the plexus are composed consecutively of roots, trunks, divisions, cords, and terminal nerves, which are formed through a complex process of combining, dividing, recombining, and finally redividing. The brachial plexus is formed by the union of the anterior primary rami of the fifth through eighth cer-

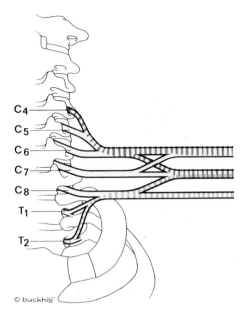

The fourth cervical nerve contributes to two thirds of all plexuses, and the second thoracic nerve contributes to more than one third.

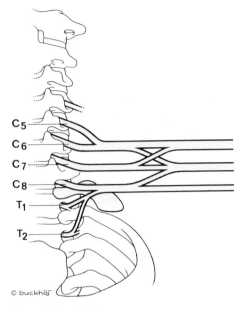

Postfixed plexus

Similarly, when the contribution from T_2 is large and that from C_4 is lacking, the plexus appears to have a caudal position and has been termed "postfixed". Usually, the prefixed or postfixed positions are associated with the presence either of a cervical rib or of an anomalous first rib.

Prefixed plexus

When the contribution from C_4 is large and that from T_2 is lacking, the plexus appears to have a more cephalic position and has been termed "prefixed".

It is doubtful whether these prefixed and postfixed variations are more common than those in which the plexus is spread out to include *both* C_4 and T_2 or contracted to exclude both.

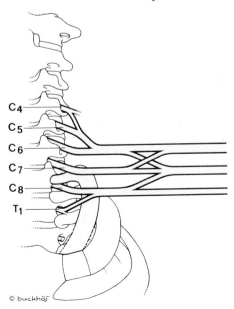

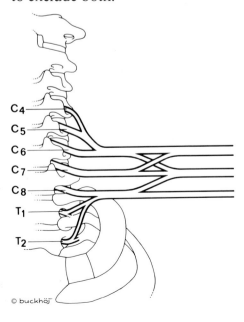

Roots

The roots of the brachial plexus represent the anterior primary divisions of the lower four cervical and first thoracic nerves. After emerging from the intervertebral foramina, the roots of the fifth to the eighth cervical nerves pass behind the vertebral artery and travel laterally in the "gutters" or through unique to the superior surfaces of the cervical transverse processes. After arriving at the distal end of the transverse processes, the roots are directed toward the first rib, above which they fuse to form the trunks of the plexus. Immediately after leaving the protection of its cervical transverse process, the root of the fifth cervical nerve may receive a twig from the root of the fourth cervical nerve. The root of the first thoracic nerve divides into a small and a large branch, the smaller branch passing along the intercostal space as the first intercostal nerve. The larger branch, may be joined by a twig from the second thoracic nerve, which then passes upward and laterally, in front of the neck of the first rib and behind the pleura over the apex of the lung to take part in the formation of the trunks of the plexus.

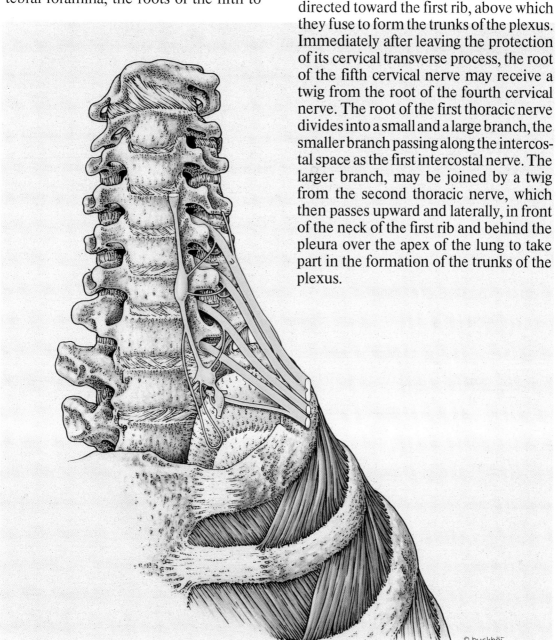

© buckhöj

15

Trunks

The five roots of the brachial plexus, after having received the contributions from above and below, combine above the first rib to form the three trunks of the plexus. The superior trunk is formed by the union of the roots of the fifth and sixth cervical nerves, the inferior trunk is formed by the union of the roots of the eighth cervical and first thoracic nerves, while the seventh cervical nerve simply continues as sole contributor to the middle trunk.

Divisions

As the trunks pass over the first rib and under the clavicle, the fibers that compose them regroup, and each trunk divides into an anterior and posterior division. While the six divisions are not particularly important to the techniques of regional anesthesia, it is at this level that the ultimate distribution of the plexus is determined, for it is the regrouping of fibers at this level that results in separation of those fibers destined for the anterior (flexor or volar) surface of the upper extremity from those destined for the posterior (extensor or dorsal) surface. However, there is some overlap in the case of the sensory, cutaneous distribution.

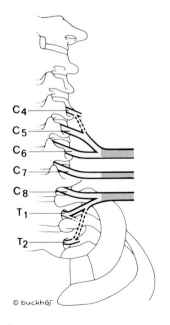

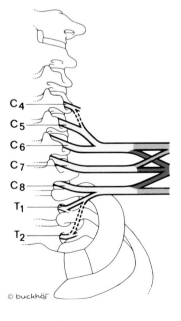

Cords

As the plexus emerges from under the clavicle, the fibers recombine to form the three cords of the plexus. The lateral cord is formed by the union of the anterior divisions of the superior and middle trunks; the medial cord is simply the continuation of the anterior division of the inferior trunk; and the posterior cord is composed of the posterior division of all three trunks. Thus, because of their derivation, the medial and lateral cords give rise to nerves that will supply the flexor surface of the upper extremity, while those nerves arising from the posterior cord will supply the extensor surface.

Major Terminal Nerves

Each of the three cords of the plexus gives off a branch that contributes to or becomes one of the major nerves to the upper extremity and then terminates as another major nerve. Thus the lateral and medial cords give off as their branches the lateral and medial heads of the median nerve and then continue as major terminal nerves, the lateral cord terminating as the musculocutaneous nerve and the medial cord as the ulnar nerve. Similarly, the posterior cord gives off, as its major branch, the axillary nerve, and then continues as the radial nerve.

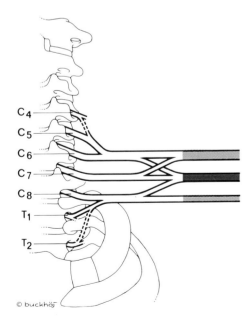

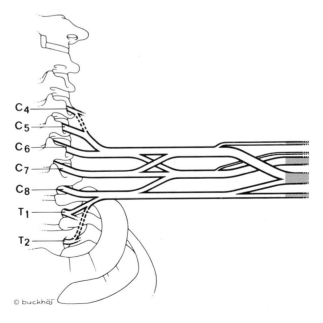

Brachial Plexus

formed and these divide into two sets of threes, the divisions which by reuniting give rise to the three cords. The three cords each give off three, lateral branches before becoming the major terminal branches of the plexus.

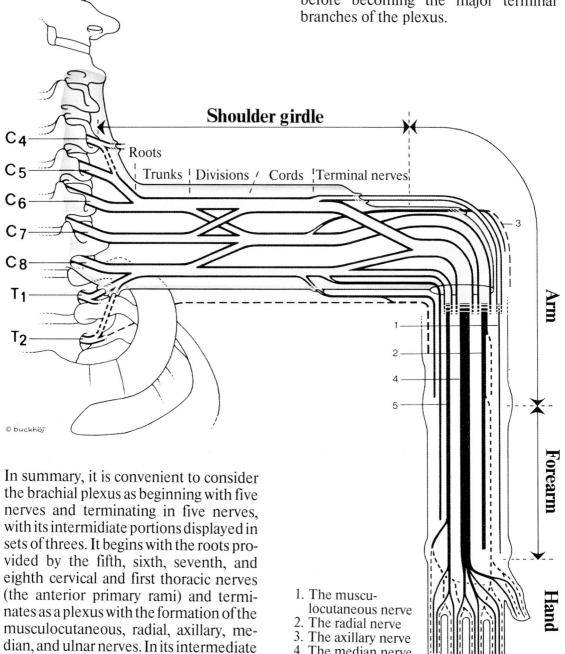

© buckhöj

In summary, it is convenient to consider the brachial plexus as beginning with five nerves and terminating in five nerves, with its intermidiate portions displayed in sets of threes. It begins with the roots provided by the fifth, sixth, seventh, and eighth cervical and first thoracic nerves (the anterior primary rami) and terminates as a plexus with the formation of the musculocutaneous, radial, axillary, median, and ulnar nerves. In its intermediate portions, first three main trunks are

1. The musculocutaneous nerve
2. The radial nerve
3. The axillary nerve
4. The median nerve
5. The ulnar nerve

18

Distribution of Brachial Plexus

It is convenient to divide the branches of the brachial plexus into those that arise above the clavicle and those that arise below it, grouping them together as supraclavicular and infraclavicular branches.

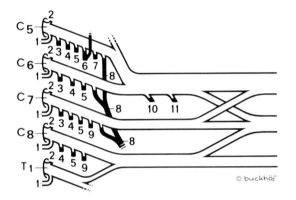

1. Ramus communicans
2. Dorsal rami
3. Nerve to the longus colli muscle
4. Nerve to the middle and posterior scalene muscles
5. Nerve to the anterior scalene muscle
6. Phrenic nerve
7. Dorsal scapular nerve
8. Long thoracic nerve
9. Nerve to the scalenus minimus muscle
10. Nerve to the subclavius muscle
11. Suprascapular nerve

Supraclavicular Branches

The supraclavicular branches, which arise from the roots and trunks of the plexus, are, with one exception, entirely motor, so for the purposes of sensory anesthesia these branches are of little interest. As a matter of fact, even the infraclavicular branches of the proximal portions of the three cords are almost exclusively motor nerves. However, while as regional anesthetists we must have complete knowledge of the distribution of the sensory nerves to the upper extremity in order to provide surgical anesthesia appropriate for the procedure, we must also have knowledge of the distribution of the motor nerves in order to provide muscular relaxation and a motionless surgical field. In addition, it is through an intimate knowledge of the motor distribution of the brachial plexus that the etiology of persistent postoperative neurological deficits can be determined, both clinically and electromyographically (Chapter V).

Branches from the Roots

The nerves to the longus colli and the scalene muscles (C_2–C_8)

Almost immediately after emerging from the intervertebral foramina (but after receiving the respective sympathetic nerve contributions), each of the lower four cervical nerves gives off branches that supply the longus colli and the scalene muscles (anterior, middle, and posterior).

1. Longus colli muscle . . . . C_2-C_7
2. Anterior scalene muscle . . . . C_4-C_6
3. Middle scalene muscle . . . . C_3-C_8
4. Posterior scalene muscle . . . . C_6-C_8
5. Scalenus minimus muscle . . . . C_7-C_8

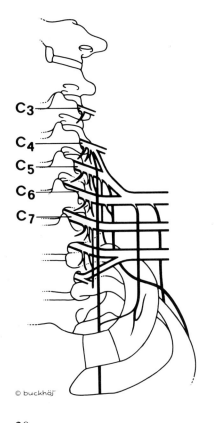

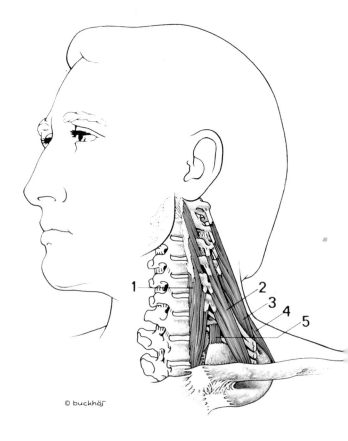

The long thoracic nerve (C_5-C_7)

Almost simultaneously, the long thoracic nerve, arising from the fifth, sixth, and seventh cervical nerves, come off, which unite to run behind the plexus to innervate the serratus anterior muscle.

Serratus anterior muscle C_5-C_7

1. Long thoracic nerve

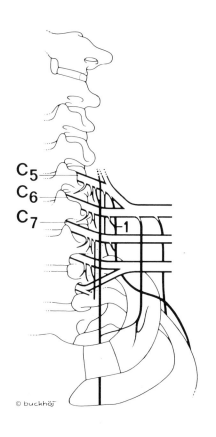

C₅
C₆
C₇

© buckhöj

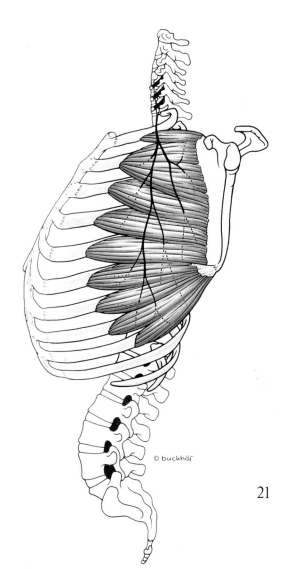

© buckhöj

21

The dorsal scapular nerve (C_5)

The dorsal scapular nerve arises from the fifth cervical nerve to supply the rhomboid major and minor and the levator scapulae muscles.

1. Levator scapulae muscle............ C_3-C_5
2. Rhomboid minor muscle.............. C_5
3. Rhomboid major muscle .... C_5

1. Dorsal scapular nerve

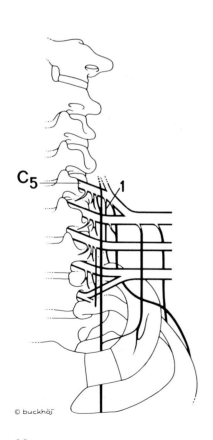

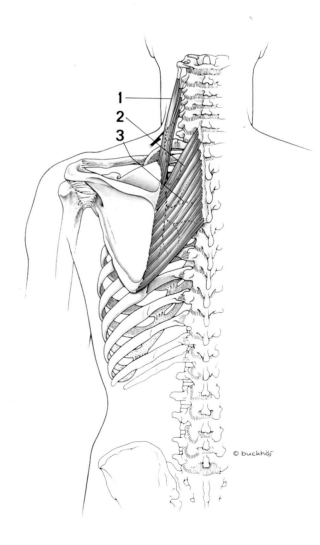

Contributions to the phrenic nerve (C_5)

Not infrequently, a branch of the fifth cervical nerve may contribute to the phrenic nerve, at its origin. Occasionally, the brachial plexus gives rise to an accessory phrenic nerve, a branch that may arise from the fifth cervical nerve (C_5) or from the nerve to the subclavius muscle (C_5-C_6), as described under that nerve. It passes ventral to the subclavian vein and joins the phrenic nerve at the root of the neck, forming a loop around the vein.

1. Phrenic nerve

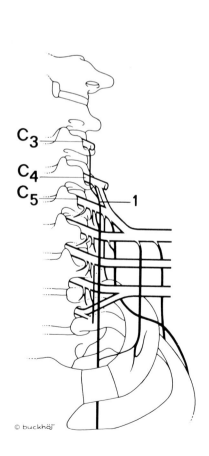

© buckhöj

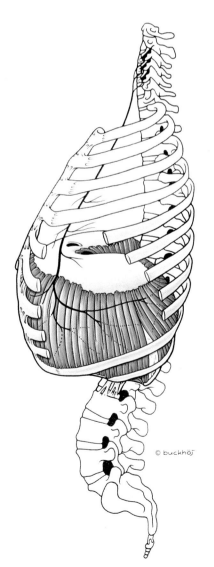

© buckhöj

Branches from the Trunks

The trunks give rise to two branches, the nerve to the subclavius muscle and the suprascapular nerve.

The nerve to the subclavius muscle (C_5-C_6)

The nerve to the subclavius muscle arises from the front of the superior trunk and passes ventral to the lower part of the plexus and the subclavian artery and vein to reach the subclavius muscle. The accessory phrenic nerve mentioned earlier may occasionally be a branch of this nerve.

1. Nerve to the subclavius muscle

Subclavius muscle C_5-C_6

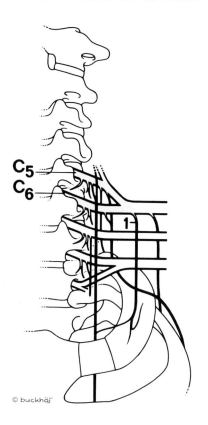

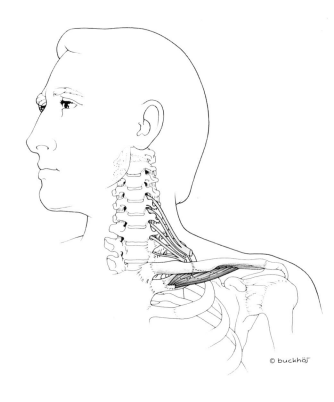

© buckhöj

© buckhöj

24

The suprascapular nerve (C_5-C_6)

The suprascapular nerve arises from the superior aspect of the superior trunk, and descends parallel to but above the plexus until, superior to the cords, it passes through the scapular notch to supply the supraspinatus and infraspinatus muscles. It also supplies sensory branches to the shoulder joint, *the only sensory fibers that arise above the clavicle*. After it has left the superior trunk, because of its position superior to the plexus, this nerve may be stimulated during the subclavian perivascular technique of brachial plexus block, giving rise to paresthesias to the shoulder.

However, because the nerve leaves the plexus and its investment of fascia shortly after arising from the superior trunk, such paresthesias cannot be relied upon as an indicator that the anesthetist's needle lies within the sheath, since a paresthesia in this distribution could indicate stimulation of fibers either before or after the nerve has left the sheath.

1. Suprascapular nerve

1. Supraspinatus muscle .... C_5
2. Infraspinatus muscle .... C_5-C_6

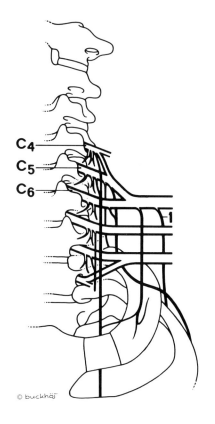

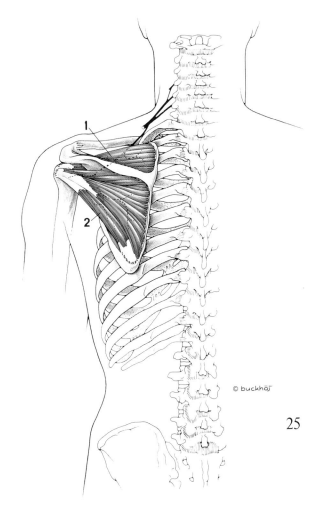

25

Infraclavicular Branches

The infraclavicular branches comprise all of the motor and sensory nerves to the upper extremity proper and hence their names must be committed to memory.

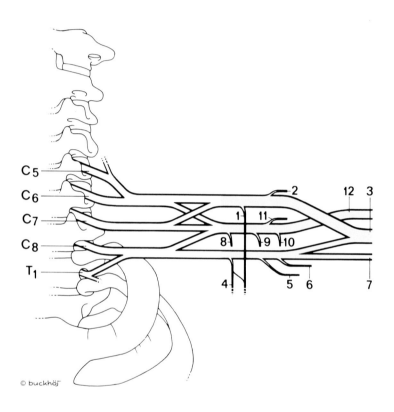

© buckhöj

1. Lateral pectoral nerve ⎤
2. Musculocutaneous nerve ⎬ Lateral cord
3. Median nerve ⎦

4. Medial pectoral nerve ⎤
5. Medial brachial cutaneous nerve ⎪
6. Medial antibrachial cutaneous nerve ⎬ Medial cord
7. Ulnar nerve ⎦

8. Upper subscapular nerve ⎤
9. Thoracodorsal nerve ⎪
10. Lower subscapular nerve ⎬ Posterior cord
11. Axillary nerve ⎪
12. Radial nerve ⎦

Branches from the Cords

Aside from some exceptions, there are no branches that arise from the level of the divisions of the plexus, so the rest of the branches of the brachial plexus arise from the three cords. These branches may conveniently be considered with reference to their cord of origin.

Lateral Cord
The lateral pectoral nerve (C_5-C_7)

The lateral cord gives rise to the lateral pectoral nerve, which passes superficial to the first part of the axillary artery and vein, communicates with the medial pectoral nerve, which arises from the medial cord, and then pierces the clavipectoral fascia to reach the pectoralis major muscle. Not infrequently it also sends fibers to the pectoralis minor muscle.

1. Pectoralis major muscle C_5-T_1

1. Lateral pectoral nerve

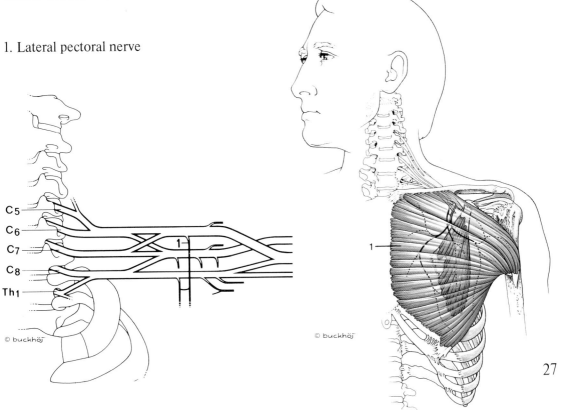

C5
C6
C7
C8
Th1

© buckhöj

© buckhöj

27

The musculocutaneous nerve C_5-C_7

The musculocutaneous nerve is the major terminal branch of the lateral cord. Shortly after giving off the lateral head to the median nerve, the musculocutaneous nerve leaves the plexus and enters the coracobrachialis muscle. The nerve courses through the axilla in this muscle and then descends obliquely and laterally between the biceps and brachialis muscles, sending motor fibers to all three of these powerful flexors of the forearm before terminating in the forearm as the lateral antebrachial cutaneous nerve.

The lateral antebrachial cutaneous nerve C_5-C_6

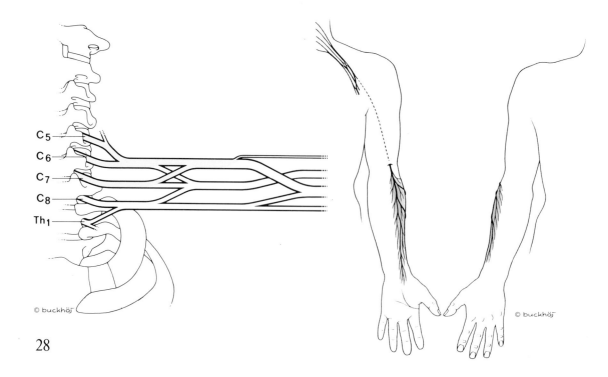

Musculocutaneous nerve injury

Paralysis of the coracobrachialis, biceps and brachialis muscles causes inability to flex the forearm.

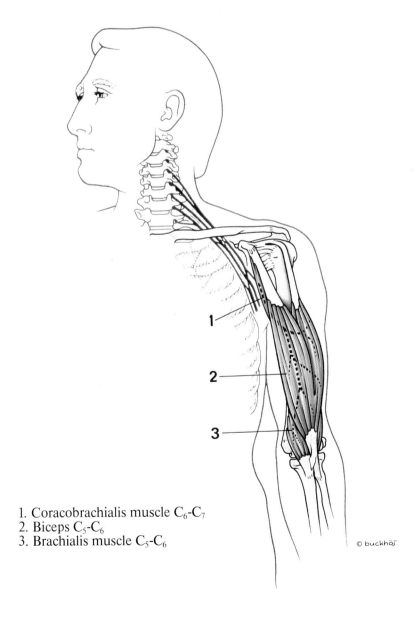

1. Coracobrachialis muscle C_6-C_7
2. Biceps C_5-C_6
3. Brachialis muscle C_5-C_6

© buckhöj

The median nerve (C_6-T_1)

Though occasionally the median nerve includes fibers originating from C_5, more frequently the motorfibers originate from C_6-T_1 and the sensory fibers from C_6-C_8. In either case, just before terminating as the musculocutaneous nerve, the lateral cord contributes the lateral head of the median nerve, which joins with the medial head, contributed by the medial cord, to form the median nerve. Thus, this nerve may be considered as a branch of both of the cords derived from the anterior divisions. The contributions from the two cords straddle the third part of the axillary artery before they unite on its ventral surface. The nerve then descends along the course of the brachial artery and passes on to the lower aspect of the forearm, where it gives out muscular branches and enters the hand to terminate in muscular and cutaneous branches. This nerve provides motor branches to most of the flexor and pronator muscles of the forearm, supplying all of the superficial volar muscles except the flexor carpi ulnaris, and all of the deep volar muscles except the ulnar half of the flexor digitorum profundus. In the hand the motor branches supply the first two lumbricales and the thenar muscles that lie superficial to the tendon of the flexor pollicis longus. Sensory branches supply the skin of the palmar aspect of the thumb, the lateral two and one-half fingers, and the distal end of the dorsal aspect of the same fingers. Rarely the median nerve may encroach upon the area usually innervated by the ulnar nerve, and when it does, then the median nerve provides the sensory innervation of the entire ringfinger. It also may encroach upon the area ordinarily innervated by the radial nerve, also providing the sensory innervation of the dorsal surface of the entire thumb and first three fingers as far as the metacarpal-phalangeal joints.

Cutaneous distribution .... C_6-C_8

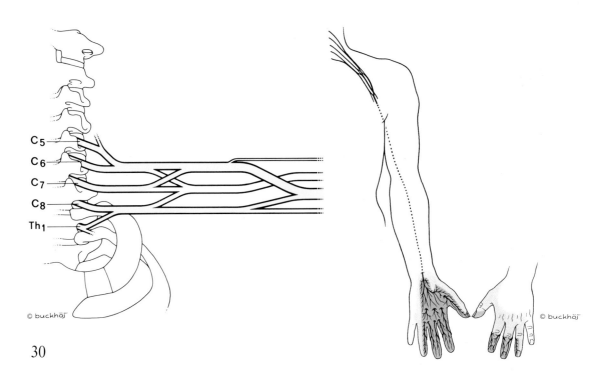

C 5
C 6
C 7
C 8
Th 1

© buckhöj

© buckhöj

30

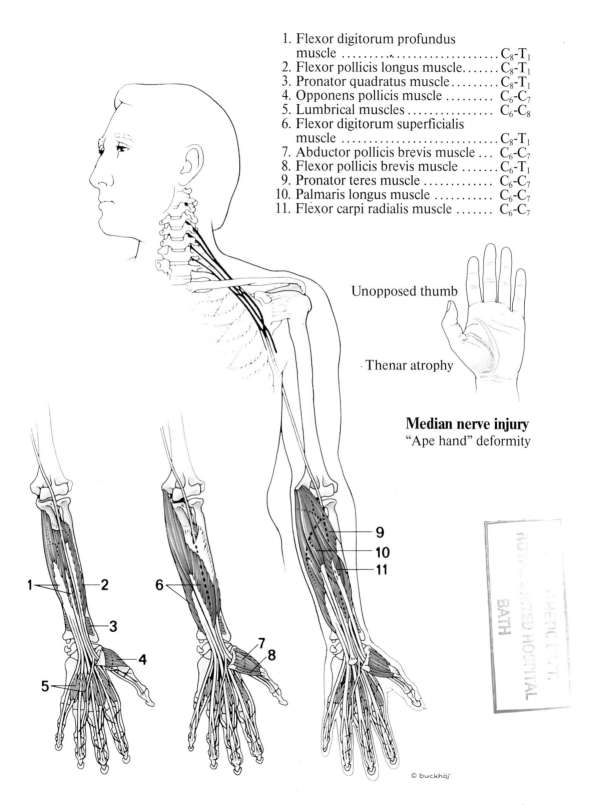

1. Flexor digitorum profundus muscle .... C_8-T_1
2. Flexor pollicis longus muscle ...... C_8-T_1
3. Pronator quadratus muscle .... C_8-T_1
4. Opponens pollicis muscle .... C_6-C_7
5. Lumbrical muscles .... C_6-C_8
6. Flexor digitorum superficialis muscle .... C_8-T_1
7. Abductor pollicis brevis muscle ... C_6-C_7
8. Flexor pollicis brevis muscle .... C_6-T_1
9. Pronator teres muscle .... C_6-C_7
10. Palmaris longus muscle .... C_6-C_7
11. Flexor carpi radialis muscle .... C_6-C_7

Unopposed thumb

Thenar atrophy

Median nerve injury
"Ape hand" deformity

© buckhöj

31

Medial Cord

Just before branching as the ulnar nerve, the medial cord contributes medial head of the median nerve, which joins with the lateral head from the lateral cord to form the median nerve, the distribution of which has already been described.

The medial pectoral nerve (C_8-T_1)

1. Pectoralis minor muscle C_8-T_1

The first collateral branch of the medial cord is the medial pectoral nerve, which passes between the axillary artery and vein, joins the lateral pectoral nerve from the lateral cord to form a loop around the artery, and then enters the pectoralis minor muscle, which it supplies. Several fibers continue through this muscle to supply the lower part of the pectoralis major muscle. The loop formed by the lateral and medial anterior thoracic nerves also gives off several branches to both of the pectoral muscles.

1. Medial pectoral nerve
2. Medial brachial cutaneous nerve
3. Medial antebrachial cutaneous nerve

1. Pectoralis minor muscle C_8-T_1

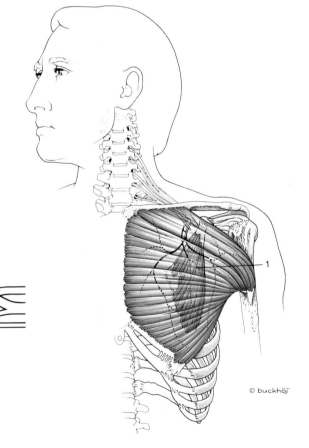

© buckhöj

© buckhöj

32

The medial brachial cutaneous nerve (C_8-T_1)

The medial brachial cutaneous nerve is the second collateral branch of the medial cord. It is a small branch which, as its name implies, supplies the medial portion of the upper arm as far distally as the medial epicondyle. It leaves the axillary sheath high in the axilla, where part of it forms a loop with the intercostobrachial nerve, with which it has a reciprocal relationship with respect to size and distribution. In some instances the intercostobrachial nerve innervates the entire medial aspect of the upper arm from the apex of the axilla to the medial epicondyle, and in other instances this entire area is innervated by the medial brachial cutaneous nerve. However, most frequently this area is innervated jointly by the two nerves, with the medial brachial cutaneous innervating the lower portion and the intercostobrachial innervating the upper portion.

1. Intercostobrachial nerve
2. Medial brachial cutaneous nerve

The medial antebrachial cutaneous nerve (C_8-T_1)

The third branch of the medial cord before it gives rise to its major terminal nerve is the medial antebrachial cutaneous nerve, which arises from the medial cord just medial to the axillary artery. The nerve travels down the arm medial to the brachial artery to supply the skin over the entire medial aspect of the forearm as far as the wrist. In addition, however, near the axilla it gives off a filament which supplies the skin overlying the biceps muscle as far as the elbow, so this nerve supplies significant brachial as well as antebrachial cutaneous innervation.

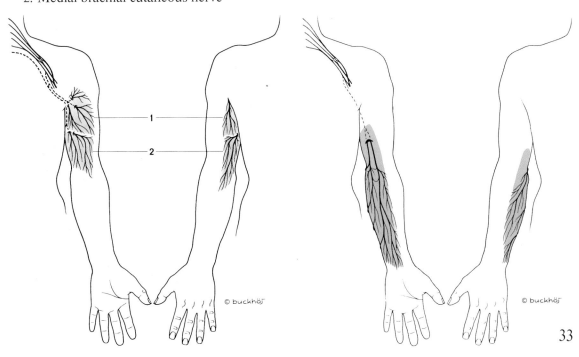

© buckhöj

© buckhöj

The ulnar nerve (C_8-T_1)

The ulnar nerve is the major terminal continuation of the medial cord after the medial head of the median nerve has separated from it already at the lower border of the pectoralis minor muscle. It descends medial to the artery as far as the middle of the arm, running parallel to and between the median and medial antebrachial cutaneous nerves. In the middle of the arm it angles dorsally and laterally to continue its descent in a groove on the medial head of the triceps. From there it passes behind the medial epicondyle of the humerus (where it is covered only by skin and fascia and can readily be palpated as the "funny bone" of the elbow) and then passes down the ulnar side of the forearm into the hand. Motor branches in the forearm supply the flexor carpi ulnaris and the ulnar head of the flexor digitorum profundus and in the hand supply all of the small muscles deep and medial to the long flexor tendon of the thumb except for the first two lumbricales. The ulnar nerve gives off no sensory branches in the forearm, but in the hand it usually supplies the skin of the little finger and the medial half of the hand and ringfinger.

Occasionally the ulnar nerve may encroach on the area usually served by the median nerve, so that it may provide the sensory innervation of the entire ringfinger and even the palm of the hand and the palmar aspect of the proximal phalanges of the index and middle fingers. It may also occasionally encroach on the area usually served by the radial nerve, providing the sensory innervation over the dorsum of most of the hand, the dorsum of the entire ring-finger, and the dorsal surface of the proximal phalanges of the index and middle fingers.

Cutaneous distribution C_8-T_1

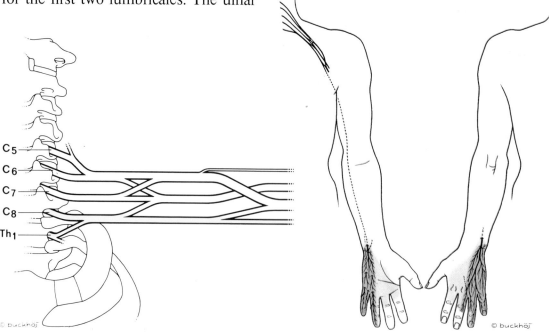

C 5
C 6
C 7
C 8
Th 1

© buckhøj

© buckhøj

34

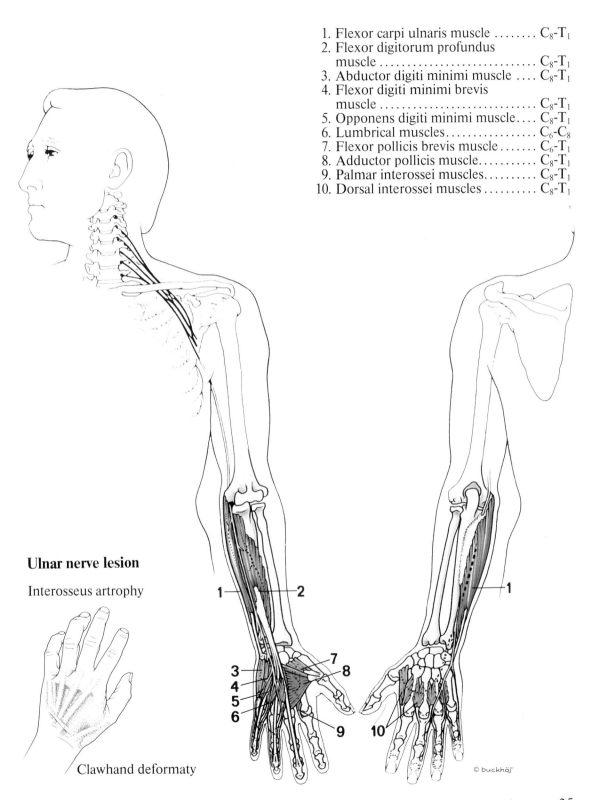

1. Flexor carpi ulnaris muscle .... C_8-T_1
2. Flexor digitorum profundus
   muscle .... C_8-T_1
3. Abductor digiti minimi muscle .... C_8-T_1
4. Flexor digiti minimi brevis
   muscle .... C_8-T_1
5. Opponens digiti minimi muscle.... C_8-T_1
6. Lumbrical muscles................. C_6-C_8
7. Flexor pollicis brevis muscle .... C_6-T_1
8. Adductor pollicis muscle........... C_8-T_1
9. Palmar interossei muscles......... C_8-T_1
10. Dorsal interossei muscles .... C_8-T_1

Ulnar nerve lesion

Interosseus artrophy

Clawhand deformaty

© buckhöj

35

Posterior Cord

Like the medial cord, the posterior cord gives off three smaller collateral branches before giving rise to two major terminal nerves. Two of the three are the subscapular nerves, one of which arises above and the other below the third nerve, the thoracodorsal nerve.

The subscapular nerves (C_5-C_6)

The upper subscapular nerve, usually the smaller of the two, enters the upper part of the subscapularis muscle, which it supplies, while the lower subscapular nerve supplies the lower portion of the subscapularis muscle and then terminates as the nerve to the teres major muscle.

1a. Upper subscapular nerve
1b. Lower subscapular nerve

1. Subscapularis muscle............... C_5-C_6
2. Teres major muscle................. C_5-C_6

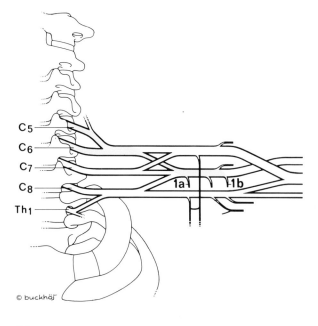

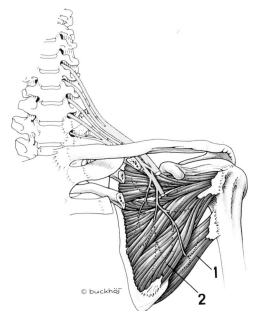

The thoracodorsal nerve (C_6-C_8)

The thoracodorsal nerve, arising between the two subscapular nerves, courses along the posterior wall of the axilla with the subscapular and thoracodorsal arteries and terminates in branches which supply the latissimus dorsi muscle.

Latissimus dorsi muscle C_6-C_8

1. Thoracodorsal nerve

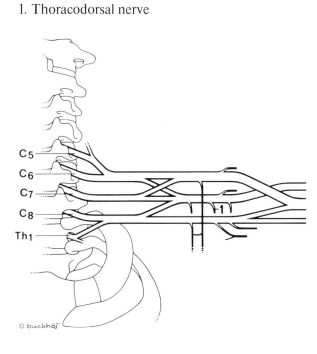

C5
C6
C7
C8
Th1

© buckhöj

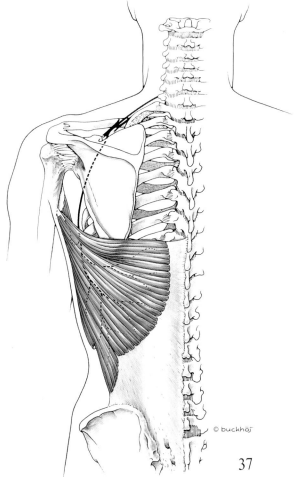

© buckhöj

The axillary nerve (C_5-C_6)

Like the lateral and medial cords, the posterior cord gives off one major terminal branch before continuing as another; thus, before the posterior cord becomes the radial nerve, it gives off the axillary nerve. This nerve leaves the axilla immediately after arising by way of the quadrilateral space, which is bounded by the surgical neck of the humerus, the teres major and minor muscles, and the long head of the triceps muscles. It then branches, sending motor fibers to the teres minor and deltoid muscles and sensory fibers, the lateral brachial cutaneous nerve, to supply the skin overlying the lower two thirds of the posterior part of the deltoid muscle. Prior to branching the axillary nerve also furnishes an articular twig to the shoulder joint.

The lateral brachial cutaneous nerve (C_5- C_6)

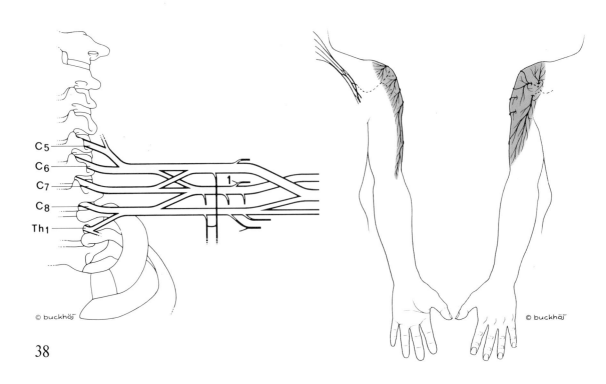

© buckhöj

© buckhöj

Axillary nerve injury

Deltoid paralysis causes inability to abduct the arm

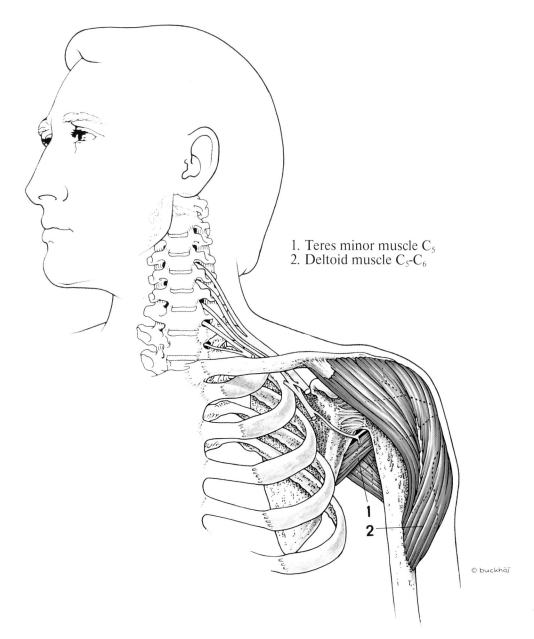

1. Teres minor muscle C_5
2. Deltoid muscle C_5-C_6

© buckhöj

The radial nerve (C_5-T_1)

The radial nerve, the largest branch of the entire plexus, is the terminal continuation of the posterior cord. In its descent down the arm, it accompanies the profunda artery behind and around the humerus in the musculospiral groove, and then reaches the lower anterior side of the forearm where its terminal branches arise. Motor branches in the arm supply the triceps, anconeus, and the upper portion of the extensor-supinator group of forearm muscles. Motor branches in the forearm supplied by the deep radial nerve pass to the rest of the extensor-supinator group of muscles.

Like the medial antebrachial cutaneous nerve, the major sensory branches of the radial nerve are misnamed in that the dorsal antebrachial cutaneous nerve innervates not only the posterior aspect of the forearm as far as the wrist but also much of the postero lateral aspect of the upper arm as well. For this reason some authorities refer to the sensory branches innervating the dorsal aspect of the arm as the dorsal brachial cutaneous nerve and

to those that supply the dorsal surface of the forearm as the dorsal antebrachial cutaneous nerve. In addition, the radial nerve supplies sensory branches to the hand by way of the superficial radial nerve, which innervates the dorsal aspect of the radial half of the hand, or more precisely, the dorsal aspect of the entire thumb and the dorsal aspect of the index, middle, and radial (lateral) half of the ring finger, but in the latter three only as far as the distal interphalangeal joint. Occasionally, the radial nerve may encroach upon the area usually innervated by the ulnar nerve so that it provides the sensory innervation over the entire dorsum of the hand and fingers as far as the distal phalanges, except for the skin over the fifth metacarpal and the entire little finger. Similar encroachment of the radial nerve

1. Dorsal brachial cutaneous nerve ... C_5-C_6
2. Dorsal antebrachial cutaneous
   nerve.............................. C_5-C_8
3. Cutaneouos distribution .... C_6-C_8

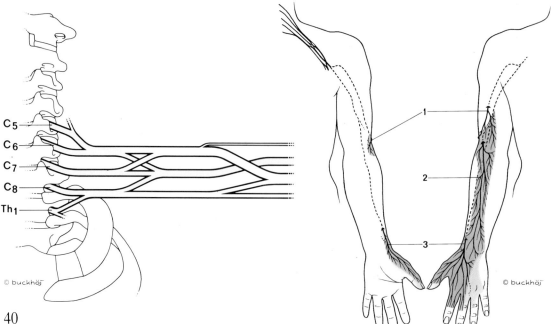

C5
C6
C7
C8
Th1

© buckhöj

© buckhöj

on the area usually innervated by the median nerve also occurs on occasion, so that the radial nerve provides the sensory innervation of the entire distal phalange of the thumb.

1. Triceps brachii muscle .... C_7-C_8
2. Supinator muscle .... C_6
3. Extensor carpi radialis brevis muscle .... C_6-C_7
4. Abductor pollicis longus muscle .... C_6-C_7
5. Anconeus muscle .... C_7-C_8
6. Extensor pollicis longus muscle .... C_6-C_8
7. Extensor indicis muscle .... C_6-C_8
8. Extensor pollicis brevis muscle .... C_6-C_7
9. Brachioradialis muscle .... C_5-C_6
10. Extensor carpi radialis longus muscle..................... C_6-C_7
11. Extensor digitorum muscle .... C_6-C_8
12. Extensor carpi ulnaris muscle ..... C_6-C_8
13. Extensor digiti minimi muscle ..... C_6-C_8

Wrist drop

Radial nerve injury

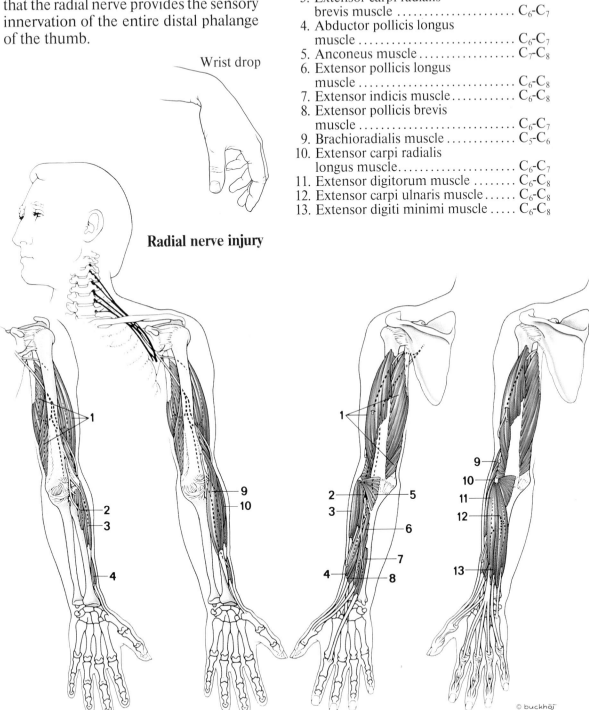

© buckhöj

Sympathetic Contributions to the Brachial Plexus

The segmental *preganglionic* sympathetic contributions to the brachial plexus are variable but generally extend considerably more caudad than one would expect. The highest segmental contribution is usually T_2, with T_1 contributing only rarely, while the lowest may be as far caudad as T_8, T_9, or even T_{10}.

The *postganglionic* contributions to the brachial plexus reach the roots of the plexus in the form of the gray rami communicantes from the sympathetic chain. This sympathetic input takes place at the point where the roots of the fifth to eighth cervical nerves, having passed posterior to the vertebral artery and between the anterior and posterior intertransverse muscles, reach the tips of the respective transverse processes to enter the space between the anterior and middle scalene muscles. At this point each of the roots of the fifth and sixth nerves receives a gray ramus communicans from the middle cervical sympathetic ganglion, while each

© buckhöj

root of the seventh and eighth nerves receives a gray ramus from the inferior cervical or, more commonly, from the stellate ganglion. The root of the first thoracic nerve receives one and frequently two rami communicantes from the stellate ganglion or from the first and even second thoracic ganglion. The sympathetic gray rami communicantes reach the roots of the brachial plexus either by piercing the prevertebral muscles or by passing beneath the medial border of the anterior scalene muscle. However, there are two other pathways by which sympathetic fibers reach the roots of the brachial plexus: the sympathetic plexus associated with the vertebral artery gives postganglionic fibers to the roots of the fourth, fifth, and sixth cervical nerves; and in those cases where the second thoracic nerve contributes a branch to the brachial plexus via the first thoracic nerve, that branch may very well contain sympathetic fibers from the second thoracic ganglion (nerve of Kuntz).

1. Ramus communicans
2. Middle cervical sympathetic ganglion
3. Stellate ganglion

Sympathetic Distribution to the Upper Extremity

It is important to appreciate that there are two distinct and separate pathways by which postganglionic sympathetic fibers are distributed to the upper extremity. The first mode of sympathetic distribution is a *distal* innervation that is carried to the peripheral vessels via the somatic nerves of the plexus. Having entered the plexus at the level of the roots as described above, these sympathetic fibers continue with the somatic fibers of the plexus as they form the roots, trunks, divisions, cords, and terminal nerves, and are distributed with them to the arterial system of the distal extremity, where – after penetrating the vascular wall, they form a nerve network surrounding the muscular coat.

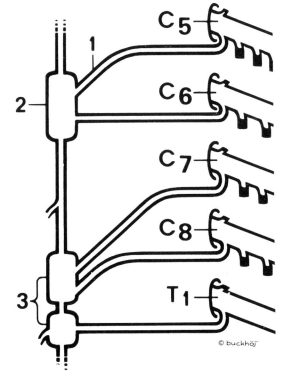

© buckhöj

The second mode of sympathetic distribution is a *proximal* innervation that arises directly from the cervical part of the sympathetic chain, particularly the middle and inferior cervical (or stellate) ganglia. The postganglionic sympathetic fibers pass directly to the subclavian artery and are conveyed in a plexiform manner along the outer coat of the vessel and its branches and into the arm along the axillary artery. The sympathetic fibers derived in this manner do not extend beyond the proximal portion of the brachial artery. Excitation or blockade of these proximal fibers alone presumably effects a change in vascular distensibility with relatively minor changes in pressure along the arterial tree.

1. Ramus communicans
2. Middle cervical sympathetic ganglion
3. Stellate ganglion
4. Second thoracic ganglion
5. Vertebral artery
6. Postganglionic sympathetic fibers
7. Subclavian artery

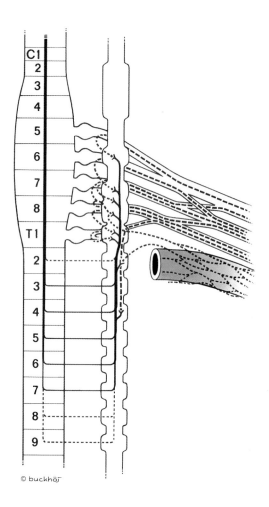

© buckhöj

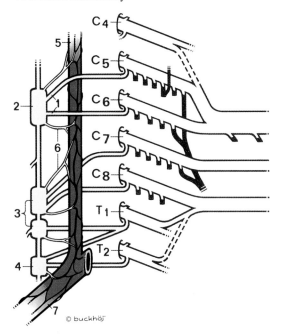

© buckhöj

Distal innervation

It appears that it is solely through the *distal* innervation that is, through the sympathetic fibers travelling with the somatic nerves derived from the brachial plexus that constrictor impulses are carried to the resistance vessels in the extremity. This is of significance to the regional anesthetist, for it implies that blockade of any peripheral nerve results in complete blockade of the vasoconstrictor fibers in the area of its distribution. It should be appreciated that these fibers also exert strong control over the capacitance vessels, namely the veins, so again peripheral block can result in considerable peripheral pooling of blood and reduce venous return to the heart.

44

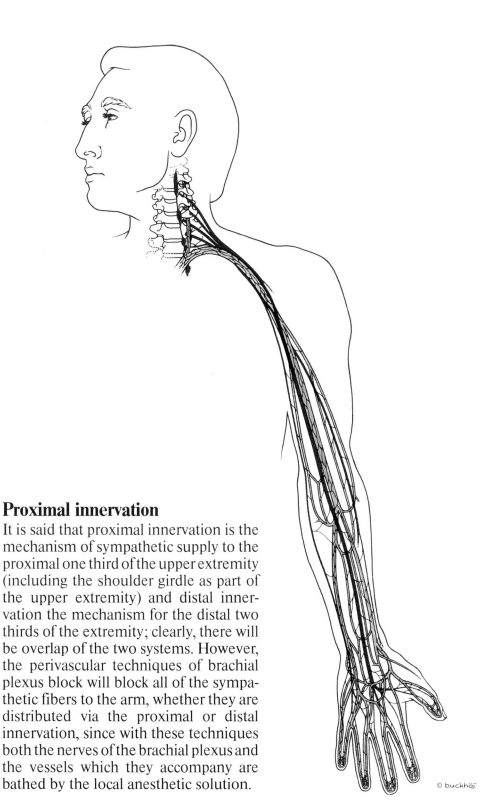

Proximal innervation

It is said that proximal innervation is the mechanism of sympathetic supply to the proximal one third of the upper extremity (including the shoulder girdle as part of the upper extremity) and distal innervation the mechanism for the distal two thirds of the extremity; clearly, there will be overlap of the two systems. However, the perivascular techniques of brachial plexus block will block all of the sympathetic fibers to the arm, whether they are distributed via the proximal or distal innervation, since with these techniques both the nerves of the brachial plexus and the vessels which they accompany are bathed by the local anesthetic solution.

© buckhöj

45

Relations of the Brachial Plexus

For the purposes of brachial plexus anesthesia, familiarity with the perineural structures that surround and accompany the plexus in its course from vertebral column to upper arm is as important as knowledge of the formation and distribution of the plexus itself. For it is an understanding of these structures and their relationships that forms the basis of the perivascular (interfascial) techniques of brachial plexus block, which like peridural techniques, allow a *predictable* level of anesthesia to be provided by a single injection.

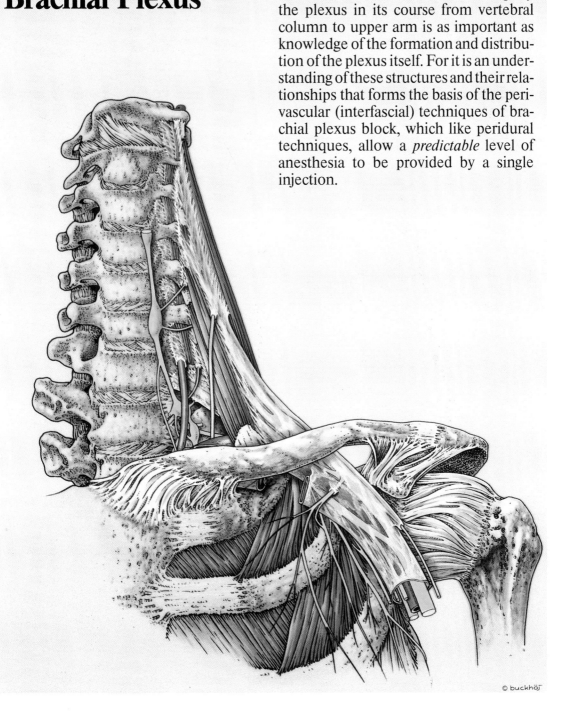

© buckhöj

The structures that are the most important to this concept are the anterior and
middle scalene muscles.

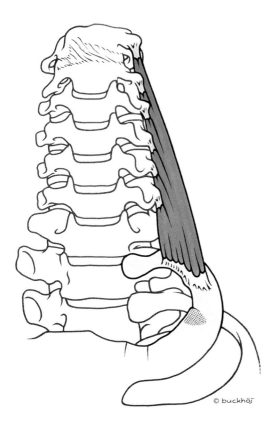 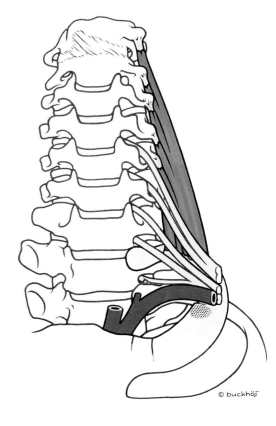

© buckhöj   © buckhöj

The middle scalene muscle arises from
the posterior tubercles of the transverse
processes of the lower six cervical vertebrae and inserts on the first rib just posterior to the subclavian groove (on top of
the first rib).

Since the subclavian artery and inferior
trunk of the plexus cross the first rib in this
groove, the insertion of the middle scalene muscle is just behind and in contact
with the trunks of the plexus as they cross
the first rib.

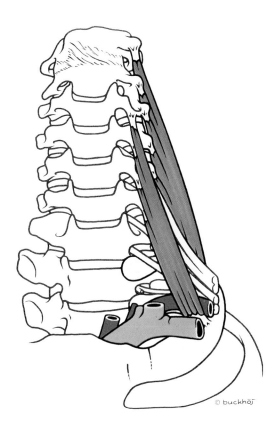

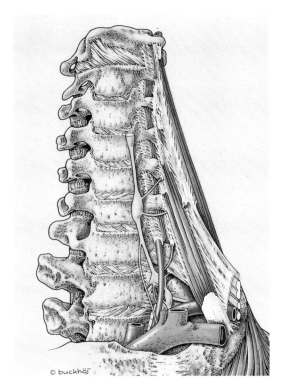

The anterior scalene muscle arises from the anterior tubercles of the transverse processes of the third, fourth, fifth, and sixth cervical vertebrae and inserts on the scalene tubercle of the first rib, separating the subclavian vein from the subclavian artery. Thus the anterior scalene muscle is just in front of and in contact with the subclavian artery as it crosses the first rib.

The fascia covering the scalene muscles is derived from the prevertebral fascia, which splits to invest these muscles and then joins again at their lateral margins to form an enclosed space, the interscalene space. Thus it is really the posterior fascia of the anterior scalene muscle and the anterior fascia of the middle scalene muscle that constitute what we, as anesthetists, conceive of as the "sheath of the brachial plexus."

In its passage from the cervical transverse processes to the first rib, the plexus, first as roots and then as trunks, may be considered to be "sandwiched" between the anterior and middle scalene muscles and hence invested by the fasciae of those muscles. The analogy to a sandwich is an appropriate one, for the dimensions of the interscalene space are akin to those of the space between the two slices of bread in a sandwich, that is, very tall or long in one dimension and very short or narrow in the other. In the case of the "scalene sandwich", the interscalene space is very tall in its vertical axis and extremely nar-

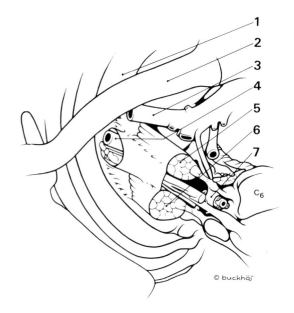

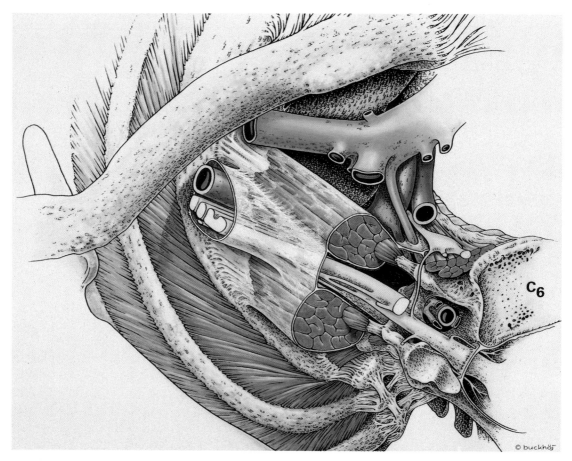

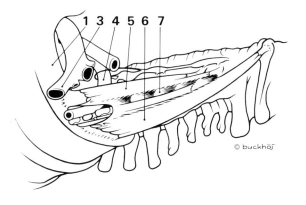

1. First rib
2. Clavicle
3. Subclavian vein
4. Subclavian artery
5. Anterior scalene muscle
6. Middle scalene muscle
7. Transverse process of C_6

row (actually only a potential space until it has been expanded by an injection) in its anteroposterior dimension.

Furthermore, it is important to note that as the three trunks cross the first rib they are "stacked" one on top of the other vertically, they lie slightly closer to the middle scalene muscle than to the anterior scalene muscle, whereas the subclavian artery, which crosses the first rib immediately in front of the trunks, lies slightly closer to the anterior than to the middle scalene muscle. If these relationships are kept in mind when one is performing an interscalene or subclavian perivascular brachial block, the chances of finding the plexus with the needle on the first attempt are greatly enhanced.

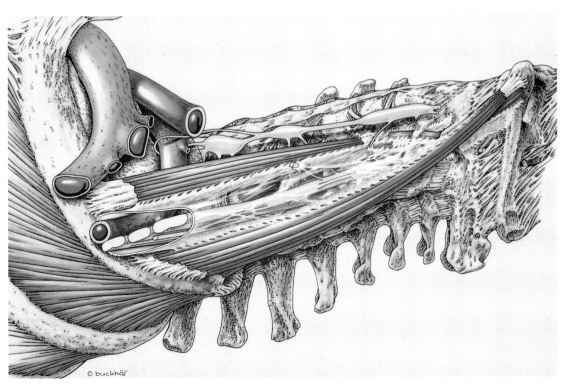

51

It is important to emphasize and re-emphasize the fact that the three trunks are "stacked" one on top of the other as they cross the first rib, and hence they were properly named by early anatomists as "superior, middle, and inferior trunks." The vast majority of textbooks of regional anesthesia, written after anesthesiologists had replaced surgeons as regional anesthetists, portray the three trunks crossing the first rib one behind the other (horizontally) rather than one on top of the other (vertically). If this was the case, early anatomists would have named the trunks anterior, middle, and posterior trunks. This misunderstanding of the anatomy at this level gave rise to several illogical clinical practices that will be discussed in subsequent sections.

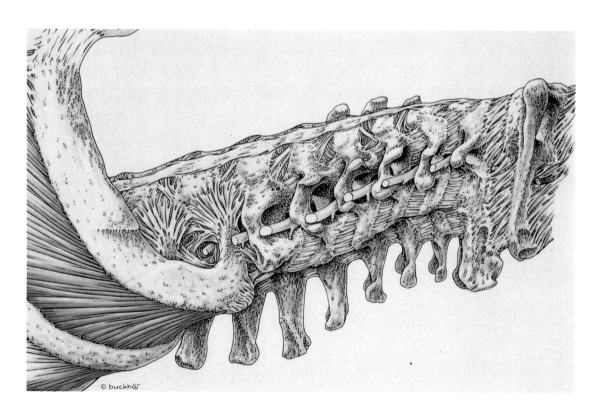

© buckhöj

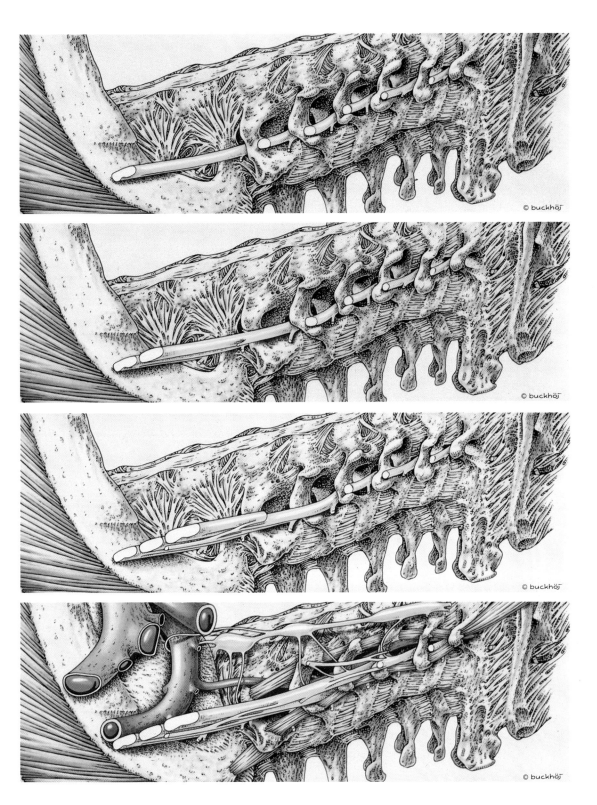

Actually, the interfascial compartment in which the brachial plexus forms and travels has its origins even proximal to the interscalene space. As stated earlier, the cervical transverse processes have been likened to short rain gutters, the troughs of which are formed by the anterior and posterior tubercles. The trough, however, is converted into a conduit by the anterior and posterior intertransverse muscles, which pass between the anterior and posterior tubercles, respectively, of the transverse processes of two contiguous cervical vertebrae. There are seven pairs of these muscles, the first pair being between the atlas and axis and the last pair between the seventh cervical and first thoracic vertebrae. Thus after leaving the intervertebral foramina, the roots of the brachial plexus actually travel in tunnels formed by the superior surface of the transverse process below, by the inferior surface of the transverse process above, and by the fascia investing the anterior and posterior intertransverse muscles anteriorly and posteriorly.

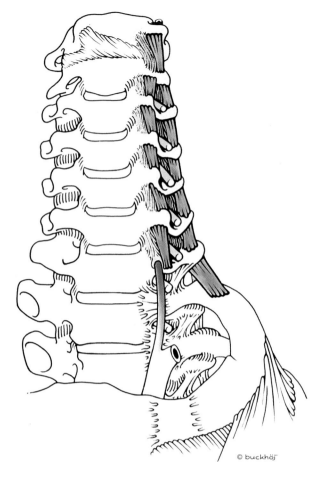

© buckhöj

The roots of the fifth through the eighth cervical nerves pass dorsal to the vertebral artery in their course through this short tunnel, but even as they emerge from the intervertebral foramina, the roots immediately pass into their respective fascia-invested intertransverse tunnel, each of which is continuous with the interscalene compartment laterally. As the roots leave their respective tunnels, they immediately enter the interscalene space, wherein they descend toward the first rib and converge to form the three trunks of the plexus.

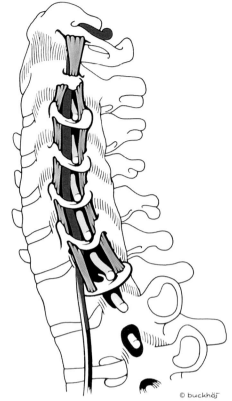

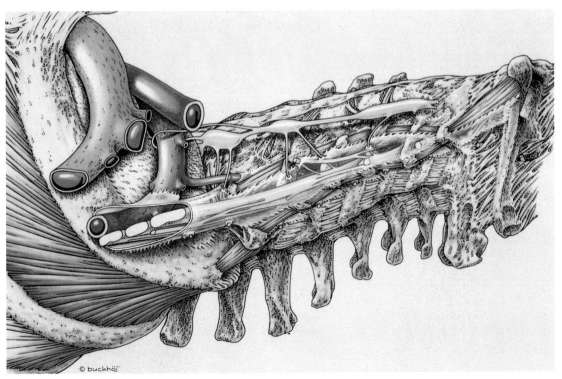

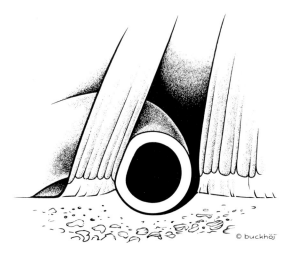 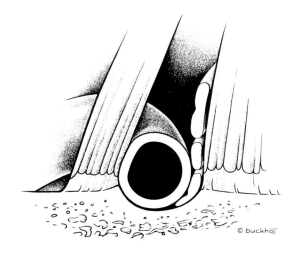

Another anatomical detail that can have immense clinical significance for the anesthetist is the fact that because the subclavian artery is a pulsatile structure that begins its pulsations early in embryologic development long before the first rib has ossified, the developing artery "erodes" a groove on the superior surface of the first rib between the insertions of the anterior and middle scalene muscles, the subclavian groove.

The clinical significance of this is that, as the artery "settles into" the groove it is creating on top of the first rib, not infrequently the inferior trunk of the brachial plexus gets trapped behind and even beneath the artery.

Years later, because of this anatomical relationship, the artery may serve as a mechanical barrier to the diffusion of local anesthetic solutions injected higher in the interscalene space. This is the reason why small (and sometimes even large) volumes of local anesthetic injected via the interscalene technique of brachial plexus block may fail to provide anesthesia in the distribution of the ulnar nerve, the fibers of which are buried deep within the inferior trunk behind or beneath the subclavian artery.

After the trunks have crossed the first rib, at about the upper border of the clavicle, they split to form the short anterior and posterior divisions of the plexus, a critical organizational step in the transition from trunks to cords and in the rearrangement of fibers into ultimate flexor and extensor distribution.

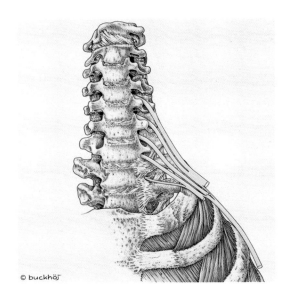

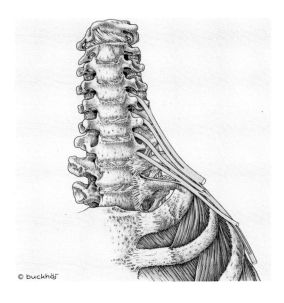

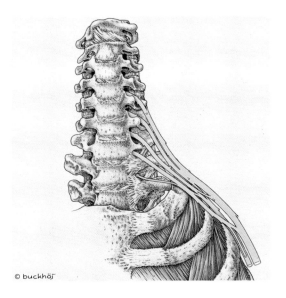

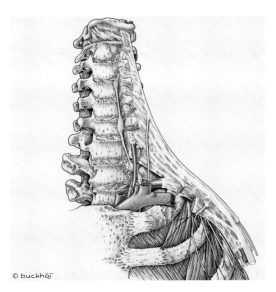

In passing under the clavicle, the subclavian artery becomes the axillary artery, and the relationship of the artery and plexus changes significantly above the clavicle:

In passing over the first rib and under the clavicle the subclavian vein also becomes the axillary vein, and its relationship with the entire neurovascular bundle changes.

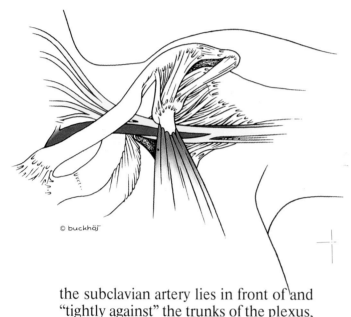

© buckhöj

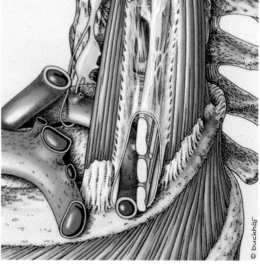

© buckhöj

the subclavian artery lies in front of and "tightly against" the trunks of the plexus,

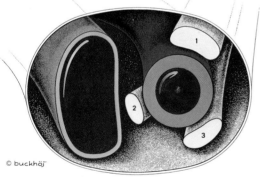

© buckhöj

1. Median nerve
2. Ulnar nerve
3. Radial nerve

whereas distal to the clavicle, the axillary artery lies central to the three cords, though they are not truly medial, lateral, and posterior with respect to their position around the artery until they pass behind the pectoralis minor muscle.

Above the first rib the subclavian vein does not lie within the neurovascular bundle as it is forming between the scalenes but rather is separated from its companion, the subclavian artery, by the insertion of the anterior scalene muscle.

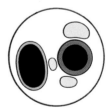

However, as it passes over the first rib and under the clavicle, the subclavian vein, in becoming the axillary vein, does join the neurovascular bundle so distal to the clavicle, parts of the plexus are sandwiched between artery and vein.

As the artery, vein, and plexus enter the axilla as the fully formed neurovascular bundle, they invaginate the prevertebral fascia at the lateral margins of the anterior and middle scalene muscles, carrying this fascial investment of the neurovascular bundle into the axilla as the axillary fascia, an extension of the prevertebral or scalene fasciae forming the axillary perivascular space, a tubular extension of the interscalene space.

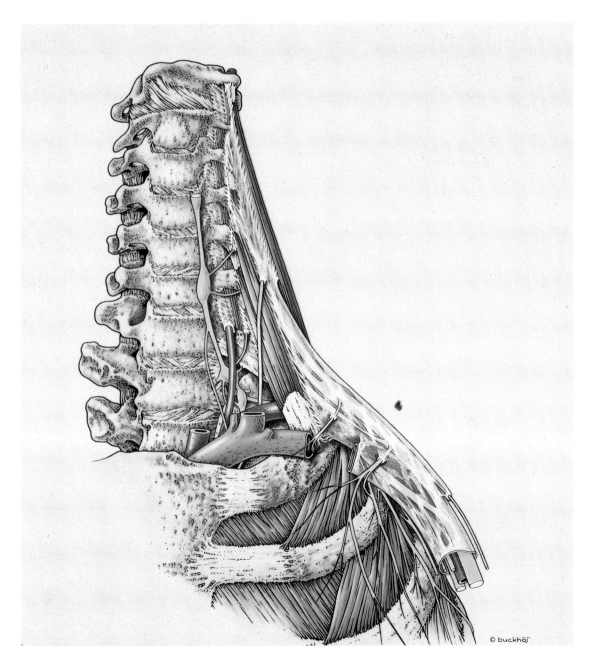

© buckhöj

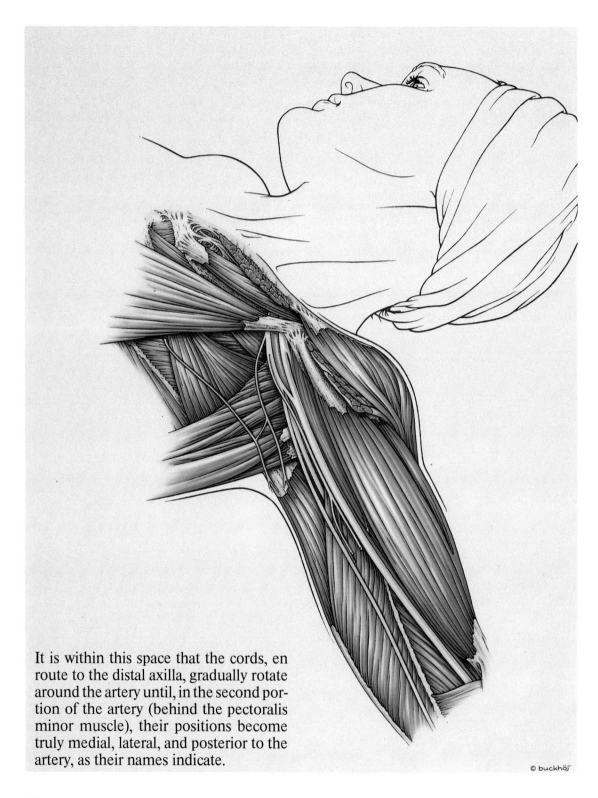

It is within this space that the cords, en route to the distal axilla, gradually rotate around the artery until, in the second portion of the artery (behind the pectoralis minor muscle), their positions become truly medial, lateral, and posterior to the artery, as their names indicate.

© buckhöj

It is approximately at the lateral edge of the pectoralis minor muscle that the cords give rise to the terminal nerves of the plexus, as described earlier. However, only the median, radial, ulnar, and medial antebrachial cutaneous nerves continue with the brachial artery and vein(s) within the axillary sheath at the level at which the various axillary block techniques are performed.

It is particularly important clinically that two of the major terminal nerves of the plexus, the musculocutaneous and axillary nerves, are not in the sheath at this level, since they leave the sheath high in the axilla under cover of the pectoralis minor muscle, at the level of the coracoid process, a useful landmark on x-ray.

As soon as it leaves the sheath, the musculocutaneous nerve enters the substance of the coracobrachialis muscle and continues down the arm within the substance of this muscle throughout most of its length, so while it travels parallel to the nerves that remain within the sheath, it is separated from them by the thick axillary sheath and by the fascial investment of the coracobrachialis muscle. The axillary nerve also leaves the sheath and the axilla immediately after arising from the posterior cord.

The intercostobrachial nerve always travels parallel to but outside the axillary sheath, and the medial brachial cutaneous nerve usually does likewise, although occasionally it remains within the sheath.

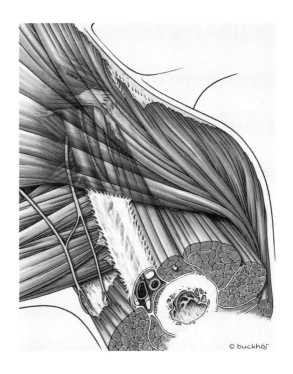

© buckhöj

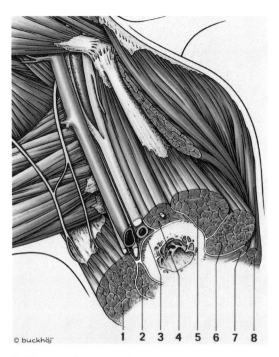

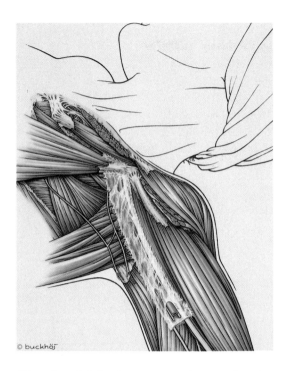

1. Triceps, long head
2. Triceps, lateral head
3. Triceps, medial head
4. Coracobrachialis
5. Biceps, short head
6. Biceps, long head
7. Pectoralis major
8. Deltoid muscle

The brachial plexus terminates in the upper arm, as it begins in the neck, that is, sandwiched between several muscles, namely the coracobrachialis muscle and the short head of the biceps above and the long head of the triceps below.

Thus, the neurovascular bundle and the plexus contained within it again lie in a protective "gutter", the walls of which are formed by these muscles and the floor by the head, neck, and shaft of the humerus.

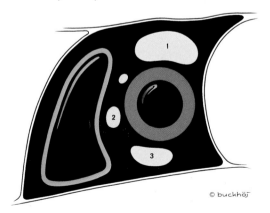

1. Median nerve
2. Ulnar nerve
3. Radial nerve

62

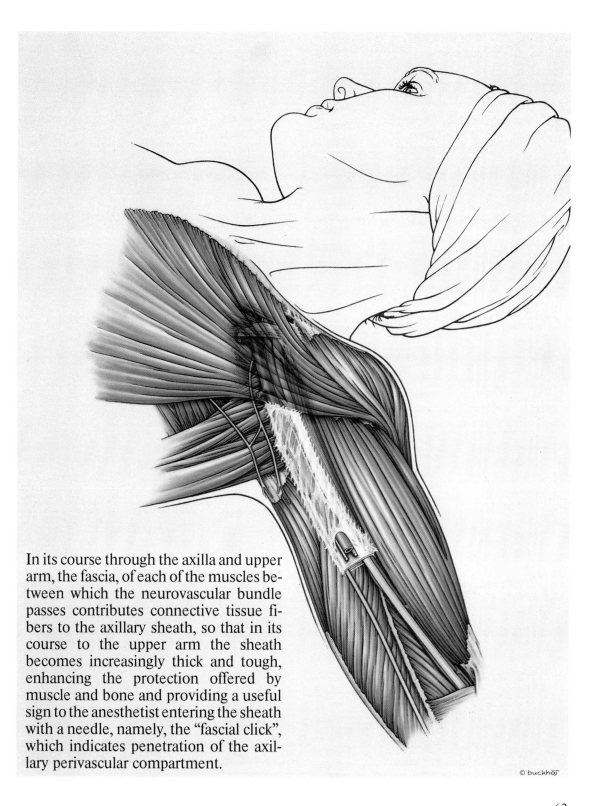

In its course through the axilla and upper arm, the fascia, of each of the muscles between which the neurovascular bundle passes contributes connective tissue fibers to the axillary sheath, so that in its course to the upper arm the sheath becomes increasingly thick and tough, enhancing the protection offered by muscle and bone and providing a useful sign to the anesthetist entering the sheath with a needle, namely, the "fascial click", which indicates penetration of the axillary perivascular compartment.

© buckhöj

63

Recently Rorie has described septa extending inward from the sheath surrounding the neurovascular bundle, and Thompson has demonstrated what appeared to be compartmentalization of dye injected into the axillary sheath on computed tomographic scans. The conclusion of both authors was that the perivascular space surrounding the brachial plexus is subdivided into multiple compartments by connective tissue septa, that these septa interfere with circumferential spread of injected local anesthetics, and that they explain the occasional occurrence (termed "not uncommon" by Thompson) of a profound block of rapid onset in one nerve and a partial or absent block in others following any perivascular technique of brachial block.

While it is difficult to refute the findings of both Rorie and Thompson, the author has not encountered such septa during the dissection of the brachial plexuses of over 50 cadavers, nor have any of hundreds of x-rays taken after the injection of radiopaque dye into the perivascular compartment at all levels indicated compartmentalization of the injection solution. Furthermore, in most series of brachial plexus blocks using any of the perivascular techniques, the incidence of partial block is the exception rather than the rule, so if such septa do exist, they are apparently of little clinical significance.

Summary

The important anatomical concept for the anesthetist is that of a continuous, fascia-enclosed, perineural, and perivascular compartment that extends from the origins of the brachial plexus at the intervertebral foramina to its termination in the upper arm. Thus, brachial plexus anesthesia can be approached conceptually and technically the way peridural anesthesia is approached. The perineural compartment can be entered at any level and the extent of anesthesia that will result from an injection of local anesthesia into the compartment will depend upon the volume of anesthetic agent utilized and the level at which it is injected. Furthermore, as with epidural anesthesia, utilizing this concept it is not necessary to find the nerves to be blocked with the needle but simply to find the space and allow the injected anesthetic solution to find the nerves. An understanding of the anatomical basis of the perivascular (interfascial) concept not only allows one to provide simpler, safer, and more successful regional anesthesia for upper extremity surgery but also gives one insight into the reasons for the problems associated with many of the techniques of brachial plexus block utilized in the past.

References & Bibliography

Anson, B. J. and Maddock, W. G.: Callanders' Surgical Anatomy. W. B. Saunders Co, Philadelphia, 1958.

Aubaniac, R. et Fortesa: The Clavipectoral fascia. Work carried out in the Anatomy Laboratory of the Faculty of Medicine of Algers [French] pp. pages 70-79, 1951.

Becker, R. F., Wilson, J. W. and Gehweiler, J. A.: The Anatomical Basis of Medical Practice. Williams & Wilkinson, Baltimore, 1971.

Callander, C. L.: Surgical Anatomy. W. B. Saunders Co., Philadelphia, 1934.

Chusid, J. G.: The Spinal Nerves. In Correlative Neuroanatomy & Functional Neurology. Chapter 5, 17th Ed., Lange Medical Publications, Los Altos, California, pp. 111-138.

Chusid, J. G.: The Autonomic Nervous System. In Correlative Neuroanatomy & Functional Neurology. Chapter 6, 17th Ed., Lange Medical Publications, Los Altos, California, pp.139-154.

Cunningham: Cunningham's Textbook of an Anatomy. 10th Ed. Edited by Romanes, G. J. Oxford University Press, London, 1964.

Cunningham: Cunningham's Manual of Practical Anatomy, 13th Ed. Volume I: Upper and Lower Limbs. Revised by Romanes, G. J. Oxford University Press, London, 1966.

Devloo, R. A.: Local Anesthesia in Chap 4, Vol I, Lewis-Walters Practice of Surgery, pp 35-39, W. F. Prior Co. Hagerstown Pa, 1966.

Ellis, H. and Mc Larty, M.: Anatomy for Anesthesists, pp. 157-185. Blackwell Scientific Publications, Oxford 1963.

Grant, J. C. B.: An Atlas of Anatomy. The Williams & Wilkins Co., Baltimore, 1951.

Gray: Gray's Anatomy, 27th Ed. Lea & Febiger, Philadelphia, 1959, pp 1011-1031.

Hollinshead, W. H.: Anatomy For Surgeons, 3: The Back and Limbs Hoerber-Harper, New York, 1958.

Jamieson, E. B.: Illustrations of Regional Anatomy, 8th Ed. Section VI, The Upper Limb. E. & S. Livingstone Ltd. Edinburgh.

Kaplan, E. B.: Variations of the Subclavian Vessels in the Region of the Scalenus Anterior Muscle Bull. Hosp. Joint Dis 8:217-218, 1947.

Kramer, J. G., and Todd, T. W.: The Distribution of Nerves to the Arteries of the Arm.: with a Discussion of the Clinical Value of Results. The Anatomical Record 8:243-255, 1914.

Kuntz, A.: Distribution of the Sympathetic Rami to the Brachial Plexus. Arch Surg. 15:87-876, 1927.

Kuntz, A., Alexander, W. F., and Furcolo, C. L.: Complete Sympathetic Denervation of the Upper Extremity. Ann. Surg. 107:25-31, 1938.

Lockhart, R. D.; Hamilton, G. F.; Fyfe, F. W.: Anatomy of the Human Body, pp. 284-295. J. B. Lippencott, Philadelphia, 1959.

Netter, F. H.: The CIBA Collection of Medical Illustrations, Volume I: Nervous System. CIBA Pharmaceutical Products, New York, 1953.

Pernkopf, E.: Atlas of Topographical and Applied Human Anatomy. W. B. Saunders Co., Philadelphia, 1980.

Rorie, D. K.: The Brachial Plexus Sheath. Anatomical Record 187:451, 1974.

Schaeffer: Morris' Human Anatomy, 11th Ed. Blakiston, New York, 1942.

Thompson, G. E. and Rorie, D. K.: Functional Anatomy of the Brachial Plexus Sheaths. Submitted for publication to Anesthesiology, 1982.

Thorek, Phillip: Anatomy in Surgery. J. B. Lippencott Co., Philadelphia, 1951.

II. Historical Considerations

"Those who do not remember the past are condemned to relive it."
Santayana

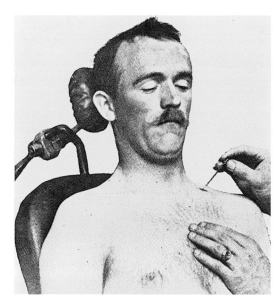

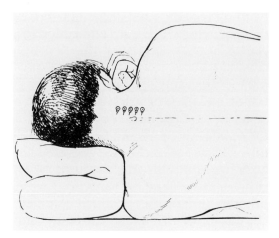

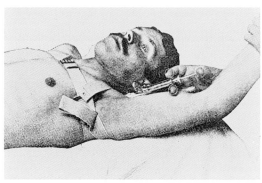

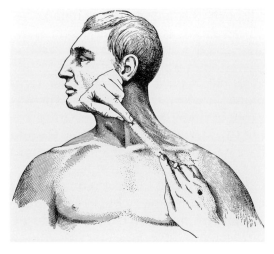

Evolution of Perivascular Techniques of Brachial Plexus Block

The first brachial block was also one of the first regional anesthetics ever administered; it was less than a year after the report by Koller in 1884 of the anesthetic properties of cocaine that Halsted injected the roots of the brachial plexus in the neck with cocaine and then surgically freed up the cords and peripheral nerves of the plexus, which were embedded in a cicatricial mass. However, this first brachial block was accomplished by exposing the roots surgically under local infiltration and injecting each of them with a small amount of dilute cocaine intraneurally under direct vision. Only about 0.5 ml of local anesthetic was required for each injection, this small volume being sufficient to distend the roots noticeably, but also sufficient to produce complete anesthesia of the upper extremity and allow painless surgical intervention; so although the anesthetic technique required almost as extensive surgery as the anticipated surgical procedure brachial plexus block was born.

In 1897 Crile utilized a similar technique, in which the brachial plexus was exposed under local anesthesia just behind the sternocleidomastoid muscle and cocaine injected into the nerve trunks under direct vision. Interestingly enough, Crile's first use of this technique was not carried out for surgery, but as a therapeutic measure in a 12 year old boy who developed tetanus three days after sustaining a compound fracture of the forearm. The tetanic spasms in the arm displaced the fractured bone, producing severe pain, but following the block, "the arm was entirely quiet and painless for four hours, and for about thirty-six hours a partial blocking was maintained." Subsequently, over the next few years Crile did use this technique to provide anesthesia for procedures on the upper extremity, and in every case, including a disarticulation of the shoulder joint, the anesthesia provided was reported as excellent; so while Halsted has chronological priority as the originator of brachial plexus anesthesia, because he failed to publish most of his work due to his subsequent addiction, this technique of "intraneural brachial plexus block" became known as "Crile's technique".

Naturally, since this technique did involve surgical exposure of the plexus, it never came into widespread use, and after the turn of the century efforts to provide regional anesthesia of the upper extremity centered around the development of percutaneous techniques. Nonetheless, as late as 1914, Allen wrote that "it is far better, safer, and surer, as well as quite simple, to resort to the free exposure of the plexus above the clavicle and injection of each individual nerve by the intraneural method." With respect to the recently introduced percutaneous techniques, Allen stated that "aside from the danger in the solution injected if injected in sufficient quantity and strength, the anatomy of the region should be sufficient to deter any but the most venturesome from this practice." It is fortunate for the subsequent development of regional anesthesia that some of these "venturesome" individuals were forthcoming.

Technique of Halstead (1884) and Crile (1897)

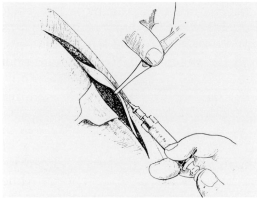

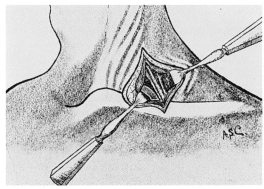

With a flat sandbag under the base of the neck and the head extended and rotated to the opposite side, a line is drawn from the middle of the sternocleidomastoid down to the middle of the clavicle. A wheal is made about the center of this line; with a long fine needle and large syringe the skin and subcutaneous tissue along this line are anesthetized with cocaine 0.1%. An incision is now made along the lower outer border of the sternocleidomastoid down to the superficial fascia, and after further infiltration with 0.1% cocaine, it is continued down through the deep fascia. It may be necessary to double ligate and divide the transversalis coli vessels to obtain a free field. With a little blunt dissection and palpation the plexus is located just above the subclavian artery; by locating the pulse of this vessel with the fingertip the exact position of the plexus is more readily located. By keeping the shoulder well depressed the plexus is easily brought into view. The trunks of the plexus thus exposed are injected, first on their outer covering and then into their substance, with a 0.5% solution of cocaine in sufficient volume to cause a localized swelling. Rapidly following the injection there is total loss of sensory and motor function of the entire arm.

From Surgical Operations With L. A. Arthur Hertzler. Surgery publishing Company N. Y. 1916.

From Jama 38, page 491-499, copyright 1902.
Reprinted by permission from American Medical Association.

Evolution of Axillary Perivascular Brachial Plexus Block

In 1911 Hirschel described the first *percutaneous* technique for blocking the brachial plexus and reported on its successful use in three patients. He made separate injections above and below the axillary artery with a 4 inch needle directed toward the apex of the axilla. He advised that the injection of local anesthetic be started as soon as the needle was inserted, and that the injection be continued as the needle was advanced "to push the vessels aside and to avoid entering them." The assumption that the continuously injected solution could push aside major blood vessels is obviously questionable, but it is of significance that Hirschel never reported encountering signs or symptoms of intravascular injection. Hirschel's percutaneous technique of blocking the brachial plexus from the axilla resulted from a multitude of axillary dissections carried out as part of radical mastectomies, and his intimate knowledge of the anatomy of the area is apparent from his emphasis on the need to continue the injection high into the axilla in order to block the musculocutaneous and axillary nerves, which leave the plexus there.

In his original report Hirschel forced a hard rubber ball as far up under the pectoral muscles as possible and fixed it to the shoulder and chest by two elastic bandages in an effort to attain a higher level of anesthesia and to prevent the anesthetic solution from being absorbed too rapidly.

Later, for practical reasons, he abandoned this practice without altering the satisfactory results obtained with his technique, though at the same time he did increase the volume of anesthetic injected to as much as 50 ml. One year after his first publication Hirschel reported 25 additional cases carried out successfully with his technique, but others were apparently unable to reduplicate his results, although his technique was included in the textbooks of regional anesthesia subsequently published in Germany, France, and the United States. Consequently, few reports appeared in the early literature concerning the axillary technique, and those that did were far from enthusiastic. Hartel, for example, stated that the technique was completely lacking in precision, since one or more of the nerves were almost always missed. Allen summarized the apparent attitude toward the axillary approach in 1914 as follows: "While the supraclavicular injection will find a place in our recognized methods of procedure, this injection within the axilla is, to say the least, unsurgical, and is not to be recommended."

Nonetheless, in 1917 Capelle in Germany described a technique, ignored by his contemporaries, that must be considered as the forerunner of the axillary perivascular technique. While Capelle was not aware of the existence of a fascial compartment, nonetheless he did demonstrate that axillary block could be simplified greatly by injecting local anesthetic around the artery in the bicipital groove perpendicular to the abducted

Technique of Hirschel (1911)

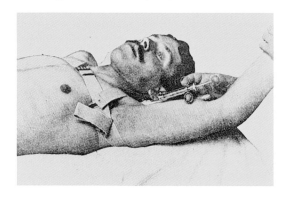

The patient lies supine on the table with the arm to be anesthetized in extreme abduction. To prevent the anesthetic solution from being absorbed too rapidly, a rubber ball is applied to the easily palpable vessels and fixed to the shoulder and chest with two elastic bandages. In order to have room enough for the injection the ball must be pushed far under the pectoral muscles. With the left hand the pulsating artery is felt for and fixed; with the right the syringe is held in the direction of the arm with the attached needle pointing towards the axilla. The needle is introduced into the skin over the artery, injecting as it is advanced to push the vessels aside and to avoid entering them. The best point to introduce the needle is near the insertion of the latissimus dorsi muscle. After about 10 ml of 2% Novocain-suprarenin solution have been injected over the artery for a distance of 3 to 4 cm, the needle is withdrawn, but not completely, and the same amount is introduced lateral and medial to the artery. As this is being done the artery may be held aside a little by the left hand. The injections above and in front of the artery surround the median and ulnar nerves with anesthetic, but to block the radial nerve the needle must be pushed under the artery, where this nerve lies. Finally, the needle should be pushed upward toward the first rib as far as possible under the pectoralis muscle in order to reach the musculocutaneous nerve. The axillary nerve is reached at the same level but below the vessel. At each of the two points about 10 ml of solution are injected. Following the injection gentle massage aids in spreading the anesthetic solution. After the onset of anesthesia, the bandages and ball are removed and the upper arm exsanguinated and tied off tightly.

From Münchener Medizinische Wochenschrift 58, page 1555-1556, copyright 1911.
Reprinted by permission from MMW Medizin Verlag GmbH, München.

arm at the level of insertion of the latissimus dorsi muscle. He pointed out accurately that all of the nerves derived from the plexus, except for the axillary and musculocutaneous, surround the artery at this level and thus will be bathed by the local anesthetic; even the musculocutaneous nerve, he said, lies near enough to the injection site to be blocked by the anesthetic. Though Capelle stated that his periarterial technique was as effective as Kulenkampff's supraclavicular technique for procedures on the distal third of the upper arm, the technique was completely ignored.

In 1921 in France, Reding described a technique that was virtually identical to the perivascular techniques of today, but his technique, like that of Capelle, was either ignored or forgotten by the surgeons and anesthetists of the day. Reding chose to block the terminal nerves with a short needle in the distal axilla, where they are "gathered into a bundle and are surrounded by a common fascial sheath which contains and directs the course of the anesthetic solution." In a classic article that might very well have been written forty years later, not only did Reding accurately describe the anatomy and the anatomical relationships of the neurovascular bundle in the axilla, including the importance of the sheath, but he also correctly pointed out that the musculocutaneous nerve leaves the sheath at a much higher level and must be blocked by a separate injection made within the substance of the coracobrachialis muscle, though because he used 40–80 ml, this probably was not necessary. It is of interest that Reding, having so carefully described the importance of the fascial sheath, still made multiple injections into

Technique of Capelle (1917)

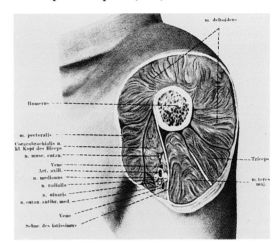

If blockade of the axillary nerve is not necessary (the peripheral cutaneous branches can always be anesthetized by a circular subcutaneous injection over the deltoid muscle), we can simplify axillary block by making an injection around the axillary artery in the bicipital groove to produce truly perineural anesthesia. With our technique the needle does not need to be advanced a great distance along the artery in a cephalad direction; the needle is simply inserted at the level of insertion of the latissimus dorsi muscle perpendicular to the abducted arm, since we are only attempting to deposit the local anesthetic around the artery as close to it as possible. As may be seen in the illustration of a cross section of the upper arm at the level at which our technique is carried out, the nerves (of the brachial plexus) surround the artery at this level, with the exception of the axillary nerve and the musculocutaneous nerve, which separate from the other nerves at a higher level, though the musculocutaneous nerve lies in the coracobrachialis muscle, which is not so far away that the local anesthetic can not reach the nerve. The remaining nerve trunks are immediately bathed in the local anesthetic solution when it is deposited around the artery, and the resultant block is as certain as with the supraclavicular technique.

We usually find 30-40 ml of 2% Novocain with adrenaline to be sufficient, though anesthesia is not complete for 30, and sometimes even 40-50 minutes after the injection. The duration of anesthesia is approximately 2 hours from the onset of complete anesthesia.

From Bruns Beiträge zur Klinische Chirurgie 104, page 122-139, copyright 1917.
Reprinted by permission from Springer-Verlag. Heidelberg.

the sheath, above, below, in front of, and in back of the artery. And yet, while it seems illogical to the author, even today many anesthetists, including those who employ large volumes with the axillary perivascular technique, presumably to reach the musculocutaneous nerve, continue the practice of entering and injecting into the sheath several times, rather than making a single injection within it. Nonetheless, Reding reported that in his first 40 cases he achieved 97% success, so one would have expected that the simplicity, safety, and high success rate of this technique would have caused it to be adopted universally as the technique of choice for performing brachial plexus block, or at least, the axillary technique of choice; but whether due to the fact that the technique was not included in any of the current textbooks and hence not perpetuated, or it was the supraclavicular approach of Kulenkampff was so overwhelmingly popular (in spite of a multitude of published complications associated with it), the technique of Reding and the concept of the neurovascular sheath were ignored and/or forgotten for almost four decades.

Technique of Reding (1921)

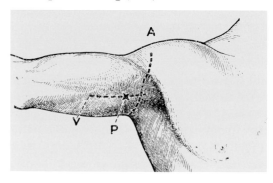

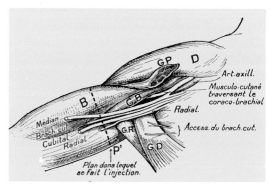

The patient is placed in the dorsal recumbent position with the arm abducted and lying on a table with the hand in supination. When the axilla has been shaved and prepared, a line is drawn over the artery (V) and a second (A) perpendicular to the first, is drawn from the insertion of the pectoralis major to the insertion of the latissimus dorsi muscle. Point P, the site of injection, is marked on line V about 2 cm lateral to the intersection with line A. At this point the median, ulnar, medial antebrachial cutaneous, and radial nerves are gathered into a bundle which lies with the vessels in the groove formed by the biceps and coracobrachialis muscles above and the triceps below. They are surrounded by a common fascial sheath which will contain and direct the course of injected anesthetic solution. The amount of anesthetic injected is 45 ml of a 2% solution of procaine.

The left thumb is placed at point P, fixing the neurovascular bundle and palpating the pulsations of the artery. The needle is then introduced perpendicular to the sheath, penetrating it and seeking successively the four nerves which at this level lie above, below, in front of and behind the artery, which it surrounds with a large cuff of the anesthetic agent. It is best to begin by looking for the median nerve because of its constant location in the upper part of the groove; the three other nerves are so close to each other that searching for paresthesias from them is unnecessary. The musculocutaneous nerve does not lie within the sheath, so it must be anesthetized by infiltrating the coracobrachialis muscle, which it enters at a considerably higher level; thus, the needle is advanced to the upper part of the inner surface of the humerus and the anesthetic is injected into the muscle fanwise between the bone and the sheath. The medial brachial cutaneous nerve is blocked by injecting a small amount of anesthetic into the subcutaneous tissue just below the sheath.

From Presse Medical 29, page 294-296, copyright 1921. Reprinted by permission from Masson, Editeur, S. A.

However, one author who include the axillary approach in his textbook was Gaston Labat, though the technique described by Labat was modified little from that of Hirschel, except that Labat deplored the practice of injecting anesthetic solution while advancing the needle. In fact, he felt that the needle should not be attached to the syringe during insertion; and he emphasized that after the needle had been placed and the syringe attached, aspiration tests should be made repeatedly prior to the injection. He did state that the anatomic features of the region are such that one should consider it good fortune to have placed the needle in its correct position without puncturing a blood vessel. Perhaps it is for this reason that the technique failed to attract much of a following, even after inclusion in the classic textbook of Pauchet in France and that of Labat in the United States.

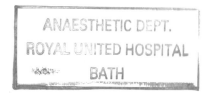
Technique of Labat (1922)

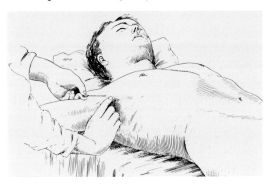

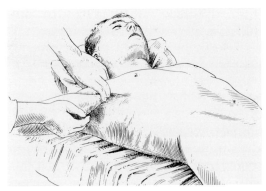

With the patient lying on his back and the upper extremity placed in 90° abduction, the axillary artery is defined by palpation and retracted downward by the index finger. A 10 cm needle is introduced through a wheal raised under the lower border of the pectoralis major muscle, close to its brachial attachment, and advanced in a direction parallel with the axis of the arm, along the outer wall of the axilla deeply beneath the muscle. After making sure that the point of the needle is not lying in the lumen of the blood vessel, the syringe is gently connected with the needle and injection made of 10-15 ml of the 2% solution. The syringe is almost completely discharged in the depth, and the rest of the solution is distributed while the needle is withdrawn. The axillary artery is then retracted upward toward the pectoralis major by the index finger, and the needle inserted through another wheal raised a little below the first site of puncture. The needle is advanced deeply behind the artery, in a direction parallel with the axis of the arm, along the outer wall of the axilla, thus aiming at its apex so as to reach the radial nerve in front of the head of the latissimus dorsi muscle. If no paresthesias are obtained, part of the solution is injected in the depth, and the rest while the needle is withdrawn, as for the first injection, using from 10-15 ml of the 2% solution. But if the needle happens to hit one of the main branches of the plexus during its progression in the axillary space, it should be stopped and the injection made without moving. The axilla is then gently massaged for a while to hasten the diffusion of the anesthetic fluid. As a rule the needle is never attached to the syringe when it is introduced in the vicinity of large blood vessels. Time is allowed before connecting the syringe, and the aspiration test made and renewed, so as to make sure that the point of the needle does not lie in the lumen of the blood vessel.

From Labat's Regional Anesthesia, page 218-220, copyright 1923. Reprinted by permission from W. B. Saunders & Co., Philidelphia.

Later in the same decade Pitkin, after experiencing failures with Hirschel's technique, injected dye into cadavers using Hirschel's technique and then made dissections to determine the relationship of the deposited dye to the nerves. On the basis of these studies Pitkin decided that the failures with this technique were due to the use of a short needle and that the plexus *could* be anesthetized more reproducibly if the nerves could be bathed anteriorly and posteriorly with anesthetic solution all the way from the cervical transverse processes to the lateral margin of the pectoralis major muscle. Thus, he developed his "improved technique" of advancing a 5, 6, 7, or even 8 inch needle from the axilla under the clavicle and over the first rib until contact was made with the transverse processes of the sixth and seventh cervical vertebrae respectively. As if this were not heroic enough, Pitkin injected 10 ml continuously during the insertion of each needle and an additional 10 ml during its subsequent withdrawal! He did concede that intermittent aspiration should be performed to prevent the occurrence of convulsions "which will not produce any real harm, but it throws a scare into the operator who is witnessing it for the first time and causes the nurse and intern staff to ask embarrassing questions which cannot be satisfactorily answered." And if convulsions did not occur immediately from intravascular injection, one would expect that they might very well occur somewhat later from systemic absorption, when one considers the fact that when using this technique in conjunction with cervical and intercostal blocks for radical mastectomy, as Pitkin did, a total volume of approximately 260 ml of 1.0 to 1.5% Novocain® was invariably injected. Nonetheless, Pitkin claimed that he never saw a toxic reaction due to systemic absorption, and felt that this was due to his routine use of epinephrine 1:360,000, which delayed absorption without impairing elimination. Certainly, his "almost 100% success" with this technique attests to Pitkin's mastery of the needle, but it is not surprising that this approach, requiring two insertions of an 8 inch needle, never became popular.

Technique of Pitkin (1927)

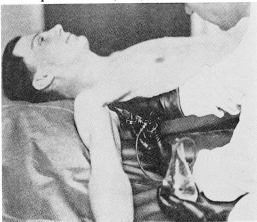

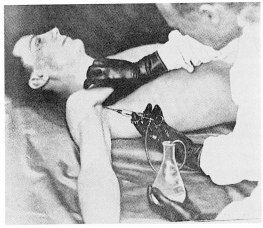

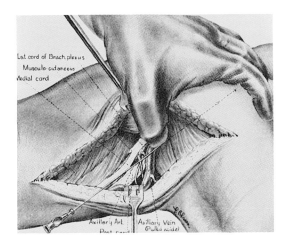

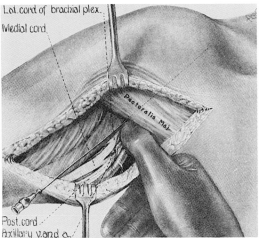

The patient is placed on the table in the dorsal recumbent position, and the arm is placed at a right angle to the body on a table having the same height as the top of the cushion on the operating table. A cutaneous wheal is raised just beneath the lateral margin of the pectoralis major muscle. The skin is manipulated by the thumb so as to draw the wheal forward over the axillary vessels, which are pressed posteriorly. A 6, 7, or 8 inch needle (depending on the size of the patient) is inserted through the wheal and carried up through the axilla under the clavicle anterior to the axillary nerves and vessels as they pass over the first rib, a small amount of anesthetic solution being projected in advance of the needle. As soon as the point of the needle emerges from under the clavicle, its progress is directed by the fingers (which can now release the axillary vessels) to the transverse process of the fifth cervical vertebra. Five ml of 1.5% Novocain solution is injected at this site, and an additional 10 ml are deposited as the needle is withdrawn, bathing the entire anterior aspect of the cervical and brachial plexuses. When the needle has been completely withdrawn, the skin is manipulated to retract the wheal posteriorly, and the axillary nerves and vessels are now retracted upward and forward by the thumb. The needle is reinserted through the wheal and passes up over the first rib to the nerve trunks, projecting a small amount of solution ahead of the advancing needle.

While still holding the vessels forward with the thumb, the fingers of the same hand guide the point of the needle to the transverse process of the sixth cervical vertebra, and 5 ml of the anesthetic solution are injected. Fifteen ml are again deposited along the posterior aspect of the cervical and brachial plexuses as the needle is withdrawn.

From Anesthesia and Analgesia Volume 21, page 83-95, copyright 1942.
Reprinted by permission from International Anesthesia Research Society.

From Pitkins: Conduction Anesthesia, page 73, copyright 1953.
Reprinted by permission from Lippencott, New York.

In 1946 Hingson described a technique in Pitkin's *Conduction Block* (published after Pitkin's death) which was technically similar to that of Reding, except that although local anesthetic was deposited above and below the artery, with a separate injection into the biceps muscle to block the musculocutaneous nerve, no mention was made of the axillary sheath or the neurovascular bundle it contains. Because Hingson's technique utilized *much* smaller volumes than that of Reding, the separate blockade of the musculocutaneous nerve was absolutely necessary, for a volume of 10 ml injected periarterially would never reach this nerve via the sheath.

Technique of Pitkin, Hingson and Southworth (1946)

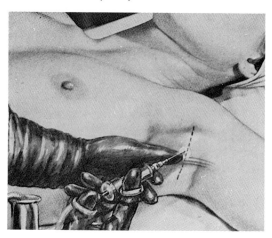

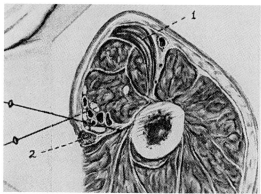

With the arm at right angles to the body, the insertion of the pectoralis major and the insertion of the tendon of the latissimus dorsi muscle are palpated. An imaginary line is drawn between these two points and injections are made through this line anterior and posterior to the brachial artery as follows: the brachial artery is palpated between the short head of the biceps and the long head of the triceps muscles. With the fingertip pressing the brachial artery against the inner surface of the humerus, the artery is retracted slightly posteriorly and a 1 inch 25-gauge needle is inserted through a subcutaneous wheal anterior to the fingertip and beneath the inner border of the short head of the biceps. After 5 ml of the 2% procaine-suprarenin solution have been injected, the needle is withdrawn to the skin surface, redirected slightly anteriorly, and inserted into the short head of the biceps muscle until the point is directly in front of the anterior surface of the humerus. Here 5 ml of the solution are injected to block the musculocutaneous nerve. Without any change in the position of the finger on the brachial artery, the artery is retracted slightly anteriorly and 5 ml of solution are injected between the fingertip and the long head of the triceps muscle.

Ten ml of a 2% procaine solution will be more than adequate to bathe all of the nerves when the injection is made as indicated above.

From Pitkins: Conduction Anesthesia, 1st Ed., page 624, copyright 1946 and 2nd ed., copyright 1953.
Reprinted by permission from Lippencott, New York.

No clinical reports appeared in the literature using Hingson's technique, and yet the technique described in 1949 by Accardo and Adriani is simply Hingson's technique, but with the production of paresthesias an essential part of the technique. This technique, considered by many to be the first axillary block, utilized four separate injections in the axilla to block the median, musculocutaneous, ulnar, and radial nerves; but in each case the injection was only made after a paresthesia in the distribution of the nerve to be blocked had been produced. Again, however, no reference is made to the existence of a fascial sheath or compartment. In spite of the rather unpleasant requirement of repeated paresthesias, the only clinical reports that subsequently appeared using this technique, those of Small in 1951 and of Clayton and Turner in 1959, concerned the use of this technique in children! Whether because of the reticence of anesthetists to evoke multiple paresthesias or because of technical problems of accomplishing complete anesthesia (Adriani himself later said that the radial nerve was not infrequently missed), this technique was not adopted by many.

Technique of Accardo and Adriani (1949)

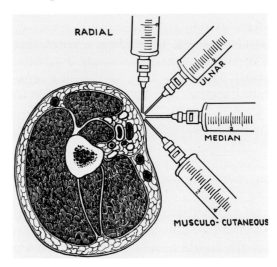

The patient is placed in the supine position with the arm abducted at 90° and resting upon a support in external rotation. A line is drawn between the insertion of the pectoralis major and latissimus dorsi muscles. The midpoint of this line lies over the brachial artery, which is easily palpable even in obese subjects. A wheal is raised at this point, the artery is retracted posteriorly with the thumb and index finger, and a ¾, 1 or 1 ¼ inch 25-gauge needle is introduced directly perpendicular to the skin and humerus toward the median nerve, which is frequently palpable along the superior surface of the artery. Paresthesias are sought to the fingertips, and when they have been evoked, 5 ml of 2% procaine are injected. The needle is then withdrawn almost to the skin and reintroduced at an angle of 45° anterior to the direction of the first injection. The point will thus be directed toward the insertion of the pectoralis major muscle; this maneuver is designed to inject the musculocutaneous nerve, which at this point invariably lies close to the artery. When paresthesias to the elbow have been produced by the needle advancing in this direction, 5 ml of 2% procaine are injected. The needle is then withdrawn almost to the skin, the artery is retracted anteriorly toward the upper surface of the arm, and the needle is directed posteriorly (downward) at an angle of 45° to the line of the original injection. The needle is advanced in this direction until paresthesias to the 4th and 5th digits are obtained, after which 5 ml of the 2% procaine are injected. The needle is once again withdrawn almost to the skin and is reintroduced at an angle of almost 90° to the direction of the original injection, and when paresthesias to the distribution of the radial nerve along the back of the hand are obtained, a final 5 ml of 2% procaine are injected.

The syringe should remain attached to the needle throughout all maneuvers. It is also imperative that the needle be at right angles to the long axis of the humerus at all times. Aspiration must be attempted before each injection, and afterward the injection site is gently massaged for 5 minutes.

From Southern Medical Journal 42, page 920-923, copyright 1949. Reprinted by permission from Southern Medical Journal, Birmingham, USA.

In 1958, while repairing a deep laceration of the apex of the axilla in a child, Preston Burnham, an orthopedic surgeon, was impressed by the compactness of the nerves at this level, where they were gathered closely about the artery and enveloped by a fascial investment. Thus, the neurovascular sheath was rediscovered 37 years after it had been described by Reding; and though Burnham was unaware of Reding's work, he immediately recognized that this sheath could simplify percutaneous anesthesia of the great nerves of the upper arm. With the technique Burnham described there was no need to identify each nerve by eliciting paresthesias; the sheath itself was identified by the characteristic "click" that could be perceived when the needle penetrated it, and the anesthetic solution was injected into the sheath, which would confine the anesthetic and bathe all of the nerves contained therein. Although Burnham is the first person in recent times to utilize the perivascular concept, like all who approached the brachial plexus from the axilla before him, he did retain the practice of making an injection above and below the artery, a practice which his new concept should have ended.

Shortly after the appearance of Burnham's first article, Eather reported that he and his associates had performed an almost identical technique of "periarterial infiltration" in several hundred patients over the preceding few years. On the basis of their experience, he pointed out that because the musculocutaneous nerve leaves the sheath high in the axilla, injecting the local anesthetic at a higher level and in larger volumes (sometimes as high as 50 ml) was essential to satisfactory anesthesia with this technique. Burnham did subsequently increase the volume of the injection he had mentioned in his original article (6-8 ml), but in view of our present knowledge, the volume he utilized was still insufficient to *reproducibly* reach the musculocutaneous nerve. It would certainly seem that if the large volume of local anesthetic Burnham utilized to encircle the arm and thus allow the use of a tourniquet were injected into the sheath instead of being wasted in the subcutaneous tissues, a considerably higher success rate could be achieved with Burnham's technique.

Nonetheless, the simplicity of the technique led many anesthetists to try it, and within a very short time reports of its successful use began to appear in the literature. Though modifications of the original technique inevitably appeared and to varying degrees served to improve the results obtained, perivascular brachial plexus block anesthesia was now here, and here to stay.

Technique of Burnham (1958)

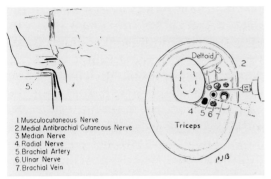

1. Musculocutaneous Nerve
2. Medial Antibrachial Cutaneous Nerve
3. Median Nerve
4. Radial Nerve
5. Brachial Artery
6. Ulnar Nerve
7. Brachial Vein

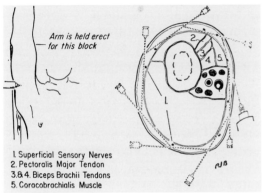

Arm is held erect for this block

1. Superficial Sensory Nerves
2. Pectoralis Major Tendon
3. & 4. Biceps Brachii Tendons
5. Coracobrachialis Muscle

The patient lies on his back with his arm abducted, the elbow flexed, and the forearm flat on the supporting table. This position externally rotates the upper arm and places the neurovascular space uppermost over the humerus. The palpating finger finds the brachial artery just under the biceps muscle and distal to the pectoralis major tendon. With the fingers on the artery, a 5/8 inch, 25-gauge needle with syringe attached is pressed through the skin into the subcutaneous tissue, where a few minims of anesthetic are injected. Now the needle and syringe are tipped slightly to one side to miss the artery and is advanced until the needle very clearly "pops" through the fascia. It is then pushed on until it is estimated that the point is next to the artery. Aspiration is attempted, and if blood appears, the needle is withdrawn slightly and angled farther away from the artery, or it is simply advanced until aspiration shows the tip to be beyond the vessel. If no blood appears on aspiration, 3-4 ml of anesthetic solution are injected, while the needle is moved in and out slightly during the injection to distribute the anesthetic throughout the neurovascular space. The needle is then withdrawn from the fascia, but not from the skin, and reinserted below the artery until the click of the fascia again indicates that the neurovascular space has been entered, at which point 3-4 ml are similarly injected.

To facilitate the tolerance of a tourniquet, a "ring" type of block is required. The 25-gauge needle is replaced by a 3 inch 22-gauge needle which is inserted through the same spot in the skin to traverse the subcutaneous tissue, where roughly 1 ml of anesthetic is deposited per insertion of the needle or to every 3 inches of circumference of the arm. This procedure effectively arrests the passage of stimuli through the superficial sensory nerves of the upper arm.

From Jama 169, page 941-943, copyright 1959.
Reprinted by permission from American Medical Association.

In 1959, for example, Hudon and Jacques presented their technique, which replaced the two sequential injections into the sheath with the insertion of two separate needles above and below the artery prior to injection. The rather disappointing 14% failure rate obtained with this modification was apparently due to the fact that their injection into the sheath was made in the distal axilla. This is substantiated by the fact that Kleinert and his co-workers were able to reduce the failure rate to 5% using a volume and technique identical to that of Hudon and Jacques, *except* that they placed that volume higher in the sheath.

The precise relationship between volume and anesthesia awaited the studies reported in 1961 by de Jong, who carried out multiple anatomical dissections to determine the diameter of the axillary sheath and the neurovascular bundle contained therein and the distance from the injection site to the level at which the musculocutaneous and axillary nerves leave the sheath. De Jong found the diameter of the average adult axillary sheath to be about 3 cm and the distance from the usual injection site to the level of the cords to be approximately 3 cm; assuming equal proximal and distal spread of local anesthetic from the site of injection, he calculated that 42 ml of anesthetic solution must be injected if the solution is to reach the level at which the musculocutaneous and axillary nerves leave the sheath. Since his dissections were carried out in healthy adult men who had died traumatic deaths, obviously this volume would be somewhat smaller in women and even less in children.

Technique of Hudon and Jacques (1959)

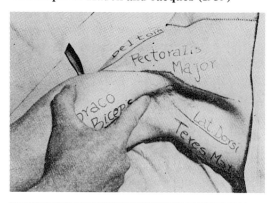

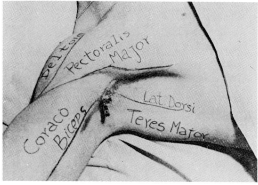

The patient lies with his arm abducted at 90° in a neutral position or in external rotation. At the level of the inferior border of the pectoralis major muscle the axillary artery is sought with the finger just below the coracobrachialis muscle. With the finger on the artery a first needle is introduced at a 30° angle just anterior to the artery and is advanced until the fascia has been penetrated, after which the pulsations of the needle are noted. A second needle is then introduced on the opposite side of the artery, also at a 30° angle with the skin, and is advanced until the fascial click and needle pulsations indicate that this needle also lies in the neurovascular space. Ten ml of lidocaine 2% or of chloroprocaine 2% with epinephrine 1:500,000 are injected through each needle, so that anesthetic is deposited on both sides of the artery and in front of the artery, the latter being accomplished by continuing to inject as the needle is withdrawn. Aspiration tests are carried out before and after each injection.

One year later Eriksson introduced the use of a tourniquet applied distal to the needle in an effort to prevent the distal spread of the anesthetic solution down the sheath during the injection. Using this simple modification, he felt he could achieve equal results with almost half the volume of local anesthetic, since the volume of the cylinder (sheath) in de Jong's calculations assumed equal flow in both directions. However, in clinical practice the use of a tourniquet is not effective in preventing retrograde flow, as indicated in Chapter III, for three reasons: first of all, because of the bulk and shape of the deltoid muscle, a tourniquet cannot be placed "immediately behind the needle" but at best, perhaps two inches distal to the needle; secondly, the tightly applied tourniquet is extremely uncomfortable for the patient, and makes identification of the axillary artery pulse much more difficult; and finally, and most importantly, as indicated in Chapter III, the tourniquet is simply ineffective in preventing retrograde or distal flow. Because of the fact that the muscles above and below the neurovascular bundle protect the sheath from the pressure of the tourniquet, the sheath is not compressed by the tourniquet and the distal flow of injected local anesthetic is therefore not obstructed.

The technique used by the author and described in detail in Chapter III is considerably simpler than all of the above techniques, and yet allows the same high incidence of successful blocks. Why? First of all, only a single injection is made into the axillary sheath. The practice of making an injection above and below the artery is as illogical as it would be to inject the front and the back of the epidural space. All techniques admit to flow up and down the sheath, but apparently not around it. Thompson has recently demonstrated the presence of fibrous tissue septa within the axillary sheath, but it would appear that these septa, if they exist, do not impair the spread of local anesthetic within the sheath, as attested to by the high success rate of single injection techniques, and by the x-ray studies presented in Chapter III. Secondly, with the author's technique the needle is inserted as high in the axilla as possible to place the tip of the needle above the humeral head, which can obstruct cephalad flow when the injection is made below it, and to place the local anesthetic as close as possible to the level at which the musculocutaneous and axillary nerves leave the sheath. Thirdly, the direction of needle insertion is as close to the long axis of the neurovascular bundle as possible, so that the thrust of the anesthetic solution will minimize retrograde and maximize central flow of the anesthetic solution. And finally, digital pressure immediately behind the injection site during the injection will prevent any retrograde flow of local anesthetic solution, allowing all of the volume injected to move centrally. To complete the technique, the digital pressure should be maintained after the completion of the injection while the arm is abducted to minimize interference with central flow caused by the humeral head *if* the injection cannot be made proximal to it. The use of a single injection *superior* to the artery also minimizes the possibility of entering the axillary vein during the performance of this technique, for the vein or veins which tend to lie in front of the artery will be compressed by the palpating finger and rolled inferiorly, out of the way of the advancing needle.

Technique of Eriksson (1962)

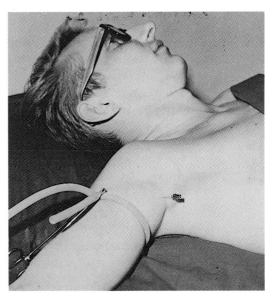

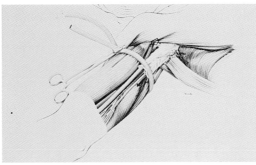

The patient is placed in the supine position with the arm abducted at an angle of about 90°. After a tourniquet has been applied to the upper arm just below the axilla to prevent the anaesthetic solution from spreading distally, the axillary artery is palpated and a *short* (4-5 cm) needle is inserted toward and slightly above it. If the needle shows marked pulsation, it indicates that its point lies near the artery in the correct fascial compartment. After careful aspiration the anesthetic solution is injected, bearing in mind the patient's body weight and general condition. Paresthesia is not sought using this technique. However, should it be encountered, the needle point is in the correct position, but injection must not be attempted until the point has been withdrawn slightly. In very obese patients it is an advantage to elicit paresthesias. The tourniquet applied to the upper arm prevents the anesthetic solution from spreading distally and forces it upward. Thus the chance of producing a successful block of the musculocutaneous nerve is considerably increased, and at the same time the volume of local anesthetic injected may be reduced. The tourniquet should remain in place for about 10 minutes.

All of the axillary perivascular techniques have in common the use of considerable volumes of local anesthetic solution. In the occasional cardiac patient in failure or in otherwise debilitated patients the use of volumes as high as 40-50 ml may be undesirable. In 1965 de Jong in this country and Clavet in Canada described modified axillary techniques which allow the use of considerably lower volumes: they injected 20-25 ml of local anesthetic into the axillary sheath to block all of the nerves except for the musculocutaneous, which they blocked just above the elbow by injecting 5 ml of local anesthetic subcutaneously along the lateral margin of the biceps tendon. Here the lateral antebrachial cutaneous nerve, the sensory continuation of the musculocutaneous nerve, becomes superficial on its way to the lateral aspect of the forearm.

However, in blocking the musculocutaneous nerve at this level, it must be appreciated that only sensory blockade will be achieved, with no blockade of the powerful flexors of the forearm, which will remain intact. For this reason, in order to assure the surgeon of a quiet operative field in patients when a low volume technique is desirable, the author utilizes a technique (Chapter III) very similar to that of Reding: after injecting 10-15 ml of local anesthetic into the sheath, as described in Chapter III, the needle is withdrawn from the sheath (but not from the skin) and is redirected into the substance of the coracobrachialis muscle, where an additional 5 ml achieves both sensory *and motor* block of the musculocutaneous nerve.

Since it is common practice today to use a pneumatic tourniquet to provide the surgeon with a bloodless field, whatever technique is utilized to provide anesthesia at the surgical site, sufficient anesthesia must be provided so that the tourniquet itself does not cause pain. If surgery is confined to the hand, the tourniquet *may* be placed just proximal to the elbow, obviating the need for a supplemental block. If the surgery involves the forearm, however, the tourniquet must be placed as high on the upper arm as possible, and this requires anesthesia of the axillary, medial brachial cutaneous, and intercostobrachial nerves. The axillary nerve will be blocked if a large enough volume of local anesthetic has been injected to reach the level where this nerve leaves the axillary sheath, but the medial brachial cutaneous nerve and the intercostobrachial nerve are not inside the sheath, but run parallel to the sheath just superficial to it, and can be blocked by simply depositing a few ml's of local anesthetic subcutaneously after injection into the sheath. The use of a large volume and separate block of the medial brachial cutaneous and the intercostobrachial nerves obviates the necessity of placing a "subcutaneous bracelet" around the arm, as Burnham did in order to prevent tourniquet pain.

Technique of de Jong (1965)

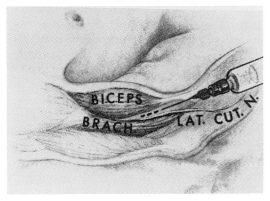

The patient lies supine, the upper arm at right-angle abduction to the body, the forearm flexed, and the hand resting on a table. The pulsations of the axillary artery are palpated and followed to their most proximal palpable location. After raising a skin wheal, a few milliliters of anesthetic solution are deposted in the subcutaneous tissues to block the intercostobrachial and medial brachial cutaneous nerves. The left hand grasps the patient's upper arm with the left thumb over the artery just distal to the site of injection and the fingers lying over the biceps and deltoid muscles. A 26-gauge needle and attached syringe are then directed inward perpendicularly to the skin toward the humerus. After advancing through the skin for only a few millimeters, the penetration of the axillary fascia will produce a characteristic "snap." Advancing a few more millimeters places the tip of the needle within the neurovascular compartment where 10-15 ml of anesthetic are deposited. Two such needle insertions are made through the axillary sheath into the neurovascular compartment, and after satisfactory placement, moderate pressure to occlude the compartment is exerted by the left thumb throughout each injection.

Following completion of the axillary block, the patient's arm is brought down and placed on an arm board with the elbow slightly flexed and the hand pronated so that the palm lies on the arm board. At the elbow crease, the lateral edge of the biceps tendon is identified by palpation and traced proximally to identify the lateral edge of the biceps muscle. A 22-gauge needle 5 cm long, with filled syringe attached, is inserted about 2.5 cm proximal to the elbow crease and is advanced subcutaneously for 4 to 5 cm along the lateral edge of the biceps tendon and muscle. Five ml of anesthetic are injected (with repeated aspiration) as the needle is slowly advanced to block the lateral antebrachial cutaneous nerve, which emerges from the lateral edge of the biceps muscle in this area.

Evolution of Subclavian Perivascular Brachial Plexus Block

Only a few months after Hirschel described his axillary approach to the brachial plexus, Kulenkampff described the first percutaneous supraclavicular approach. In his original article Kulenkampff pointed out that above the clavicle, where the plexus has just emerged from the scalene tringle, it lies just under the skin as it passes over the first rib and under the clavicle and thus is very accessible to a percutaneous technique. Since with his technique the midpoint of the clavicle and subclavian artery provided seemingly constant and easily identifiable landmarks and because the first rib provided a safe backstop to limit the progress of the needle, Kulenkampff felt that his technique offered far greater accuracy and safety than Hirschel's technique.

Kulenkampff performed his first attempts at this technique on himself, attempts in which he used only 5 ml of Novocain®. Even this small volume caused paresis of the arm, though the anesthesia was incomplete, as would be expected. Continuing his studies in patients, Kulenkampff increased the volume to 10 ml and was able to obtain complete anesthesia in the vast majority of cases. However, the crucial point emphasized by Kulenkampff, but subsequently forgotten by many who attempted his technique, was that the purpose of the technique was *not* to hit the first rib with the needle but to find the trunks of the plexus with the needle. He stated that if the landmarks were identified correctly and the needle was inserted in the proper direction, paresthesias would result as soon as the deep fascia had been penetrated. The only purpose the rib served, according to Kulenkampff, was to prohibit pleural penetration and to confine the injected solution somewhat; he even went on to state that if the first rib was reached, the needle was deep to the plexus, so the solution should not be injected at this point. Furthermore, unlike many subsequent modifications, Kulenkampff's was a *single injection* technique, for as he quite accurately stated, the nerves lie very close together between the scalene muscles in loose areolar tissue, which the injected local anesthetic solution can easily penetrate; so once a paresthesia was obtained, the entire contents of the syringe were to be injected. Multiple injection techniques were subsequent modifications of Kulenkampff's technique, and the practice of "walking the rib" was not introduced for almost thirty years. However, the later modifications of Kulenkampff's technique did *not* increase the success rate and served only to increase the incidence of complications. As is so often the case in medicine, it would take almost half a century before the simplicity of the original technique would be rediscovered.

In the first few years following Kulenkampff's original report, the literature was filled with clinical case reports. The earliest of these were enthusiastic about the efficacy of the technique and proclaimed emancipation from general anesthesia. Before long, however, the reports began to concern themselves with an increasing array of complications: phrenic nerve paralysis, pneumothorax, hemopneumo-thorax, prolonged paralysis of the arm, mediastinal emphysema, and even death. But in spite of these the technique remained popular, perhaps because of its obvious utility in treating the casualties of the first World War, which began only a few years after its introduction.

Except for the attempt of Perthes to improve the success rate of the technique by locating the plexus with an electric stimulator, a concept which never gained popularity, the technique remained unaltered for about a decade, though virtually everyone (including Kulenkampff) increased the volume of local anesthetic to at least 20 ml. The first significant modification was that of Labat, published in the first edition of his book in 1922. Labat advocated the injection of the local anesthetic at three separate points, but offered his technique only as an *alternative* to be utilized when paresthesias could not be produced by Kulenkampff's technique. Nonetheless, this alternative became known as Labat's technique and was adopted by many who preferred it to Kulenkampff's technique. The anatomical basis for Labat's second injection was the fact that the seventh cervical nerve, which emerges from just below Chassaignac's tubercle, forms the axis of the brachial plexus. He felt that if the anesthetic solution were distributed at that point, it would diffuse up and down along the spine in the loose areolar tissue surrounding the roots, blocking them and any branches originating high in the plexus. He felt that the third injection was necessary to complete the block in case one of the trunks joins the plexus beyond the first rib after passing in front of the anterior scalene muscle and subclavian artery. Such an anatomical variation is virtually unheard of, but with a technique in which

Technique of Kulenkampff (1911)

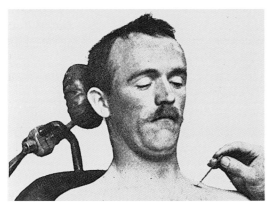

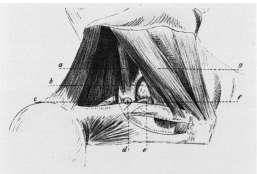

a) Musc. scalen. med. — b) Lungenspitze. — c) M. omohyoid. — d) Quaddel. — e) Art. subclav. mit Art. transvers. colli. — f) M. scalen. ant. — g) M. sternocleidomast.

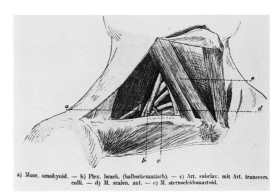

a) Musc. omohyoid. — b) Plex. brach. (halbschematisch). — c) Art. subclav. mit Art. transvers. colli. — d) M. scalen. ant. — e) M. sternocleidomastoid.

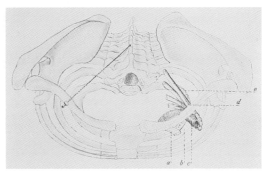

If possible, the patient is in the sitting position with the head turned slightly to the opposite side. The position of the subclavian artery is determined by palpation, the most frequent location being the point where a projection of the course of the external jugular vein intersects the clavicle. A wheal is raised just lateral to the artery and just above the clavicle. A thin 4 cm needle is inserted through the wheal in a direction that is backward, downward, and inward, as though one were aiming at the spinous process of the second thoracic vertebra. The needle is advanced until a paresthesia to the arm occurs or until the first rib is contacted. However, the objective is to hit the trunks, not the rib. Thus if the plexus is not encountered before the first rib is reached, the needle must be withdrawn and the direction altered somewhat, usually more medially and closer to the vessel. When a paresthesia has been definitely obtained, a syringe is carefully attached to the needle, and 10 ml of 2% Novocain-adrenaline are injected. It is to be emphasized that no solution should be injected until paresthesias have been evoked; when the needle lies on the first rib, it is deep to the plexus, and injection at this point will be ineffective.

An understanding of the relationship between the plexus, the artery, the clavicle, and the rib is essential. Injection is at a point that roughly corresponds to the middle of the clavicle: at this point the plexus has just emerged from between the anterior and middle scalene muscles and lies close to the skin in loose areolar tissue, where it may easily be infiltrated. The area into which the solution is injected is bounded medially by the subclavian artery, laterally by the clavicle, and inferiorly by the first rib.

From Beiträge zur Klinische Chirurgi 114, page 666-680, copyright 1919 and 79, page 550-572, copyright 1912.
Reprinted by permission from Springer-Verlag, Heidelberg.

paresthesias were *not* sought, the additional injection undoubtedly improved the statistical chances of making at least one of the three injections within the sheath, and thus improved the incidence of successful block.

In 1926 Livingston described a technique that is probably the earliest ancestor of the subclavian perivascular technique. Though few details were given, the technique appeared to be Kulenkampff's technique carried out *without* the production of paresthesia. The landmarks were the same, and only a single injection was made. The difference lay in the fact that Livingston rigidly *avoided* contact with the nerve trunks: as soon as the deep cervical fascia had been penetrated, 30 ml of 2% procaine were injected. In Livingston's words, "the solution rather than the needle found the plexus." Two years later Labat included Livingston's technique in the second edition of his book *Regional Anesthesia,* and Labat's discussion of the anatomical basis for Livingston's "subfascial technique" might well have been written some forty years later: "The plexus and the artery are separated from the surrounding structures by a fascial investment which represents two walls; the one in front belonging to the scalenous anticus muscle and the other behind to the scalenus medius. These walls proceed laterally and slightly forward to meet the deep cervical fascia."

Technique of Labat (1922)

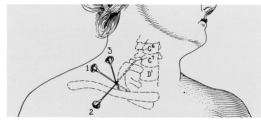

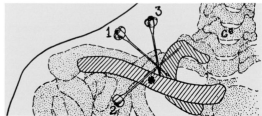

With the patient lying on his back, and the arm alongside of the body, the shoulder on the side to be injected is depressed so as to lower the clavicle. The midpoint of the clavicle is determined, a point that frequently corresponds to a projection of the course of the external jugular vein. The subclavian artery is defined by palpation, and a wheal raised just lateral to it, 1 cm above the clavicle. In most cases the wheal will be just above the midpoint of the clavicle, so if the pulse cannot be felt, it is sufficient to raise the wheal 1 cm above the midpoint of the clavicle. The patient is informed about the procedure and is instructed to signal as soon as he feels a paresthesia. With the index finger the subclavian artery is retracted inward and downward, and a 5 cm needle (unattached to a syringe) is inserted through the wheal close to the tip of the index finger. It is introduced in a direction that is backward, downward, and inward toward the first rib, and when the deep fascia has been penetrated, it should be advanced very gradually, as the plexus lies just beneath the fascia at that point. If paresthesias have not been obtained after the needle has been inserted 2 to 3 cm, it ordinarily comes in contact with the first rib, unless the direction of insertion has been incorrect. Absence of paresthesias is proof that the needle has passed between the branches of the plexus without contacting them, so the needle should be withdrawn and reinserted in a slightly different direction. As soon as paresthesias have been produced, 10 ml of 2% procaine are injected. However, if after two or three attempts no paresthesias have been obtained, it is not advisable to continue to try repeated punctures in different directions. Instead 10 ml of anesthetic are injected beneath the deep fascia in the direction of the first rib, followed by two supplemental injections made as follows: after partially withdrawing the needle, it is reinserted toward Chassaignac's tubercle, where 5 ml of anesthetic are injected, whereupon the needle is again withdrawn and again reinserted, this time towards the lateral margin of the first rib behind the clavicle, where an additional 5 ml are injected. Thus, with this technique the anesthetic has been deposited at three levels. Following the last injection the entire region is lightly massaged to hasten diffusion of the procaine, and 10 minutes are allowed before surgery is begun.

In order to obtain complete anesthesia, including the shoulder, it is necessary to infiltrate the axilla fanwise along its thoracic wall to block the intercostobrachial nerve and to make subcutaneous injections along the clavicle and acromion, so as to block the sensory nerves from the cervical plexus.

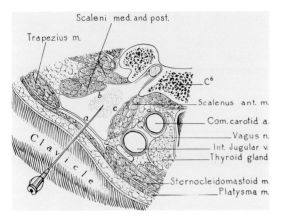

He went on to point out that if the needle was properly placed the fascia would confine the injected local anesthetic solution to the space in which the nerves lie. On the other hand, if the injection is made outside the fascial compartment containing the plexus, the injection will be into the substance of the scalene muscles, and there is little hope that the solution will diffuse to the plexus, because fascias are impermeable.

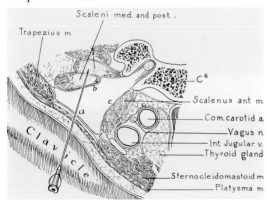

However, Labat went on to say that Livingston's technique represented "the ideal", and that he felt that the technique demanded unique skill and a highly developed tactile sense to find the deep fascia, which in some cases doesn't offer even a blunt needle much resistance.

Although Livingston's technique resulted in Labat's premature statement of the perivascular concept, the technique (and the concept) went virtually unnoticed. Perhaps this was due in part to the fact that the very next year Kulenkampff's technique was published *in English* by Kulenkampff himself. Whatever the reason, over the next decade and a half all of the reports in the literature pertained to either Kulenkampff's or Labat's technique.

Then in 1940 Patrick described a technique that represented a complete departure from previously described techniques, which he termed "unsatisfactory and dangerous." Although he was not unaware of the fascial investment of the plexus, Patrick made no attempt to identify either the fascia or the plexus, but instead chose to "lay down a wall of anesthetic" through which the plexus must pass in its course over the first rib. In spite of the fact that much of the solution was undoubtedly injected outside the fascial investment of the plexus (and was thus ineffective) with volumes of 60-70 ml of solution being injected during 5 to 6 insertions and withdrawals of the needle, a considerable volume was certain to be deposited within the sheath during the passage of the needle through it. It is thus *not* surprising that Patrick achieved a high degree of success with his technique; but it *is* surprising that the incidence of systemic effects from the large amounts of local anesthetic required was not equally high.

87

Though it lacked anatomical precision, Patrick's technique had a profound impact on almost all subsequently developed supraclavicular techniques; for it is his anatomical drawing that seems to be the source of the erroneous concept that the three trunks of the brachial plexus cross the first rib one behind the other (horizontally), a concept that lent apparent anatomical logic to the practice of walking the rib to evoke consecutive paresthesias. Nonetheless, the results achieved with this technique were such that Macintosh and Mushin felt it to be "the first technique in the history of brachial plexus anesthesia which enabled the procedure to be undertaken with the assurance that anesthesia would result." Consequently, their splendid little monograph "Local Anesthesia: Brachial Plexus" is based on Patrick's technique and represents an effort to popularize it. The success of this monograph is attested to by the fact that it went through four editions over a period of twenty years, with many printings of each edition in both England and the United States, though perhaps a better testimonial to its success was the fact that Patrick's technique, or slight modifications thereof, quickly became "the standard technique" of supraclavicular brachial block, subsequently referred to by many as the "classical supraclavicular technique".

Technique of Patrick (1940)

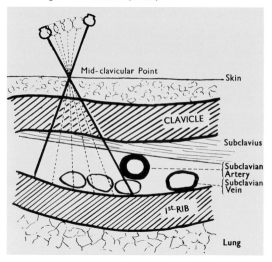

The patient lies supine on the operating table with the shoulder depressed and the head turned to the opposite side. A small intradermal wheal is raised just above the midpoint of the clavicle. A 2⅜ inch 20-gauge needle is inserted through the wheal, aimed roughly in the direction of the second or third dorsal spine. The needle is inserted slowly without the syringe attached, and its direction is altered as required until its point can be felt to impinge on the first rib. The needle now lies well above and lateral to the brachial plexus. Should any blood appear in the needle during any of its insertions, it must be withdrawn and repositioned.

A syringe loaded with 2% procaine with adrenalin is then attached, and 5-10 ml are injected as the needle is withdrawn until its point lies in the subcutaneous tissues. The syringe is now detached and the needle reinserted so as to contact the rib 5 mm nearer its sternal end. When the rib has again been contacted, the syringe is reattached, and again 5-10 ml of anesthetic are injected as the needle is withdrawn to the subcutaneous tissue. The injections are repeated in this manner, altering the needle axis each time so that the needle point progresses 5 mm nearer the sternal end of the rib. Thus, on each insertion, by systematically working one's way down the rib, the sector of tissue between the midclavicular point and the first rib, through which the brachial plexus passes, is thoroughly infiltrated.

If the needle puncture in the skin is made at the midclavicular point, it will be found that as the injections proceed, the obliquity of the needle has to be gradually altered in order that the needle point may contact the rib each time; thus a point is finally reached at which the needle penetrates or lies close to the lower trunk of the brachial plexus. The shaft of the needle now lies against the upper and outer aspects of the third part of the subclavian artery, and the pulsation of the artery is transmitted to the needle, so that the hub can be seen to be beating synchronously with the pulse. When this is observed, the final injection is made. In all, 5 or 6 injections are required before the artery is reached, using a volume of 60-70 ml of the 2% procaine solution.

From British Journal of Surgery 27, page 734-739, copyright 1940. Reprinted by permission from John Wright & Sons Ltd.

An interesting modification of Patrick's technique was that of Knight, which Lundy stated to be "the most satisfactory technique of infiltrating the plexus." Knight utilized Patrick's "wall of anesthetic" concept, but modified it by making the three injections through three separate needles placed parallel to one another. Furthermore, Knight's was the first technique to utilize a directly caudad direction of needle insertion; and since the scalene muscles and the interscalene space run directly caudad, it would seem likely that *at least one* of the three injections would remain in the space and give highly successful results. Unfortunately, Knight never described his technique in a professional journal, but did allow its inclusion in the textbook *Clinical Anesthesia* by John Lundy, and later in *The Management of Pain* by John Bonica. Thus we have no way of knowing the rationale for the change in landmarks and for the change in the direction of needle insertions, but it would seem to imply a new look at or better understanding of the anatomy.

In 1944, two years after Knight's technique appeared, Murphey pointed out that on the basis of anatomical dissections, the usual landmark utilized for supraclavicular techniques, i.e., the midpoint of the clavicle, was unreliable in locating the plexus, but that there was a very constant relationship between the position of the easily palpable anterior scalene muscle and the plexus. Therefore, he described a technique wherein the primary landmark was the lateral border of this muscle and the direction of insertion of the single needle was directly caudad, as with Knight's technique, not mesiad or dorsad, as with most other techniques. According to Murphey, with this

Technique of Knight (1942)

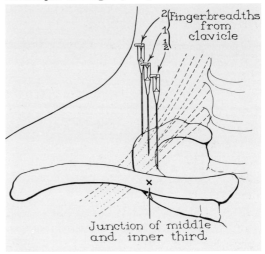

The beginning landmark is a point at the junction of the inner and middle thirds of the clavicle and a wheal is raised one fingerbreadth above this point. After this wheal has been raised, a needle is inserted through it in a caudad direction and is advanced until contact is made with the first rib. Then a second needle is inserted parallel to the first only one-half fingerbreadth from the clavicle (halfway between the clavicle and the first needle). And finally, a third needle is inserted parallel to the first but one fingerbreadth posterior to the first needle (or two fingerbreadths from the clavicle). With these three needles resting on the superficial surface of the first rib, a 2% solution of procaine or metycaine is injected through each of the needles, so that 2 or 3 ml are deposited on top of the first rib, and the remainder of the solution is deposited as each needle is slowly withdrawn. For the average adult a total of 10 ml are injected through each needle, but if the patient is very large and robust, and if the operation is to be of long duration, it is advisable to use all of the 50 ml that are usually prepared. The result of this procedure is that the subcutaneous tissue that overlies the first rib, and the tissue that surrounds the brachial plexus, becomes infiltrated with the solution; anesthesia, although it may be 20 minutes or more in appearing, usually ensues. If the operation is high in the arm, it is necessary to make a bracelet-like injection, intradermally and subcutaneously, around and under the arm near the shoulder, for the purpose of blocking some of the intercostal nerves as they end in the upper part of the arm. For the best results this bracelet type of injection should be used routinely with brachial plexus block.

From Lundy: Clinical Anesthesia, page 105 fig. 27, copyright 1942. Reprinted by permission from W. B. Saunders & Co., Philadelphia.

Technique of Murphey (1944)

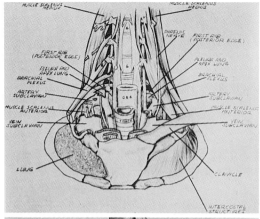

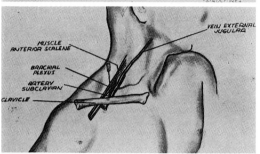

The patient's head is turned toward the opposite side and flexed toward the shoulder. The fingers of the examiner's hand are drawn medially from the edge of the trapezius muscle just above the clavicle; and just lateral to the clavicular head of the sternocleidomastoid muscle, the lateral edge of the anterior scalene muscle is identified. About 2 cm above the clavicle, immediately over the lateral edge of this muscle, a small wheal is made in the skin. An ordinary fine caliber intravenous needle is inserted through the wheal and directed caudad, parallel to the midline, thus making a 30-45° angle with the skin of the neck. After a little experience, the anesthetist can detect the presence of the needle in the fascia surrounding the nerves because of the increased resistance to the needle. The needle is advanced until a paresthesia is obtained, at which time 15-30 ml of 2% procaine with adrenalin are injected. If the first rib is encountered without the production of paresthesias, the needle should be withdrawn and reinserted at a slightly different angle. If anesthesia of the upper arm is necessary, one must encircle the upper arm with a subcutaneous injection of the anesthetic solution.

From Ann. Surg. 119, page 935-943, copyright 1944.
Reprinted by permission from J. B. Lippencott Company, Philadelphia.

technique, once a paresthesia was obtained, which he stated would usually occur on the first insertion of the needle, anesthesia was accomplished *by a single injection.* Certainly this technique represents somewhat of a historical step backward but a giant clinical step forward!

In spite of the simplicity of Murphey's much more anatomical technique, it was virtually ignored, and over the subsequent twenty years the most frequently utilized supraclavicular technique was that described in 1949 by Bonica and Moore, one that would seem to be a synthesis of Kulenkampff's and Patrick's techniques: the technique begins by utilizing the classical landmarks and direction of needle insertion and demands a definite paresthesia prior to the first injection. Thereafter, the technique continues as Patrick's technique, in which a wall of anesthetic solution is laid down from rib to fascia by "walking the rib" and making multiple injections during each withdrawal of the needle. These authors describe in detail "the fascia ensheathing the plexus and artery which makes possible the deposition and retention of anesthetic solutions within a relatively closed space" and yet while they do identify the sheath during the first insertion of the needle, they do not attempt to make subsequent injections within the sheath, in spite of the fact that by their own statement, "this would afford the best means of anesthetizing the plexus."

Technique of Bonica and Moore (1949)

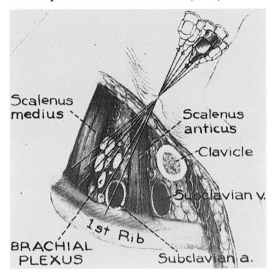

Scalenus medius

Scalenus anticus

Clavicle

Subclavian V.

1st Rib

BRACHIAL PLEXUS

Subclavian a.

The patient lies in the supine position with a small pillow under the upper thoracic spine, allowing the neck to hyperextend and the shoulders to fall back. The head is rotated to the opposite side, and the shoulders are depressed caudad. A skin wheal is raised 1 cm above the clavicle just posterolateral to the subclavian artery. This usually corresponds to the midpoint of the clavicle, and in patients in whom the artery cannot be palpated, the midpoint may be used as a landmark. A 5 cm, 22-gauge, short bevel needle is inserted through the wheal and is directed caudad, mesiad, and dorsad toward the spinous process of the third thoracic vertebra. If the needle is introduced slowly and gently, the operator is able to discern penetration of the deep fascia, denoting that the needle is within the fascial compartment which encloses the plexus. Proceeding slowly, the needle is advanced until a paresthesia is obtained or until the needle point has advanced 3 cm. If the needle direction is right and the patient is not fat, this is deep enough to contact the upper surface of the first rib. If paresthesias have not been obtained when the rib is contacted, the needle should be withdrawn and reinserted until a paresthesia is produced. When it is, the needle is frozen; and following aspiration, 15 ml of anesthetic are injected. After the injection the syringe is detached and the needle advanced until it contacts the rib. The full syringe is again attached, and 10 ml of solution are injected as the needle is progressively withdrawn, depositing the last ml as the needle point emerges from the deep fascia. The needle is then reinserted and directed so it will strike the rib 1 cm nearer its sternal end. This will place it immediately posterolateral to and in contact with the artery, a fact that is evidenced by the synchronous oscillations of the needle with the arterial pulse. Upon contacting the rib, the syringe is reattached, and again, 7 to 10 ml of anesthetic are injected as the needle is withdrawn. A final insertion of the needle is made, this time directing it so it will strike the rib surface 1 cm posterolateral to the first injection, and the maneuver of injection during withdrawal is repeated. If during the second and third insertion of the needle a different paresthesia is produced, the needle is arrested and 5 ml of anesthetic are injected. If a tourniquet is to be used or if surgery involves the upper arm, a subcutaneous ring is made around the upper arm to block the branches of the superficial cervical plexus and those of the intercostobrachial nerve.

From Bonica: The Management of Pain, page 307, copyright 1953. Reprinted by permission from Lea & Febiger Publishers, Philadelphia.

It was not until 1958 that the potential of the sheath in brachial plexus anesthesia was fully realized in the technique of Lookman, who like Livingston, relied completely on the fascial investment of the plexus to accurately guide the injected local anesthetic to all parts of the plexus. As with earlier anatomically precise techniques, Lookman's technique was based on careful dissections that clearly indicated that the plexus lies in a closed, watertight compartment and which Lookman termed the "paravertebral space." According to his studies this space lies between the anterior and middle scalene muscles and is pyramidal in shape, with its apex pointing upward and medially toward the exit of the fourth cervical nerve. However, though his description of the space was exceedingly accurate, and though his entire technique depended upon injection into the space, Lookman did not attempt to verify the needle's proper placement within the space prior to injection. He felt that since the relationship between the brachial plexus, the subclavian artery, and the first rib is fairly constant, if a needle is placed on the first rib immediately behind the artery, it *must* be within the paravertebral space. Though Lookman admitted that there was a definite tendency for the point of the needle to pass too far posteriorly and hence to come to lie within the substance of (or even behind) the middle scalene muscle, nonetheless, in his hands the technique provided excellent results with only a single injection.

Once again, though Lookman's technique appeared at a time when the importance of the axillary perivascular space to the axillary approach was first being appreciated, a similar importance was not attached by others to Lookman's paraver-

91

tebral space in the supraclavicular approach. Thus, the simplicity and safety of the axillary perivascular technique continued to attract increasing numbers of anesthetists, who were unaware of this equally simple and safe supraclavicular approach and welcomed a means of avoiding the threat of pneumothorax that was always a possibility with supraclavicular techniques.

In an attempt to minimize this threat with these techniques, Fortin and Tremblay advocated the use of a short needle, one that was long enough to reach the plexus but too short to reach the lung should the plexus be missed. In the meantime, also for greater safety, Ball modified Lookman's technique by directing the needle downward and inward but not backward, so that if the rib should be missed, the needle's position would then be anterior to the rib and outside the thoracic cage, rendering pleural puncture improbable, if not impossible. However, these were simply technical maneuvers to avoid complications due to anatomical inconsistencies. What was needed was more precise and constant landmarks to allow localization of the sheath and plexus with minimal chance of pneumothorax.

In 1964 the author described his technique, which allowed accurate percutaneous location of the plexus and at the same time applied the concept upon which the axillary perivascular technique was based to the supraclavicular approach. As an extension of the axillary perivascular concept, it was appropriately named the subclavian perivascular technique (Chapter III). This technique is the result of numerous anatomical dissections that showed that the relationship of the plexus and subclavian artery to the midpoint of the

Technique of Lookman (1958)

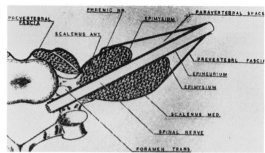

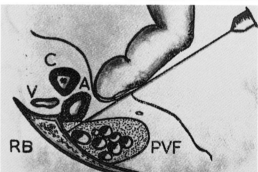

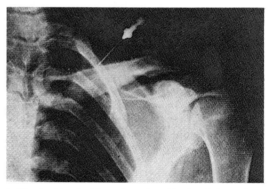

A skin wheal is raised 1 cm above the mid-point of the clavicle, lateral to the palpable pulsations of the subclavian atery. The index finger of the operator's free hand guards and retracts the subclavian artery downward. A 0,8 mm hypodermic needle whose hub is occluded by the index finger is inserted just above the retracting finger (over the subclavian artery) in a downward, inward, and backward direction, aiming toward the upper surface of the first rib, with the needle lying in between the subclavian artery and the trunks of the brachial plexus. The point of the needle then touches the upper surface of the rib.

The needle is steadied in this position and, in adults, one injection only of 30 ml is made. The solution is then close to the plexus, and within the space. The needle is not manipulated in different directions, and no attempt is made to elicit paresthesia. As soon as the injection is completed, the arm is supported by a triangular bandage.

From Anaesthesia 13, page 5-18, copyright 1958.
Reprinted by permission from Dr. J. N. Lunn, Department of Anaesthetics, The Welsh National School of Medicine.

first rib is not constant enough to allow this to be utilized as the primary landmark in *any* supraclavicular technique. More important, these dissections showed that there *is* a constant relationship between the anterior and middle scalene muscles, the plexus, and the first rib: the trunks of the plexus are always sandwiched between the two scalene muscles, and these muscles are always found to insert on the first rib. Thus, if a needle is inserted between the two scalene muscles and in the direction of the space between them, the plexus is almost certain to be encountered as the needle is advanced; but even if the plexus should be missed, the needle will certainly "insert" on the first rib with the anterior and middle scalene muscles.

These same anatomical studies showed that the axillary sheath is simply a lateral extension of the paravertebral (scalene) fascia which is carried out to the upper arm by the neurovascular bundle, forming a continuous perineural and perivascular space that surrounds the plexus from cervical vertebrae to distal axilla. Thus, as with Kulenkampff's original technique, once a paresthesia has been obtained to verify the presence of a needle within the space, a single injection is made and the fascia will confine the anesthetic solution to the perineural and perivascular compartment.

In short, with its anatomical precision and conceptual logic, the subclavian perivascular technique finally provides a supraclavicular approach that can truly equal the simplicity, safety, and high degree of success that are achieved with the axillary perivascular technique.

Evolution of Interscalene Perivascular Brachial Plexus Block

During the same year in which Hirschel and Kulenkampff described their percutaneous approaches to the brachial plexus via the axillary and supraclavicular routes respectively, Kappis was attempting to develop techniques for blocking the spinal nerves at all levels where they emerged from the vertebral column. The following year he published his technique for producing "paravertebral conduction anesthesia of the thoracic and lumbar nerves", in which he utilized a lateral approach and injected the nerves just lateral to the intervertebral foramina, where the nerves and all their branches could be blocked with a high degree of certainty. Shortly thereafter, he extended the use of this "paravertebral conduction anesthesia" to include the cervical and brachial plexuses; but in the cervical area, because of the presence of the vertebral artery and vein in front of the intervertebral foramina, Kappis chose to block the nerves more laterally, where they emerge from the sulcus of the transverse processes, and to block them by a posterior rather than a lateral approach.

In spite of Kappis' claim that the technique was easy to perform, it lacked precision and was undoubtedly extremely painful to the patient, requiring as it did, multiple injections. The fact that they could be made through a single wheal was most likely of little consolation to the patient, since blockade of each nerve

Technique of Kappis (1912)

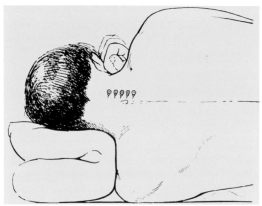

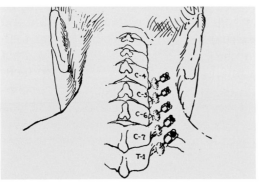

The patient is in the lateral recumbent position with the head on a pillow so as to obtain complete relaxation of the muscles. To block C_5 and C_6 a needle is inserted lateral to the spinous processes and is advanced in a slightly medial direction until at a depth of 3 to 4 cm the lateral border of the articular process is contacted. If the patient is thin, a finger palpates the transverse process as the needle is walked off the articular process laterally and is advanced until the transverse process is reached. If the neck is too muscular to feel the transverse process, the needle is simply walked off the articular process and advanced 1 ½ cm where 5 ml of 1.5% procaine are injected at each nerve.

One hits C_7 and C_8 better if the needle is directed slightly caudad so as to circumvent the transverse processes of the seventh cervical and first thoracic vertebrae, in front of which lie the nerves. The technique of needle insertion is the same as for C_5 and C_6. However, because the nerves in the neck lie in close proximity to each other, a separate skin puncture is not needed for each nerve; one can raise a single wheal and simply alter the direction of the needle to reach the various transverse processes.

Ordinarily, each time a transverse process is contacted by the needle 5 ml of local anesthetic are deposited to block each nerve. However, if one cannot find the individual transverse processes with the needle, then one injection of 30 ml may be made along the lateral border of the vertebral column.

From Bonica: The Management of Pain, page 308, copyright 1953. Reprinted by permission from Lea & Febiger Publishers, Philadelphia.

From Macintosh, R. R. & Mushin, W. W.: Local Analgesia. Brachial Plexus, 4th ed. page 8, copyright 1967. Reprinted by permission from E. & S. Livingstone Ltd., Edinbourgh and London.

required a separate thrust of the needle. The most fortunate patients would seem to be those in whom the individual transverse processes could not be found, for in this situation Kappis advocated a single injection of 30 ml just lateral to the spinal column; and if this injection happened to be into the interscalene space, the chances of obtaining complete anesthesia were undoubtedly better than with the more typical (and traumatic) technique wherein the transverse processes could be identified.

Four years later Santoni outlined "a paravertebral approach never before described," but the technique differed from Kappis' technique only in that each injection had to be made through a separate skin wheal; clearly, this technique was even more traumatic to the patient than that advocated by Kappis. It is no small wonder that a posterior paravertebral approach, whether that of Kappis or of Santoni, never became popular.

Technique of Santoni (1916)

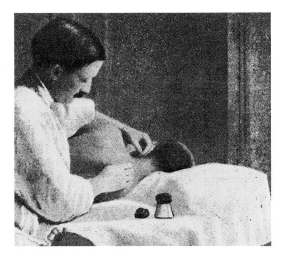

We have come to inject the five roots of the brachial plexus by the following procedure: the first four injections are made along a vertical line that is 3 cm lateral to the interspinous line. The transverse process of the sixth cervical vertebra is located, and a needle is inserted at this level and advanced directly anteriorly until contact is made with bone. The point of the needle is then reinserted more laterally; and when it clears bone, it is advanced an additional 1 cm where it reaches the fifth cervical nerve. The same maneuver is repeated at points that are 15, 30 and 45 mm below the site of the first injection in order to inject the sixth, seventh and eighth cervical nerves. Injection of the first thoracic nerve is accomplished by inserting the needle 3.5 cm lateral to the midline and 2 cm above the level of the spinous process of the first thoracic vertebra; after contacting the first rib, the needle is redirected inferiorly and slightly medially.

This technique has not been described previously. We have had occasion to use it only four times on patients, but in each case with complete success.

From Santoni: Thèse pour le Doctor en Mèdecine, L'Anesthésie regionale des nerfs rachidiens, copyright 1916.

In 1919 in an effort to avoid the dreaded complication of pneumothorax associated with Kulenkampff's technique, Mulley described a technique that must be considered to represent the first *lateral* paravertebral approach, if not the first interscalene approach; for although Heidenhain had utilized a similar approach at a higher level to anesthetize the cervical plexus, he never attempted to utilize his technique to block the brachial plexus. Mulley's objective was simply to block the plexus at a level higher than that at which Kulenkampff carried out his block, so that pleural injury was impossible and no major vessels could be damaged. Certainly this technique represents a great simplification over the posterior techniques, although the landmarks described by Mulley appear to be somewhat vague. Nonetheless, in his first fifty-four cases Mulley obtained complete success in fifty-one, which represents a 95.5% success rate. This compares favourably with the interscalene technique of brachial plexus block which it anticipates. It is difficult to explain why Mulley made a second injection of 10 ml lateral to his primary injection of 20 ml at the site of his initial paresthesia, but it may be because of his high degree of success with this technique that Labat simply added Mulley's two injections, one medial and one lateral, to Kulenkampff's original technique in coming up with his own modification of supraclavicular brachial block.

95

Technique of Mulley (1919)

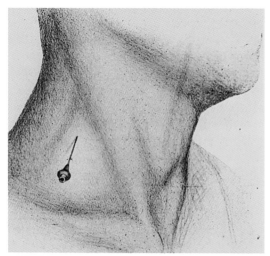

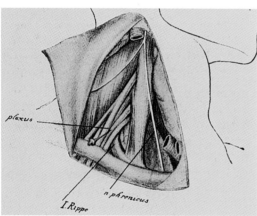

With the patient in the supine position, if the neck is turned sharply to the opposite side, a distinct triangle is formed by the clavicle inferiorly, the sternocleidomastoid muscle medially, and the neck muscles laterally. The central point of this triangle is the site of needle insertion. Should the triangle be indistinct, the point may be located by measuring three fingerbreadths above the clavicle and about ½ cm posterior to the external jugular vein. The needle is inserted through this point as illustrated. The plexus can hardly be missed here, and the patient will usually experience paresthesias to the fingertips immediately. When such paresthesias have been obtained, 20 ml of 2% procaine are injected, after which another 10 ml are injected by a small lateral excursion of the needle. The sensation of a heavy extremity usually occurs within 10-15 minutes after the injection, and in another 5 minutes anesthesia is complete.

From Beiträge zur Klinische Chirurgie 114, page 666-680, copyright 1919.
Reprinted by permission from Springer-Verlag, Heidelberg.

In spite of its apparent effectiveness and its freedom from complications, Mulley's technique was not widely utilized. In 1925 Hilarowicz attempted to improve upon the technique, which he felt had not been adopted because of the inaccurate or imprecise landmarks provided by Mulley. Hilarowicz felt that Mulley's point one-half centimeter behind the external jugular vein and three fingerbreadths above the clavicle is an inexact and variable landmark, that in most people this point lies posterior to the plexus and that therefore a needle inserted here might simply pass into muscle and the search for paresthesias might be in vain. Furthermore, he pointed out, the midpoint of Mulley's "triangle" was even more vague and less accurate.

Hilarowicz felt that what was needed to perfect Mulley's technique of "high plexus anesthesia" was the introduction of fixed guidelines, and this he attempted to do: he chose Chassaignac's tubercle as his fixed point of reference, and the direction of the spinous processes as the pathway to each of the transverse processes. However, he complicated Mulley's technique by returning to the practice of injecting 5 ml at each of the transverse processes. As a result, Hilarowicz's technique more closely resembled a lateral version of Kappis' technique than it did Mulley's, so if it did actually provide the lateral technique with greater precision, it also added to its complexity. Nonetheless, in a report published three years later Hilarowicz reported no failures in over fifty cases. He attributed this success to the fact that with his technique he distributed the anesthetic solution parallel to the cervical spine from the transverse process of C_6 to the neck of the first rib. What he did not appreciate was that Mulley had accomplished the same objective with one or two injections using larger volumes.

Technique of Hilarowicz (1925)

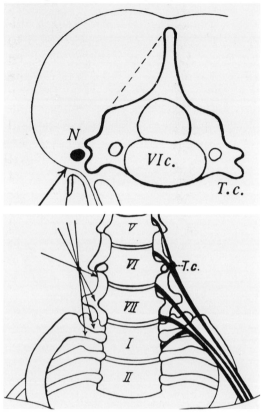

The patient is placed in the supine position with the head hyper-extended and turned to the opposite side. With the index finger Chassaignac's tubercle is palpated at the posterior border of the sternocleidomastoid muscle. On the outer aspect of this promi-nence and directly behind it lies C_6, separated from it only by the narrow insertion of the scalenus anticus muscle. In descending from above, C_5 lies immediately lateral to C_6. A thin 8 cm needle is inserted over the tubercle and is advanced in the direction of the spinous process of the same vertebra. At a depth of about 1 cm (or even more superficially) paresthesias of C_5 and C_6 to the thumb and shoulder region are achieved following which 5 ml of 2% procaine are injected. The needle is then withdrawn some-what and redirected more toward the sagittal plane; and again, aiming at the spinous process of C_7 and C_8 will result in pares-thesias to the hand and little finger, after which 10 ml of the anes-thetic solution are deposited. Finally, the needle is inclined still more, this time aiming at the spinous process of T_2. At a depth of 5-7 cm the neck of the first rib is contacted at the point where C_8 and T_1 join; this results in strong paresthesias in the ulnar region, and with this the final 5 ml of procaine are injected.

The effect of the injections is first noted as motor weakness, and after about 15 minutes anesthesia is complete. This tech-nique seems to be complicated, but every anesthetic has this disadvantage when it has to be given deep and in the vicinity of important structures. It can only be performed without danger by the use of a precise technique; and with much practice, it becomes easy to do.

From Zentralblatt für Chirurgie 52, page 2349-2351, copyright 1925. Reprinted by permission from Johan Ambrosius Barth, Verlags-buchhandlung, Leipzig.

More amazing than Hilarowicz's 100% success is the fact that he did not *routinely* penetrate the pleura during at least one of his last two injections.

In the meantime in Paris, also in 1925, July Etienne, as a part of his doctoral thesis, described a technique of brachial plexus block which was technically and perhaps *conceptually* the first true inter-scalene approach: Etienne observed that in the space limited by the omotrapezoid triangle formed by the lateral edge of the sternocleidomastoid muscle and the anterior edge of the trapezius muscle, "the scalenes stand out, and going down between them are the roots that make up the brachial plexus." Etienne's technique consisted of simply inserting a needle at the level of the intercricothyroid space, halfway between the lateral border of the sternocleidomastoid and the anterior border of the trapezius, and advancing it toward the opposite shoulder parallel to the plane of the table. Etienne did not attempt to elicit paresthesias, but when he contacted bone, which he said was usually the sixth or seventh cervical trans-verse process, he slowly injected 20 ml of anesthetic solution, withdrew the needle, and massaged the injection site to pro-mote diffusion of the liquid. Etienne stat-ed that anesthesia of the brachial plexus was complete within 15 minutes in all of his 33 cases, and he reported no complica-tions whatsoever.

While the technique of Etienne, like so many others, was never mentioned by subsequent authors, in 1928 in the fourth edition of his famous book, *L'Anesthésie Régionale,* Victor Pauchet described a slight modification of the technique as a "new technique" without giving any cred-it to Etienne, who had been his pupil.

Technique of Etienne (1925)

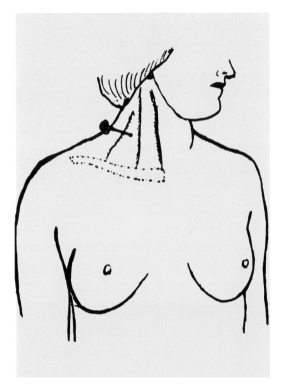

The patient lies in the decubitus supine position with his head turned away from the operator. With the left hand, the space between the posterior border of the sternocleidomastoid and the anterior border of the trapezius is identified. Then the inter-cricothyroid space is marked, and a line is drawn laterally to a point halfway between the sternocleidomastoid and trapezius muscles, where a skinwheal is raised.

Using a 4 or 6 cm needle, one punctures over the dermic wheal, directing the needle toward the opposite shoulder and keeping it parallel to the plane of the table stopping when contact with bone is made (generally the sixth or seventh cervical transverse process) 20 ml of the anesthetic solution are slowly injected at this point. The needle is then withdrawn and the area massaged to enhance diffusion of the liquid. Plexus anesthesia will be complete within 15 minutes.

From Etienne: Thèse L'Anesthésie Régionale, copyright 1925.

Technique of Pauchet (1928)

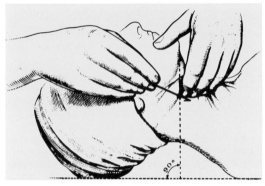

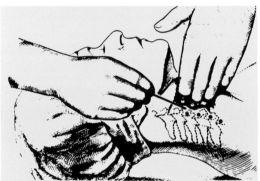

With the patient lying on his back, a line is drawn laterally through the inferior border of the mandible which corresponds to the fourth cervical vertebra, and separates the cervical plexus from the brachial plexus. A finger's breadth below this level the transverse process of the fifth cervical vertebra is palpated with the forefinger of the left hand. Without losing contact with the bone, the palpating finger is moved medially pushing the muscles and the vascular bundle toward the front.

A 6 cm needle is then inserted at about a finger's breadth above the stated point directing it obliquely downward to avoid the risk of damage to the vertebral artery, and slightly forward, between the tranverse process and the palpating finger pushing away the muscles and the vascular bundle. In this way we make the slanting plane, into which we inject 30 ml of a 1% concentration of anesthetic solution.

From Pauchet, V., Sourdat, P., Labat, G. et al.: Regional Anesthesia, 4th ed., copyright 1928 Doin et fils.
Reprinted by permission from W. B. Saunders & Co., Philadelphia.

Except for this description, the technique was totally ignored at the time of its publication and it would have been forgotten forever if it had not been rediscovered and reported recently by Vidal-Lopez.

Yet 20 years later, in 1946 the famous American surgeon-anesthetist Pitkin stated in his textbook of regional anesthesia that the lateral, paravertebral approach unquestionably yielded the highest percentage of satisfactory anesthesia of all of the approaches to the brachial plexus, especially when compared with the old posterior paravertebral approach, which yielded the highest percentage of failures. However, in his technique Pitkin made no reference to the fascial investment of the plexus, either as a landmark or as a useful means of containing the injected anesthetic agent. Pitkin's technique was somewhat similar to that of Hilarowicz in that both used multiple injections of anesthetic placed at the transverse processes of the appropriate cervical vertebrae, and both achieved a fantastic degree of success with their techniques. However, like Hilarowicz, Pitkin was unable to popularize the technique.

This approach is not mentioned in the literature again except in Bonica's classic, *The Management of Pain,* where it is described as an alternative to the supraclavicular technique. The advantage of the lateral approach described by Bonica would appear to be one of safety, for the original skin wheal was somewhat higher than with previously described techniques, so that all insertions of the needle were in a slightly caudad direction, thus minimizing the possibility of penetrating the epidural or subdural spaces with a needle that has failed to contact a nerve root. Because this seemingly minor modification would also decrease the

Technique of Pitkin (1946)

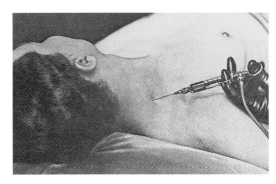

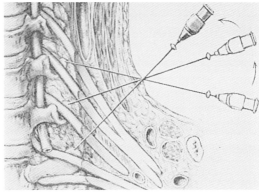

The patient is placed in a dorsal recumbent position with the head rotated to the opposite side. The degree of rotation should be sufficient to elevate the transverse processes so that they may be easily palpated along the posterior border of the sternocleidomastoid muscle. The upper border of the first rib is mapped out, and the transverse processes of the fifth, sixth, and seventh cervical vertebrae are palpated and their positions marked.

An imaginary line is drawn laterally at right angles to the long axis of the cervical spines opposite the seventh cervical vertebra. A second line is drawn from the upper border of the first rib parallel to the cervical vertebrae. At the intersection of these lines a wheal is raised. This will be about 1½ inches above the superior border of the clavicle directly over the first rib and approximately the same distance lateral to the body of the seventh cervical vertebra.

A 2½ inch 22-gauge needle attached to a continuous flow syringe is inserted through the wheal and directed toward the posterior tubercle of the transverse process, which is palpated with the other hand. When the needle point contacts bone, the operator aspirates, and if no fluid appears in the syringe, he injects 5 ml of 2% procaine with adrenaline. The needle is then withdrawn to the skin surface and redirected toward the transverse process of the sixth cervical vertebra, where another 5 ml of anesthetic are injected. The needle is again withdrawn to skin and directed toward the transverse process of the first thoracic vertebra. Similarly, if aspiration yields no blood, 5 ml of solution are deposited at this site. Usually these three 5 ml injections should be sufficient to anesthetize all the roots of the brachial plexus, but if there is any doubt in the operator's mind about the accuracy of his injections, the volume may be increased to 10 ml per injection.

From Pitkins: Conduction Anesthesia, page 498-499, copyright 1946, 2nd ed. 1953.
Reprinted by permission from Lippencott/Harper & Row, New York.

chances of penetrating the vertebral artery or vein in performing the block, this technique would seem to obviate all three of the complications most likely to occur with any lateral approach.

Having achieved such a high degree of success by applying the perivascular concept to the supraclavicular approach in developing the subclavian perivascular technique of brachial block, the author also applied this concept to the lateral approach (Chapter III): with the interscalene technique of brachial plexus block, as with the subclavian perivascular technique, the interscalene groove is the primary landmark. The cricoid cartilage is used to determine the level of the sixth cervical vertebra to avoid the discomfort imposed by palpating for Chassaignac's tubercle at a time when patient cooperation is critically important. The needle is inserted into the interscalene groove at this level in a slightly caudad direction, which is critically important for safety, as indicated in Bonica's lateral paravertebral approach to the brachial plexus. However, with the interscalene technique, when a paresthesia indicates that the perivascular space has been entered, the appropriate volume of anesthetic is injected and the needle withdrawn (see Chapter III). At this level paresthesias may occur at an extremely superficial depth, particularly in asthenic individuals.

Obviously, the degree of success achieved with interscalene brachial plexus block and the lack of complications depend on the correct location of the interscalene groove and the subsequent placement of the needle therein. To facilitate location of the groove between the anterior and middle scalene muscles, in 1976 Sharrock and Bruce recommended that patients be asked to breathe deeply and slowly while the anesthetist is trying to locate the interscalene groove, since the scalene muscles are accessory muscles of respiration and are activated by slow, deep, inspiration. These authors felt that this maneuver, because it increases the tone in the scalene muscles, makes location of the interscalene groove easier and more certain, since the muscle margins will be firmer and the palpating finger will then "sink into the groove" between them. On the other hand, Bahar, Magora, and Rousso pointed out that while the scalene muscles are indeed accessory muscles of respiration, their main function is to incline the neck to the side. They therefore proposed that in carrying out an interscalene brachial block, during the actual palpation of the landmarks, the patient be asked to incline his head to the ipsilateral side in order to make the scalene muscles contract, a maneuver that would also make the groove between them more readily palpable. While both of these maneuvers may be useful in particularly difficult cases, as a rule they defeat the original objective of the interscalene technique of brachial plexus block introduced as a means of simplifying brachial plexus anesthesia by unnecessarily complicating it.

A modification of the interscalene approach was reported in 1979 by Vongvises and Panijayanond, who approached the brachial plexus in the interscalene compartment 1.5 to 2 cm above the clavicle. However, with their "parascalene technique" the needle is inserted in a directly anteroposterior direction, so that the needle enters the space in its narrowest diameter. As with the original interscalene technique, the needle is advanced

Technique of Bonica (1953)

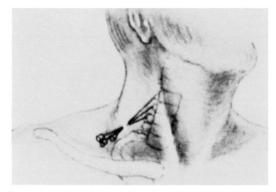

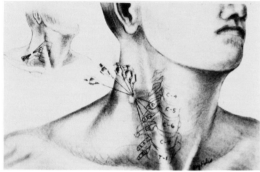

With the patient in the supine position, a small pillow is placed under the upper thoracic vertebrae, and the head of the patient is rotated to the opposite side. This position makes the transverse processes more superficial and consequently more prominent by displacing the sternocleidomastoid muscle and the blood vessels anteriorly. The transverse process of the fifth cervical vertebra is identified and a wheal raised over it. A 22-gauge 8 cm needle is introduced through the wheal and advanced until the transverse process is contacted and/or a paresthesia is elicited, whereupon aspiration is attempted; and if no blood is obtained, 5 ml of local anesthetic are injected without moving the needle. The needle is then withdrawn to the subcutaneous tissue and reinserted more caudad, toward the transverse process of the sixth cervical vertebra, which is usually easily palpable about 1.5 cm caudad to the process of the fifth. When contact is made with the process, the aspiration test is performed, and if negative, 5 ml of the anesthetic are injected. The needle is again withdrawn and redirected, this time toward the transverse process of the seventh cervical vertebra, where 5 ml of local anesthetic are again deposited. This maneuver is repeated a last time with the needle directed toward the transverse process of the first thoracic vertebra, where 7 ml of anesthetic are deposited to block the eighth cervical and first thoracic nerves. In the event the needle is too short to reach the first thoracic vertebra from the skin wheal over the transverse process of C₅, a second wheal is raised over the transverse process of C₆, and the last injection is made through it. The author prefers introducing all the needles in a caudad rather than cephalad direction in order to avoid the possibility of subarachnoid injection. The entire block is done with a total of 30 ml of local anesthetic solution.

From Bonica: The Management of Pain, page 308, copyright 1953. Reprinted by permission from Lea & Febiger Publishers, Philadelphia.

until a paresthesia indicates contact with a nerve; but obviously, because the antero-posterior dimension of the interscalene compartment is so small, the slightest movement of the needle during injection will cause it to leave the space, so that all of the volume injected may not be injected within the interscalene compartment. Vongvises and Panijayanond reported a 97% success rate with this technique, but in 11 of their 100 patients, a second injection was required because anesthesia failed to develop following the first injection, so the true success rate of the parascalene technique is 89%. Even this degree of success is amazing when one considers that the direction of needle insertion is such that it increases the likelihood that part, or even all, of the injection may be made outside the "brachial plexus sheath" because of movement of the needle during the injection.

Interscalene brachial plexus block, as described by the present author, is probably the easiest of all the perivascular techniques to learn and to carry out and provides a success rate comparable to that of both the axillary and subclavian perivascular techniques. In addition, it is particularly useful in those patients who present the greatest difficulty with the other techniques, namely, in extremely obese or uncooperative patients. In the appropriate patient undergoing appropriate surgery and with appropriate volumes of local anesthetic, this technique is a valuable addition to the perivascular techniques of providing brachial plexus anesthesia, extending the utility of this type of anesthesia to surgical procedures on the upper arm and even on the shoulder.

Technique of Vongvises and Panijayanond (1979)

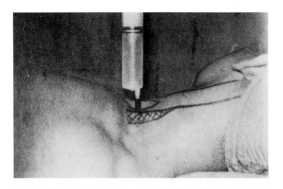

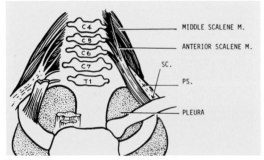

The patient lies in the dorsal recumbent position with a pillow under his head. His arms rest at his sides, and his head is turned to the side opposite that to be blocked. The patient is instructed to raise his head to bring the lateral border of the sternocleidomastoid muscle into view. The patient is then requested to relax his head and neck. The anesthesiologist then places his index finger immediately lateral to the sternocleidomastoid muscle just above the clavicle. The finger should now lie on the belly of the anterior scalene muscle from which it is moved laterally into the interscalene groove. The lateral border of the anterior scalene muscle is then marked with an "X" at a point, 1.5-2.0 cm above the clavicle. The "X" mark, if properly placed, is above the subclavian artery and medial to the external jugular vein.

A skin wheal is made at this point, and a 22-gauge 4 cm needle attached to a syringe filled with local anesthetic solution is inserted vertically through the skin wheal in an anteroposterior direction. A paresthesia is usually elicited while inserting the needle. If so, the local anesthetic solution is injected after careful aspiration. If no paresthesia is elicited, the needle will come into contact with the first rib. The needle is then withdrawn and redirected in an attempt to elicit a paresthesia. If, after several attempts, no paresthesia is obtained, the local anesthetic solution is injected along the lateral edge of the muscle a few millimeters above the first rib in a fanlike manner.

From Anesthesia and Analgesia Volume 58: No. 4, page 267-273, copyright 1979.
Reprinted by permission from International Anesthesia Research Society, Publishers.

102

Evolution of Infraclavicular Brachial Plexus Block

Although Hirschel is considered to have carried out the first axillary block because he approached the brachial plexus from the axilla, what he was really trying to do was to place the local anesthetic on top of the first rib *via the axilla*. He knew from a multitude of axillary dissections carried out as part of radical mastectomies that if the injection was not made high enough, the important musculocutaneous and axillary nerves would not be blocked. And yet needle technology at that time was such that needles long enough to reach the first rib from the axilla were simply not available. As a result, while Hirschel was enthusiastic about his technique, others did not share his enthusiasm, mostly, as stated by Hartel, because one or more of the nerves were almost always missed.

Hirschel never even considered placing the local anesthetic above the first rib by approaching the plexus from above the clavicle, because he felt the possibility of pleural damage was too great. Kulenkampff, on the other hand, felt that because the midpoint of the clavicle and subclavian artery provided constant, easily identifiable landmarks and because the first rib provided a safe backstop to limit the progress of the needle, his technique offered both greater accuracy and greater safety than Hirschel's technique. There can be no doubt that Kulenkampff's technique did provide greater accuracy, for the success rate was such

that this technique was readily adopted by most surgeons, virtually all of whom were enthusiastic about its efficacy. Before long, however, reports of complications, particularly those of pulmonary damage, indicated that this approach was not without risk.

A logical compromise or alternative to the two techniques that might preserve the advantages and overcome the disadvantages of both would be to approach the plexus at a level that is higher than that of the axillary approach, to assure blockade of all of the nerves derived from the plexus, but lower than that of the supraclavicular approach, to minimize the risk of pleural injury. Such a compromise was first suggested by Bazy in France about five years after Hirschel and Kulenkampff had described their respective techniques: according to his infraclavicular technique, the needle was inserted below the clavicle just medial to the coracoid process and advanced along the "line of anesthesia", i.e., a line connecting the coracoid process and Chassaignac's tubercle, the anterior tubercle of the sixth cervical vertebra. Thus, while the needle was inserted below the clavicle, the actual injection was made just above the clavicle and first rib.

In carrying out his technique Bazy placed the patient in the supine position with a cushion between the shoulder blades and abducted his arm 45° while it was hanging over the edge of the table, because he felt that this maneuver causes the upper portion of the plexus to be pulled away from the axillary artery and thus minimizes the possibility of vascular injury during the insertion of the needle. After an initial injection, he adducted the arm without moving the needle to "bring the plexus closer to the needle" and made a second injection before removing the needle. Bazy felt that the course of the needle, which was aimed at Chassaignac's tubercle and advanced until the tip was just above the superior edge of the clavicle, "grazing the posterior surface en route," virtually abolished the possibility of pleural damage.

Minor modifications of Bazy's technique were proposed by Babitzki, who simply used the point where the clavicle crossed the second rib, instead of the coracoid process, as the "lower point" to identify the course of the plexus, and by Balog, who altered the direction of the needle so that it actually impinged on the second rib. Balog said that his failure rate was no greater than that achieved with Kulenkampff's technique, and theorized that this could be reduced significantly by increasing the volume of local anesthetic injected from 10-30 ml. It was ultimately documented by Kim that the increase in volume did indeed increase the success rate. Nonetheless, to put these modifications into perspective, it must be appreciated that both Babitzki and Balog emphasized that their techniques were not intended to be replacements for Kulenkampff's supraclavicular technique, but only as alternatives "to be used when anatomical obstacles impair or prevent the easy and safe execution of the Kulenkampff method." Babitzki stated, "I have been a fervent disciple of the Kulenkampff technique since the first days of its publication," but, he went on, "there are cases where the Kulenkampff method can not be used because of deformities, scars, or injury in the subclavian area." Similarly, Balog stated, "Kulenkampff's technique is the one of choice, if it is feasible, and the infraclavicular approach is only to be regarded as a substitute."

Technique of Bazy (1914)

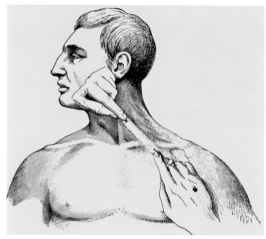

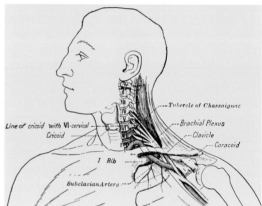

The patient lies supine on the table with a cushion between his shoulders. The arm hangs down in moderate abduction to make the coracoid process more prominent and the plexus more superficial. The anesthetist places himself beside the patient between his arm and trunk. He finds the top of the coracoid process and depresses the soft tissue just medial to it, to make it still more apparent. At the same time the assistant finds Chassaignac's tubercle with his index finger. With the arm in moderate abduction, the index finger of the anesthetist and that of his assistant point toward each other, and the line between them marks the path of the brachial plexus, i.e., the "line of anesthesia".

Along this line of anesthesia a 9 cm needle is inserted immediately below the clavicle and is advanced in the direction of Chassaignac's tubercle so that it just grazes the posterior border of the clavicle. When the needle has just passed the level of the superior surface of the clavicle, 10 ml of 2% Novocain solution are injected. At this time the arm is flexed and adducted to relax the brachial plexus and bring it in close contact with the needle, at which point a second injection is made similar to the first.

From Bazy, L., Pouchet, V. Sourdat, P. & Labouré, J.: Anesthesie Regionale, page 222-225, copyright 1917.
Reprinted by permission from W. B. Saunders & Co., Philadelphia.

Technique of Babitszky (1918)

Technique of Labat (1922)

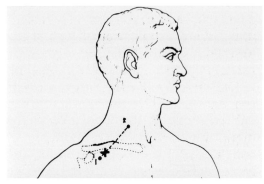

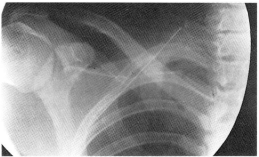

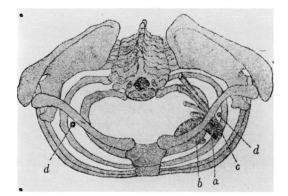

In cases where the Kulenkampff method cannot be used because of deformities, scars, or injuries in the subclavian area, it would seem advantageous to have a method available that is as easy and certain to execute as the Kulenkampff method, i.e., a different technique that also leads directly to the plexus. My technique provides just such an alternative: as in shown in the diagram the point of insertion of the needle (d) is below the clavicle at the angle formed by the clavicle and the second rib, as the former crosses the latter. The clavicle and second rib are two bony landmarks that can be easily palpated. The needle is advanced until a paresthesia is encountered (about 1½-3 cm), and the same quantity and concentration of local anesthetic are injected as with Kulenkampff's technique. The onset of anesthesia following the injection (tingling sensation followed by anesthesia of the whole arm) differs in no way from the Kulenkampff method.

To discuss the anatomical relationship and the technique more fully would be superfluous, as it is customary to familiarize one's self with the anatomy of the field in question on the cadaver any time one tends to use an unfamiliar technique. It is not my intention to advocate the use of my method exclusively as a replacement for the Kulenkampff method, which has proved itself to be excellent in thousands of cases. During my imprisonment since 1914, I have used my method when indicated in over 100 cases, and on this basis I feel justified in advising the use of it in instances where the Kulenkampff method is not practicable.

From Zentralbl. f. Chir. 45, page 215-217, 1918.
Reprinted by permission from Johan Ambrosius Barth, Verlags-buchhandlung, Leipzig.

The patient is placed in the recumbent dorsal position with a suitable hard cushion under the spine between the shoulders, so that his arm may hang backward over the edge of the table, in extension and 45° abduction. The coracoid process thus becomes more prominent and the brachial plexus more superficial. The abduction of the arm should be such that its medial aspect, if prolonged upward to meet the anterior tubercle of the transverse process of C_6 (tubercle of Chassaignac), passes one fingerbreadth medial to the coracoid process. This condition exists when the arm is in about 45° abduction.

The operator stands on the side to be operated upon, between the arm of the patient and the table. The tip of the coracoid process is defined by palpation, and the depression just medial to it is traced on the skin. The tubercle of Chassaignac is likewise defined and traced on the skin by a dot made with an applicator moistened with tincture of iodine. The straight line joining the two dots marks the direction of the brachial plexus. An 8 cm needle is inserted through a wheal raised on this line just above the lower dot and advanced upward in the direction of the upper dot. After making contact with the clavicle, the needle is withdrawn a little and passed behind the bone tangentially to its posterior aspect. As soon as the point of the needle has reached the level of the upper surface of the clavicle, injection is made of 10 ml of the 2% solution without altering the position of the needle; the arm is then flexed and drawn toward the chest, thus relaxing the brachial plexus, which, in becoming more superficial, naturally advances toward the point of the needle. Another injection is finally made of 10 ml of the same solution without displacing the needle.

From Labat's Regional Anesthesia, page 223, copyright 1923.
Reprinted by permission from W. B. Saunders & Co., Philadelphia.

From Anesthesia and Analgesia, Volume 52, page 897-904, 1973.
Reprinted by permission from International Anesthesia Research Society, Publishers.

The infraclavicular approach did not gain any degree of popularity, even as an alternative to Kulenkampff's technique, though it was included in the several editions of Labat's textbook, *Regional Anesthesia,* and also as late as 1939 in Dogliotti's textbook, *Anesthesia: Narcosis, Local, Regional, Spinal.* However, it was the original technique of Bazy, not one of the modifications, that was presented virtually unchanged in both textbooks, and the technique was still offered with an obvious lack of enthusiasm and only as an alternative to Kulenkampff's supraclavicular technique.

In 1973 Raj reintroduced the infraclavicular approach to the brachial plexus; but the technique that he described differed from previous infraclavicular techniques in that the needle was introduced more medially (just under the midpoint of the clavicle) and was directed laterally from the point of entry, so that "needle penetration to any depth would be safe and always outside of the thoracic cavity." Thus, with this technique, there is really no danger of pneumothorax, an obvious advantage over supraclavicular and previously described infraclavicular techniques. Furthermore, with this technique the local anesthetic solution, according to Raj, is deposited inside the brachial plexus sheath *above* the level of the formation of the musculocutaneous and axillary nerves, an apparent advantage over the axillary perivascular techniques. Raj also pointed out two additional advantages of his technique: one that "the ulnar segment of the medial cord is readily blocked," which is an advantage over the interscalene technique; and the other that the intercostobrachial nerve will also be blocked, so there is no need for additional infiltration, an advantage over all techniques.

The theoretical advantage, then, of the infraclavicular technique of Raj, which is really an axillary block that is performed higher in the axillary perivascular compartment, is that the injection is made at a level within the sheath that is higher than the level of exit of the musculocutaneous and axillary nerves. Therefore, less volume should be required using this technique, as compared with the traditional axillary approach, to produce anesthesia over the entire distribution of the brachial plexus. To determine how much higher in the sheath the infraclavicular technique actually deposits the anesthetic, the author and his coworkers compared Raj's technique with the axillary perivascular technique roentgenographically: two needles were placed in the same patient, one by the infraclavicular technique of Raj and one by the author's axillary perivascular technique.

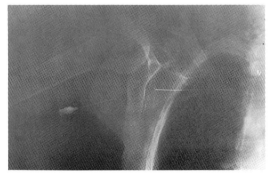

The first x-ray shows clearly that the tips of the two needles are only a few centimeters apart.

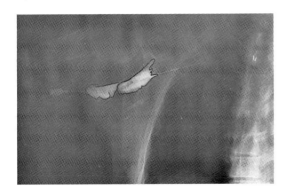

In fact, as may be seen in the second x-ray, so small is the distance between the needles that the injection of only 2 ml of dye, 1 ml through each needle, results in complete intermixing of the solutions.

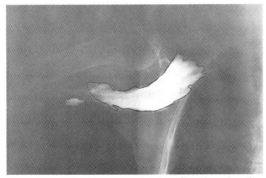

But more important is the finding in the third x-ray that when 40 ml are injected through the needle placed by the infraclavicular technique, the majority of the injected solution moves *distally down the sheath,* with little of the injected solution moving proximally. Thus, if the needle has "overshot" its mark and the tip lies *lateral* (distal) to the coracoid process, the majority of the injected solution could still miss the axillary and musculocutaneous nerves. Therefore, it appears that with the infraclavicular technique as described by Raj, the level of the needle tip may be more important in determining the upper level of anesthesia than the volume of anesthetic injected.

Hence, while Raj's modification of the infraclavicular technique has some appealing *theoretical* advantages, clinical experience and clinical studies have indicated several disadvantages that have prevented the technique from being widely accepted: first of all, although the lateral course of the needle obviates the likelihood of pneumothorax, because the palpating finger cannot identify the arterial pulse at such a high level, the needle is advanced "blindly" with respect to the vessels, and the likelihood of vascular puncture is certainly greater with this technique than with any other, although vascular puncture itself is usually without serious sequelae. Secondly, because the plexus is blocked with this technique as it passes behind both the pectoralis major and minor muscles, a long needle is required to penetrate both of these muscles, causing significantly greater discomfort to the patient than with the other perivascular techniques that block the plexus at points where it is very superficial. And finally, because the needle is directed laterally, as illustrated by the x-rays above, both the direction of the needle and the thrust of the injected solution cause most of the solution to move distally *down* the axillary sheath. Thus, if the tip of the needle is lateral (distal) to the coracoid process, the majority of the injected solution may miss the musculocutaneous and axillary nerves, which in this situation, would have left the sheath *above* the level of the tip of the needle.

An additional disadvantage, though some might not consider it such, is that with this technique a nerve stimulator must be used *routinely,* because the block is carried out where the plexus is very deeply situated; and since Raj has stated that in using a stimulator the needle should be advanced *beyond* the point of maximal response and then withdrawn back to that point, this maneuver almost invariably punctures the sheath anteriorly and posteriorly, and this can result in significant loss of local anesthetic agent from the sheath. This is illustrated vividly in the last x-ray, which was actually taken as part of a study to evaluate the efficacy of digital pressure applied high in the axilla during an infraclavicular block in preventing distal flow and enhancing central (retrograde) flow of the injected anesthetic.

And while the x-ray does show that digital pressure can increase central flow with this technique, just as it does with the axillary perivascular technique, it also demonstrates clearly the leakage of dye from the holes made in the sheath by multiple needle punctures using a nerve stimulator to place the needle. Contrast this x-ray with the first in this series in which the needle was placed on the first attempt by eliciting a paresthesia, with no further manipulation and consequently no leakage of local anesthetic.

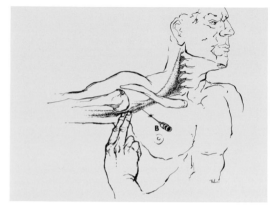

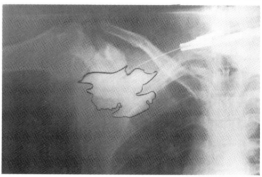

The x-rays and the illustration on page 106-108 are from Anesthesia and Analgesia, Volume 58: No: 3, page 225-233, copyright 1979. Reprinted by permission from International Anesthesia Research Society, Publishers.

Technique of Raj (1973)

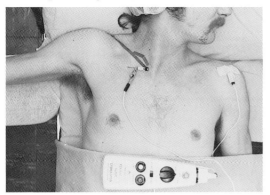

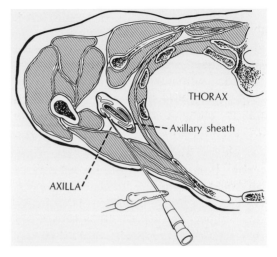

THORAX

Axillary sheath

AXILLA

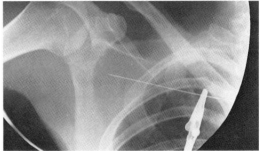

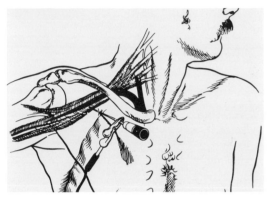

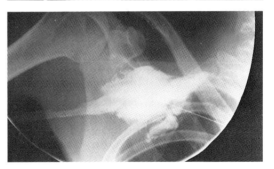

The patient lies supine with his head turned away from the arm to be blocked. The arm is abducted to 90° and allowed to rest comfortably. The physician stands on the opposite side from the arm to be blocked.

The whole length of the clavicle is marked after palpation. The subclavian artery is palpated where it dips under the clavicle and marked; it is usually at the midpoint of the clavicle. If the subclavian artery is not palpable, the midpoint of the clavicle is marked. The brachial artery is palpated in the arm and marked, and the C_6 tubercle on the same side is palpated and marked. A line is drawn from the C_6 tubercle to the brachial artery in the arm. This line goes through the midpoint of the clavicle and is the surface marking of the brachial plexus.

The ground electrode of a peripheral nerve stimulator is attached to the opposite shoulder. A skin wheal is raised one inch below the inferior border of the clavicle at its midpoint or where the subclavian artery dips under the clavicle. A 22-gauge, unsheathed, standard 3½ inch spinal needle is introduced through the skin wheal. The needle point is directed laterally toward the brachial artery. The exploring electrode is then attached to either the stem or the hub of the needle with a sterile alligator clip. The voltage control of the peripheral nerve stimulator is set to deliver 6-8 volts, and the needle is advanced at an angle of 45° to the skin. As the needle approaches the fibers of the brachial plexus, movements of the muscles supplied by those fibers will occur. The forearm and hand are carefully observed for these movements. Flexion or extension of the elbow, wrist, or digits confirms that the needle point is in close proximity to nerve fibers of the brachial plexus. The voltage is now decreased to 2-4 volts. The needle is then advanced. The muscle movements previously seen increase as the needle tip moves closer to the brachial plexus, so the needle is advanced until the muscle move-

ments start to decrease. When this happens, the needle tip has passed the nerve. Withdraw the needle slowly until the maximum muscle movements are again observed.

Hold the needle in that position as 2 ml of 2% lidocaine are injected through the needle, with the one impulse per second button on the peripheral nerve stimulator turned on. If the needle is located correctly there is an immediate loss of previously seen muscle movements (within 30 seconds). If not, the needle may have been pushed through the nerve. It should then be withdrawn slightly and the process repeated. Twenty to thirty ml of local anesthetic are then injected at that site.

From Anesthesia and Analgesia, Volume 52, page 897-904, copyright 1973.
Reprinted by permission from International Anesthesia Research Society, Publishers.

109

In 1977 Sims introduced a modification of the infraclavicular technique in an effort to overcome some of the disadvantages of Raj's technique, which he described as "difficult to master, due to lack of distinct landmarks and the thickness of the pectoralis major and minor muscles." He also stated that the technique described by Raj, because of "the long needle... and the frequent necessity of multiple attempts to locate the plexus, decreases patient acceptance of the procedure." Sims' modification moved the injection site to a point where the plexus is much more superficial, namely, in the groove between the coracoid process of the scapula and the inferior border of the clavicle. This point is lateral and superior to all but the thinnest part of the pectoralis major muscle and is medial to the pectoralis minor muscle, so the technique can be carried out with a standard 1½ inch needle, which is advanced inferiorly, laterally, and posteriorly toward the apex of the axilla. According to Sims, the plexus is usually contacted 2-3 centimeters beneath the skin. Having worked with Raj, Sims also utilizes the nerve stimulator in carrying out his modified infraclavicular block, but with his technique multiple attempts to locate the plexus are rarely necessary. Certainly, with this technique it would seem much less likely for the needle to end up lateral (distal) to the coracoid process and hence for the injection to miss the musculocutaneous and axillary nerves.

Technique of Sims (1977)

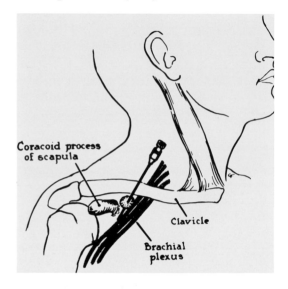

The patient is in the dorsal recumbent position with the head turned to the side opposite that on which the block is to be carried out. The index finger is placed in the groove between the coracoid process of the scapula and the inferior border of the clavicle. The finger tip is then advanced inferiorly and medially with moderate pressure of the skin. It will fall into a depression bordered inferiorly and medially by the superior portion of the pectoralis major, laterally by the coracoid process, and superiorly by the clavicle. This point is medial to the pectoralis minor muscle and superficial to the finished part of the pectoralis major. A skin wheal is raised at this point and through this wheal a 3.8 centimeter "B" bevel needle is introduced and advanced inferiorly, laterally, and posteriorly toward the apex of the axilla.

At no time should the needle be pointed medially or directed posteriorly toward the lung. The plexus will usually be reached within 2-3 cm from the skin wheal. These landmarks are distinct even in obese patients, but a longer needle may be required. The tip of a standard unsheathed needle is localized within the plexus by use of a nerve stimulator, with stimulus frequency set at one per second. Clinically, the needle should be positioned at the point of maximum stimulation.

A test dose of 2 ml of an anesthetic agent with a rapid onset is used, since agents with a slow onset may produce a vague endpoint if used for the test dose. During injection, nerve stimulation at the rate of one per second is continued. Immediate, dramatic cessation of muscle movement should ensue. Response less than this means that the needle tip is too far from the nerve and should be repositioned. If less than a perfect result is accepted at this step, the quality of the block is in jeopardy; it is here that most anesthetists fail to use the nerve stimulator properly.

Once the needle is in proper position and aspiration has been performed, 35 ml of an appropriate local anesthetic solution are injected. The needle and other hardware may then be removed from the patient.

From Anesthesia and Analgesia, Volume 56, page 554-555, copyright 1977.
Reprinted by permission from International Anesthesia Research Society, Publishers.

In 1981 Whiffler proposed a modification in which the injection site was not far from that proposed by Sims, but the technique of injection was totally different. In preparation for this technique, which he terms "coracoid block", the patient is placed in the supine position with the head turned to the side opposite that on which the block is to be performed. The patient's shoulder should be depressed and the arm abducted approximately 45° from the chest wall, a maneuver that Whiffler feels brings the axillary sheath and its contents closer to the coracoid process. Having identified the coracoid process, Whiffler estimates the depth of the anticipated injection by palpating the axillary artery as high as possible in the axilla and placing the thumb of the same hand on the anterior surface of the chest wall over the site at which the index finger palpates the artery. This point in most instances lies in the deltopectoral groove, just below the head of the humerus. The distance between the thumb and the palpating index finger is used as an indication of the depth to which the needle has to be inserted.

With Whiffler's technique, the needle is inserted just inferior and medial to the coracoid process to the depth estimated as indicated above, at which point an initial injection of 12 ml of local anesthetic is made. In ectomorphic individuals, a second injection of 12 ml is made after withdrawing the needle one centimeter from the point of the initial injection, and in muscular individuals a third injection of 12 ml is made after withdrawing the needle an additional one centimeter. Whiffler feels that one of the primary advantages of his technique is that he does not need to utilize a nerve stimulator to locate the plexus precisely, since his objective is not to locate the perivascular compartment and make an injection therein but rather to "bathe the whole of the axilla and its contents in the local anesthetic agent." In other words, this technique is akin to Patrick's supraclavicular technique carried out in the axilla in that no attempt is made to locate the plexus but rather to lay down a "wall of anesthetic" through which the plexus must pass. In Whiffler's own series there was only a 92.5% success rate, and although there was no discernible evidence of adverse sequelae, the rate of arterial puncture was 50%. Thus, there seems to be little advantage to the technique except that "flooding the axilla" as it does, it is unnecessary to block the intercostobrachial nerve separately.

In short, none of the infraclavicular techniques appears to offer significant enough advantages over the more established perivascular techniques of brachial plexus block to utilize it as the technique of choice, except in rare, unique clinical situations, but certainly, the techniques of Raj and Sims expand the utility of the perivascular concept and document once again that the sheath can be entered at any level, and at that level definite volume-anesthesia relationships can be established.

Technique of Whiffler (1981)

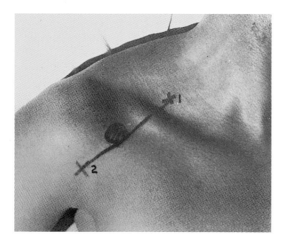 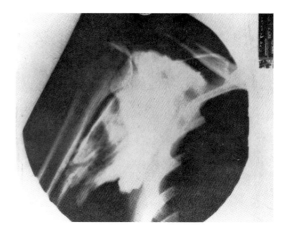

The patient is supine with the head turned to the side opposite to that on which the block is to be performed. The relevant shoulder is depressed and the arm abducted approximately 45° from the chest wall. The midpoint of the clavicle is identified and the subclavian artery palpated. The artery is followed laterally until it disappears under the clavicle and this point is marked with a skin pen (X1).

The coracoid process is identified and marked with a skin pen. The axillary artery is palpated with the index finger as high as possible in the axilla. The thumb is placed on the anterior surface of the chest wall over the site at which the index finger palpates the axillary artery. This point is marked with a skin pen (X2). In most instances this point will be found to lie in the deltopectoral groove, just below the head of the humerus. The depth at which the axillary sheath and the contents lie can be gauged by estimating the distance between the thumb and the index finger and gives an indication of the depth to which the needle has to be inserted. Points X1 and X2 are joined by a line with a skin pen. In most cases this line passes immediately inferior and medial to the coracoid process.

The skin over the coracoid process is cleaned and, using a 21-gauge 51 millimeter needle attached to a 20 ml syringe, the skin is punctured inferomedial to the coracoid process, and the line adjoining X1 and X2 transected at the depth which had pre-viously been estimated by the distance between the thumb and index finger. The needle is usually at right angles to the skin. Because of the depth at which the axillary sheath and contents lie, it is often necessary to insert the needle almost up to its hub. After aspiration, approximately 12 ml of local anesthetic agent are injected. The needle is then withdrawn 1 cm and the procedure of aspiration and injection repeated. This maneuver is repeated twice in a muscular person (36 ml total volume) and once in an ectomorphic patient (24 ml). This distributes the local anesthetic solution around the neurovascular bundle. When doubt exists about striking the axillary sheath and contents with the first injection, the needle is withdrawn until the bevel lies just beneath the surface of the skin, and it is then advanced in a slightly angled direction either inferior to the first injection or superior to the first injection, depending on where the plexus is thought to lie. The procedure of withdrawal, aspiration, and injection is then carried out as described previously. Care must be taken not to exceed the total calculated safe dose of local anesthetic drug. With this procedure the local anesthetic spreads to involve the whole axilla, as may be seen when a radiopaque dye is added to the local anesthetic agent.

From Br. J. Anaesthesia 53, page 845, copyright 1981.
Reprinted by permission from Kurt Whiffler, M. D. and Macmillan Press Ltd. London.

Textbooks & Reviews

Adriani, J.: Nerve Blocks, pp. 112-120. Charles C. Thomas, Springfield, 1954.

Adriani, J.: Labat's Regional Anesthesia, 3rd Ed. W. B. Saunders Co., Philadelphia 1918.

Allen, C. W.: Local and Regional Anesthesia, 224-245, W. B. Saunders Co., Philadelphia, 1918.

Babcock, W. W.: A Textbook of Surgery for Students and Physicians. 2nd Ed., pp. 542-544, 1937.

Berry, F. R. and Bridenbaugh, L. D.: The Upper Extremity: Somatic Blockade. Chapter 10 pp. 296-319 in Neural Blockade in Clinical Anesthesia and Management of Pain. Edited by Cousins, M. J., and Bridenbaugh, P. O., J. P. Lippencott Company, Philadelphia, 1980.

Bohler, L.: Treatment of Fractures. William Wood Co. Baltimore, 1936.

Bonica, J. J.: The Management of Pain. Lea & Febiger.Philadelphia, 1953.

Bonica, J. J.: Modern Trends in Anesthesia, Chapter 6: The Place of Regional Anesthesia (Evans, F. T. & Gray, T. C.). Butterworth & Co. London, 1958.

Bonica, J. J.: Clinical Applications of Diagnostic and Therapeutic Blocks. Charles C. Thomas, Springfield, 1959.

Braun, H.: Local Anesthesia, pp. 347-355. Lea & Febiger, Philadelphia, 1914.

Bridenbaugh, LD.: Regional Anesthesia for Surgery of the Extremities. Edited by JJ. Bonica.; Philadelphia, F. A. Davis, 1969 pages 194-205.

Collins, V. J.: Principles of Anesthesiology.Lea & Febiger, Philadelphia, 1966.

de Takats, G.: Local Anesthesia. W. B. Saunders Co. Philadelphia, 1928.

Dogliotti, A. M.: Anesthesia: Narcosis, Local, Regional, Spinal. S. B. Debour, Chicago, 1939.

Estella, J.: Manual of Surgical Anesthesia, 2nd Ed., [Spanish]. Editorial Alhambra, Madrid, Spain, 1953.

Farr, R. E.: Practical Local Anesthesia. Lea & Febiger, Philadelphia, 1923.

Galindo, A.: Illustrated Regional Anesthesia, R. M. Scientific Publications, Miami, 1982.

Gwathmey, J. T.: Anesthesia pp. 508-510, Macmillan, New York, 1929.

Hartel, F.: Local Anesthesia [German]. Neue Deutsche Chirurgie 29: 149-171, 1916.

Hartel, F.: Local Anesthesia [German] pp. 168-192. Ferdinand Enke, Stuttgart, 1920.

Hertzler, A. E.: Local Anesthesia, 4th Ed. pp. 252-255. C. V. Mosby Co., St. Louis, 1928.

Hirschel, G.: Handbook of Local Anesthesia [German]. J. F. Bergman, Wiesbaden, 1913.

Hirschel, G.: Textbook of Local Anesthesia, pp. 130-133, Translated by Krohn. E. S. William Wood and Company 1915.

Labat, G.: Regional Anesthesia, 1st Ed. pp. 181-237. W. B. Saunders Co. Philadelphia, 1922.

Labat, G.: Regional Anesthesia, 2nd Ed. W. B. Saunders Co., Philadelphia, 1928.

Lee, J. A. and Atkinson, R. S.: A Synopsis of Anesthesia, 5th Ed., Williams & Wilkins Co., Baltimore, 1964.

Lee, J. A.: Regional Anesthesia. International Anesthesia Clinics 5 (1):69-89, 1967.

Lundy, J. S.: Clinical Anesthesia. W. B. Saunders Co., Philadelphia & London, 1942.

Löfström, B.: Useful Nerve Blocks of the Arm. Symposium on Local and Conduction Anesthesia. pp. 67-73, (Sep 16) 1968.

Macintosh, R. R. and Mushin, W. W. Local Anesthesia: Brachial Plexus. Blackwell Scientific Publications, Ltd. Oxford, 1944.

Moore, D. C.: Block of the Brachial Plexus. Chapter in Regional Block: A Handbook for Use in Clinical Practice of Medicine and Surgery 1st Edition. Charles C. Thomas Publisher, Springfield, Illinois, pp. 171-188, 1953.

Moore, D. C.: Block of the Brachial Plexus. Chapter in Regional Block: A Handbook for Use in Clinical Practice of Medicine and Surgery 2nd Ed., Charles C. Thomas Publishers, Springfield, Illinois, pp. 183-201, 1957.

Moore, D. C.: Block of the Brachial Plexus. Chapter in Regional Block Anesthesia: 3rd Ed., Charles C. Thomas Publishers, Springfield, Illinois, pp. 183-201, 1962.

Moore, D. C.: Regional Block, 4th Ed., Charles C. Thomas Publishers, Springfield, 1965.

Mousel, L. H.: Local, Regional, and Spinal Anesthesia in Nelson New Loose Leaf Surgery pp. 542-543. Thomas Nelson and Sons, New York, 1941.

Pauchet, V., Sourdet, P., Labat, G.: Regional Anesthesia 3rd Ed. [French] (pp. 149-170). Librarie Octave Doin. Gaston Doin, Editeur, Paris, 1921.

Reese, C. A.: Conduction Anesthesia of the Upper Extremity – A Literature and Technique Review. AANA Journal 45: 267-278, 1977.

Shaw, W. M.: Brachial Plexus Anesthesia: A Review of the Literature Thesis for New York University Post Graduate Medical School Graduate Program In Anesthesia, 1946.

Sherwood-Dunn, B.: Regional Anesthesia (Victor Pauchet's Technique). F. A. Davis Company, Philadelphia, 1920.

Southworth, J. L. and Hingson, R. A.: Pitkin's Conduction Anesthesia. J. B. Lippencott Co. Philadelphia, 1946.

Southworth, J. L., Hingson, R. A. & Pitkin, W. M.: Pitkin's Conduction Anesthesia, 2nd Ed. J. B. Lippencott Co. Philadelphia, 1953.

Touny, E. B.: Local Anesthesia, in Lewis' Practice of Surgery, pp. 41-64. W. F. Prior Co., Hayerstown, Pa., 1945.

Winnie, A. P.: The Perivascular Technics of Brachial Plexus Anesthesia. Middle East Journal of Anesthesia 3: 239-260, 1972.

Winnie, A. P.: Regional Anesthesia. Surgical Clinics of North America 54: 861-892, 1975.

Winnie, A. P.: Regional Anesthesia of the Upper and Lower Extremities. Chapter 6 in "Anesthesia for Orthopaedic Surgery". Zauder, H. L. (Editor). F. A. Davis Company, Philadelphia, Pennsylvania, pp. 89-117, 1980.

Winnie, A. P. and Ramamurthy, S.: Clinical Considerations: Perivascular Technics of Brachial Plexus Block. ASRA Workshop, San Antonio, Texas, (Nov 20-22) 1981.

Winnie, A. P.: Plexus Anesthesia: A System of Single Injection Techniques.

Scientific Exhibits

Bosomworth, P. P. and Hamelberg, W.: An Exhibit of Perivascular, Axillary Brachial Plexus Block: Anatomy, Technique and Complications. Scientific Exhibit, ASA Annual Meeting, Los Angeles, 1961.

de Jong, Rudolph H.: Axillary Block of the Brachial Plexus Scientific Exhibit, ASA Annual Meeting, Bal Harbour Florida, (Oct 12-14) 1964.

Winnie, A. P. and Collins, V. J.: The Perivascular Techniques of Brachial Plexus Anesthesia. Scientific Exhibit, ASA Annual Meeting, Denver, (Oct 23-27) 1965.

113

References & Bibliography

The evolution of axillary
perivascular brachial plexus block

Abadir, A.: Anesthesia for Hand Surgery. Orthopedic Clinics of North America 1:205-212, 1970.

Accardo, N. J. and Adriani, J.: Brachial Plexus Block: A Simplified Technic Using The Axillary Route. South Med. J. 42: 420-923, 1949.

Bosomworth, P. P., Egbert, L. L., Hammelberg, W.: Block of the Brachial Plexus in the Axilla: Its Value and Complications. Ann. Gurg: 154: 911-914; 1961.

Brand, L. and Papper, E. M.: A Comparison of Supraclavicular and Axillary Techniques for Brachial Plexus Blocks. Anesthsiology 22: 226-229, 1961.

Brinkman, P. A. & Lincoln, J. R.: Axillary Block – A plea for Wider Use. J. of the Maine M. A. 54: 190-192, (Sept) 1963.

Bromage, P. R.: Local Anesthetic Procedures for the Arm and Hand Surg. Clin. N. America 44: 919-923, (Aug) 1964.

Burnham, P. J.: Regional Block of the Great Nerves of the Upper Arm. Anesthesiology 19:281-284, 1958.

Burnham, P. J.: Simple Regional Nerve Block for Surgery on the Hand and Forearm. JAMA 169: 941-943, 1959.

Capelle: Anesthesia of the Brachial Plexus: The Dangers and How to Avoid Them [German]. Beitr. z. klin. Chir. 104:122-139, 1917.

Clavet, M.: Anesthesia of the Upper Extremity [French Canad]. Laval Medical 34:45-56, 1965.

Clayton, M. L. and Turner, D. A.: Upper Arm Block Anesthesia in Children with Fractures. JAMA 169:327-329, 1959.

de Jong, R. H.: Axillary Block of the Brachial Plexus. Anesthesiology 22:215-225, 1961.

de Jong, R. H.: Modified Axillary Block: With Block of the Lateral Ante brachial Cutaneous (Terminal Musculo- Cutaneous) Nerve. Anesthesiology 26: 615-618, 1965.

Dales, J. W., Curtis, E., Toms, A. A., O'Reilly, K. S., Ohlke, R. F.: Axillary Arm Block with Emphasis on its Use in Children. Canad. M. A. J. 82:1160-1162, 1960.

Dudley, W. R., Dolan, P. F. and Cohen, E. N.: Correspondence ("Axillary Sheath Distention: A Useful Sign in Performing Axillary Block"). Anesthesiology 49: 302-304, 1978.

Eather, K. F.: Axillary Brachial Plexus Block. Anesthesiology 19: 683-684, 1958.

Eggers, G. W. N., Metzgar, M. T., and Plumlee, J. E.: Axillary Block and Sedation for Cardiac Catherization. Anesth. 28: 936-982, 1967.

Eriksson, E. & Skarby, H-G.: A Simplified Method of Axillary Block [Swedish]. Nord. Med. 68: 1325, 1962.

Eriksson, E.: A New Modification of Axillary Plexus Block; Movie 1964. Astra Film Library.

Eriksson E.: Axillary Brachial Plexus Anesthesia in Children with Citanest. Acta Anaesth. Scandinav. Supplementum XVI, 291-296, 1965.

Jacques, A.: Regional Anesthesia of the Brachial Plexus by the Axillary Route. Anesthesia & Analgesia 47: 160-162, 1968.

Hamelberg, W., Dysart, R., Bosomworth, P.: Perivascular Axillary Versus Supraclavicular Brachial Plexus Block and General Anesthesia. Anesth. & Analg. 41:85-90, (Jan-Feb) 1962.

Hingson, R. H.: In Southworth, J. L. and Hingson, R. H.: Chapter 14, Conduction Anesthesia of the Extremities in Pitkin's Conduction Anesthesia. J. B. Lippencott Company, Philadelphia, 1946.

Hirschel, G.: Anesthesia of the Brachial Plexus for Operations on the Upper Extremity [German] München. Med. Wochenschr. 58: 1555-1556, (July 18) 1911.

Hirschel, G.: The Use of Local Anesthesia in Extensive Procedures on the Breast and Thorax [German]. München Med. Wochenschr. 58:497-9, 1911.

Hirschel, G.: Anesthesia of the Brachial Plexus via the Axilla for Surgical Procedures on the Upper Extremity. München Med. Wochenschr. 22:1218-1220, (May 28) 1912.

Hollmen, A.: Axillary Plexus Block: A Double Blind Study of 59 cases Using Mepivicaine and LAC-43. Acta Anaesth. Scandinav. 10: 53-65, Supp. 21, (Sept) 1966.

Hollmen, A., and Mononen, P.: Axillary Plexus Block with Etidocaine. Acta Anaesth. Scand. (Suppl.) 60:25-28, 1975.

Hudon, F. and Jacques, André: Block of the Brachial Plexus by the Axillary Route. Can. Anaes. Soc. J. 6:400-405, 1959.

Högström, S.: Axillary Block – A Comparison Between Lidocain and L 67 [Prilocain] [Swedish]. Nord. Med. 69:153, 1963.

Kleinert, H. E., De Simone, K., Gaspar, H. E., Arnold, R. E., and Kasdan, M. L.: Regional Anesthesia For Upper Extremity Surgery. J. Trauma 3:3-11, 1963.

Leahey, E. B., Buscicchi, E. J., Noto, A., Rooney, J. J.: Upper-Arm Block Anesthesia: A Critical Analysis. J. Bone & Joint Surg. 46-A: 593, 1964.

Manriques, R. G. and Pallares, V.: Continuous Brachial Plexus Block for Prolonged Sympathectomy and Control of Pain. Anesth. & Analg. 57: 128-130, 1978.

Mathews, W. A.: Axillary Block. International Anesthesiology Clinics 1:707-715, (May) 1963.

Mazzacane, W. D.: Axillary Brachial Plexus Block – A Review. West Virginia Medical Journal 65:109-111, 1969.

Modell, J. H. and Smith, B. E.: Regional Anesthesia of the Upper Extremity. GP 30: 120-122, 1964.

Moir, D. D.: Axillary Block of the Brachial Plexus. Anaesthesia 17: 274-283, (July) 1962.

Moore, D. C., Bridenbaugh, L. D., Eather, K. F.: Block of the Upper Extremity: Supraclavicular Approach Versus Axillary Approach. Arch. Surg. 90: 68-72, 1965.

Pitkin, George P.: Prolonged Local or Block Anesthesia with Regulated Cell Reception. Current Researches in Anesth. & Analg. 21: 1-12, 1942 and 21: 83-95, 1942 (in two parts).

Pollock, M. & Rawstron, R. E.: An Upper Arm Nerve Block. New Zealand Med. Journal 59: 547-549, 1960.

Reding, M.: A New Method of Anesthesia of the Upper Extremity [French]. Presse Med. 29: 294-296, (April 13) 1921.

Rosenblatt, R. M., Zauder, H. L., Stevens, J. J., Lee, J. J., et al: Correspondence ("The Air Test for Regional Blocks"). Anesthesiology 51: 95-98, 1979.

Shanahan, P. T. and Kleinert, H. E.: Anesthesia Management of Upper Extremity Replantation Surgery. Anesthesiology Review 1:10-22, 1983.

Small, J. A.: Brachial Plexus Block in Children. JAMA 147: 1648-1651, 1951.

Spillar, B. R. & Spillar, E. M.: The Axillary Approach to Anesthesia of the Upper Extremity. Amer. Surg. 28: 600-603, 1962.

Thompson, G. E.: A Study of Axillary Block Using Computed Tomography. ASA Abstracts. Anesthesiology (Supplement) 55: A 146, 1980.

Urban, B. J., McDonald, H. P. Jr., Steen, S. N.: Axillary Block and Dialysis. JAMA 199: 889-891, 1967.

Vidal-Lopez, F.: Contributions to the Axillary Perivascular Anaesthetic. (Oct) 1976.

Wu, W.: A Double-Needle Technique via the Axillary Route. JAMA 215: 1953-1955, 1971.

The evolution of subclavian
perivascular brachial plexus block

Ansbro, P.: A Method of Continuous Brachial Plexus Block. Am. J. Surg. 71: 716-722, (June) 1946.

Ansbro, F. P., Blundell, A. E., Hernandez, W. E., and Carter, J. V.: Brachial Plexus Block. Am. J. Surg. 95:953-962, 1958.

Arnold, G. H., and Gibson, L. V.: Brachial Plexus Anesthesia. Southwest. Med. 23: 249-250, (Aug) 1939.

Ashwort, H. K.: Local Anaesthesia. Practioners 89: 162-168, 1962.

Atkins, H. J. B.: The Effect of Brachial Plexus Block on Patients Suffering from Secondary Traumatic Shock. Brit. J. Surg. 24: 717-727, (April) 1937.

Babitzky, P.: The Brachial Plexus Anesthesia of Kulenkampff [German]. Deutsche Med. Wochenchr. 39: 652-653, (April 3) 1913.

Balas, G. I.: Regional Anesthesia for Surgery on the Shoulder. Anesth. & Analg. 50: 1036-1041, 1971.

Ball, H. C.: Brachial Plexus Block. Anaesthesia 17: 269-273, (July) 1962.

Boit, H.: Anesthesia of the Brachial Plexus Using Kulenkampff's Technique, a Report of Over 200 Cases [German]. Beitr. s. klin. Chir. 93:336-340, 1914.

Bone, J. R.: Regional Nerve Block Anesthesia. Anesthesiology 6: 612-616, (Nov) 1945.

Bonica, J. J., Moore, D. C. and Orlov, M.: Brachial Plexus Block Anesthesia. Am. J. Surg. 78: 65-79, 1949.

Bonica, J. J. and Moore, D. C.: Brachial Plexus Block Anesthesia. Current Research in Anesth. & Analg. 29: 241-253, 1950.

Borchers, E.: Supraclavicular Anesthesia of the Brachial Plexus [German]. Zentralbl. f. Chir. 39: 873-879, (June) 1918.

Braun, H.: The Use of Local Anesthesia in Setting Closed Fractures and Dislocations [German]. Deutsche Med. Wochnchr. 39: 17-18, 1913.

Cairo, J. A.: Rev. med. latino-am. 132: 2123-2127, (Sept) 1926 (Regional Anesthesia of the Brachial Plexus) [Spanish].

Carter, S. J., Burman, S. O., and Mersheimer, W. L.: Supraclavicular Brachial Block Anesthesia. N. Y. J. Med. 66: 1315-1317, 1966.

Crile, G. W.: Anesthesia of Nerve Roots with Cocaine. Cleveland Medical Journal 2: 355, 1897.

Crile, G. W.: "Blocking" the Brachial Plexus in Tetanus Following Compound Fracture of the Forearm. In Report of the Surgical Service of Dr. G. W. Crile, at St. Alexis Hospital, for 6. Months Ending January 1897. Reported by G. J. Ashby, M. D., House Surgeon. Cleveland J. Med. 2:343-357, 1897.

Damarjian, E.: Brachial Plexus Block – One Hundred Cases. Rhode Island Med. J. 29: 271-277, 1946.

DeKrey, J. A., Schroeder, C. R., and Buechel, D. R.: Continuous Brachial Plexus Block. Anesthesiology 30: 332, 1969.

Eberle, D.: The Practical Application of Local Anesthesia [German]. Arch. f. Klin. Chir. 99: 1020-1056, 1912.

Fortin, G. and Tremblay, L.: The Short-needle Technique in Brachial Plexus Block. Canad. Anaesth. Soc. J. 6: 32-39, (Jan) 1959.

Greene, B. C.: Brachial Plexus Anesthesia: A Report of 150 Cases. M. Bull. North African Theat. Op. 2: 102-104, (Nov) 1944.

Griswold, H. A. and Woodson, W. H.: Brachial Plexus Block Anesthesia of the Upper Extremities. Am. J. Surg. 59: 439-443, (Feb) 1943.

Halperin, P. H.: Brachial Plexus Block. Wisconsin M. J. 38: 21-24, 1939.

Halsted, W. S. (reported by Matas, R.): In Memorium: William Stewart Halsted. Johns Hopkins Hospital Bulletin 36: 8, 1925.

Halsted, W. S.: Surgical Papers. Ed. by W. C. Burket, 1: 167-176. Johns Hopkins Press, Baltimore, 1925.

Hanrahan, B. M.: Brachial Plexus Block. Virginia M. Monthly 55: 305-306, (Aug) 1928.

Hanrahan, E. N.: Brachial Plexus Nerve Block. JAMA. 90: 529-530, (Feb 18) 1928.

Hartel, F. and Keppler, W.: Experience with Kulenkampff's Technique of Brachial Plexus Anesthesia with Special Regard to Complications During and after the Block [German]. Arch. f. Klin. Chir. 103: 1-43, 1913.

Hay, I. M.: Brachial Plexus Anesthesia. J. Florida M. A. 15: 601-602, (June) 1929.

Heile, H.: Symposium On Local Anesthesia [German]. Zentralbl. f. Chir. 40: 98, 1913.

Heinert, H. E., DeSimone, K., Caspar, H. E., Arnold, R. E., and Kasdan, M. L.: Regional Anesthesia for Upper Extremity Surgery. J. of Trauma 3: 3-11, 1963.

Highsmith, J. D.: Regional Anesthesia in the Treatment of Fractures and Dislocations. South. Med. J. 23: 807-813, (Sept) 1930.

Hohmeier: Mid-Rhine Surgical Convention [German]. Zentralbl. f. Chir. 40: 98-99, (Jan 18) 1913.

Hohmeier: Local Anesthesia of the Extremities [German] Zentralbl. f. Chir. 41 (supl 32): 28-29, (Aug 8) 1914.

Hollingworth, R. K.: Regional Anesthesia by the Nerve Block in Reduction of Fractures and Dislocations. J. Tennessee M. A. 24: 294-299, (Aug) 1931.

Hurley, O. A. P.: Regional Anesthesia: Its Advantages in Emergency of the Extremities. Am. J. Surg. 72: 219-228, (Aug) 1946.

Koller, C.: On the Use of Cocaine for Producing Anesthesia of the Eye. Lancet 2: 990-992, 1884. (Translation and review by Bloom, J. N.).

Knight, R.: Quoted by Lundy, J. S. in Clinical Anesthesia, p. 105. W. B. Saunders Co. Philadelphia, 1942.

Kulenkampff, D.: Anesthesia of the Brachial Plexus [German]. Zentralbl. f. Chir. 38: 1337-1350, (Oct 7) 1911.

Kulenkampff, D.: Anesthesia of the Brachial Plexus [German]. Deutsche Med. Wochenschr. 38: 1878-1880, (Oct 3) 1912.

Kulenkampff, D.: Anesthesia of Brachial Plexus [German]. Zentralbl. f. Chir. 79: 550-552, 1912.

Kulenkampff, D.: Anesthesia of the Brachial Plexus [German]. Zentralbl. f. Chir. 40: 849-852, (May 31) 1913.

Kulenkampff, D. and Persky, M. A.: Brachial Plexus Anesthesia: Its Indications Technique, and Dangers. Ann. Surg. 87: 883-891, 1928.

Labat, G.: Brachial Plexus Block: Details of Technique. Anesth. & Analg. 6: 81-82, 1927.

Labat, G.: Brachial Plexus Block. Brit. J. Anesth. 4: 174-176, (Jan) 1927.

Lippens, A.: Anesthesia of the Brachial Plexus [German]. Zentralbl. f. Chir. 41: 1294-1295, (Aug 1) 1914.

Livingston, E. M., Wertheim, H.: Brachial Plexus Block: Its Clinical Application. Anesth. & Analg. 6: 149-154, 1927.

Livingston, E. M. and Wertheim, H.: Brachial Plexus Block: Its Clinical Application. Brit. J. Anesth. 4:209-220, (April) 1927.

Livingston, E. M., Wertheim, H.: Brachial Plexus Block: Its Clinical Application. JAMA. 88: 1465-1468, (May 7) 1927.

Livingston, E. M.: Regional Anesthesia: Its Place In Medicine. Am. J. Surg. 23: 210, 1934.

Lookman, AA.: Brachial Plexus Infiltration. Anaesthesia 13: 5-18, (Jan) 1958.

Lundy, J. S. and Tovell, R. M.: The Technique of Nerve Blocking for Various Orthopedic Operations. Brit. J. Anesth. 12: 52-61, (Jan) 1935.

Mage, S.: The Use of Regional Anesthesia by the Nerve Block Method for the Reduction of Fractures And Dislocations. Ann. Surg. 85: 765-777, (May) 1927.

Matas, R.: In Memoriam: William Stewart Halsted Johns Hopkins Hosp. Bull. 36: 2-27, (Jan) 1925.

Matas, R.: Local and Regional Anesthesia: A Retrospect and Prospect. Am. J. Surg. 25: 189-196 & 362-379, 1934.

Matthes, H.: Research and Results of the Supraclavicular Block of the Brachial Plexus. Der Anaesthesist 14: 361, 1965.

Miltner, L. J. and Chao, C. L.: Brachial Plexus Anesthesia. J. Iowa Med. Soc. 29: 94-98, (March) 1939.

Molesworth, H. W. I.: Experiences with Regional Anesthesia. Brit. M. J. 1: 13-14, (Jan 4) 1930.

Moore, D. C.: The Use of Pontocaine Hydrochloride for Nerve Block and Infiltration Analgesia, Therapeutic, and Diagnostic Blocks: 1004 Cases. Anesthesiology 11: 65-75, 1950.

Moore, D. C., Bridenbaugh, L. D., Eather, K. F.: Block of the Upper Extremity: Supraclavicular Approach Versus Axillary Approach. Arch. Surg. 90: 68-72, 1965.

Moore, D. C., Balas, G. I., Minuck, M. and Penrose, B. H.: Correspondence. Anesth. & Analg. 51: 483-488, 1972.

Murphey, D. R., Jr.: Brachial Plexus Block Anesthesia, An Improved Technique. Ann. Surg. 119: 935-943, (June) 1944.

Neil, W. F. and Crooks, F.: Supraclavicular Anesthetization of the Brachial Plexus. Brit. Med. J. 1: 388-389, (Feb 22) 1913.

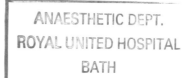
115

Neuhof, H.: Supraclavicular Anesthetization of the Brachial Plexus. JAMA 62: 1629-1631, 1914.

Næraa, A.: Anesthetizing The Brachial Plexus with Kulenkampff's Technique [Dansk]. Ugeskrift f. Læger 96: 246-248, 1934.

Patrick, J.: The Technique of Brachial Plexus Block Anesthesia. Brit. J. Surg. 27: 734-739, (April) 1940.

Patrick, J.: Brachial Plexus Block Anesthesia in Operations on the Upper Extremity. Tr. Roy. Med. Chir. Loc. Glasgow in Glasgow M. J. 18: 39-45 (Nov) 1941.

Perthes, G.: Conduction Anesthesia with the Help of Electrical Stimulation [German]. München Med. Wochenschr. 59: 2545-2548, (Nov 19) 1912.

Phillips, R. S.: How to Obtain Good Results with Brachial Plexus Block Anesthesia. Mil. Surg. 95: 197-199, (Sept) 1944.

Rhone, T. B.: Brachial Plexus Anesthesia. Ann. Surg. 101: 1153-1170, 1935.

Shaw, W. M. and Root, B.: Brachial Plexus Anesthesia: Comparative Study of Agents and Technics. Am. J. Surg. 81: 407-410, (April) 1951.

Siebert, K.: A Newer Anesthetic Technics with Special Consideration of Plexus Anesthesia [German]. Med. Klinik 8: 1945-1948, (Dec 1) 1912.

Simpson, J. K.: Supraclavicular Brachial Plexus Block. J. Florida M. A. 2: 161-165, 1915.

Small, G. A.: Brachial Plexus Block Anesthesia in Children. JAMA 147: 1648-1651, 1951.

Storzer, A.: War Surgery Reports of World War I (1914-1918) No. 107: Battle Casualty Operations on the Extremities with Special Emphasis on Plexus Anesthesia of Kulenkampff [German]. Deutsche Zeitschr. f. Chir. 147: 1-26 1918.

Strachauer, A. C.: Brachial Plexus: Anesthesia: A Complete Local Anesthesia of the Upper Extremity Permitting of All Major Surgical Procedures. The Journal-Lancet 34: 301-303, 1914.

Strode, J. E.: Brachial Plexus Block Anesthesia: Its Advantages in Treatment of Fractures of the Arm: Report of Cases. California West. Med. 31: 17-20, (July) 1929.

Tatlow, W. F. T. and Oulton, J. L.: Chantom Limbs (With Observations on Brachial Plexus Block). Canad. M. A. J. 73: 170-177, (Aug 1) 1955.

Tarsey, J. M. and Steinbrocker, O.: Supraclavicular Brachial Plexus Block: An Accessory Measure in Arthritis of the Shoulder Joint and Allied Conditions. N. Y. State J. M. 37: 1275-1278, 1937.

Thurlow, J. F.: Brachial Plexus Anesthesia. Am. J. Surg. 77: 338-343, 1949.

Touhy, E. B.: Brachial Plexus Block. Am. J. Surg. 34: 544-546, (Dec) 1936.

Veen, J.: Anesthesia of the Brachial Plexus [Dutch]. Nederl. tijdschr. v. geneesk. 84: 598-804, (Feb 17) 1940.

Villafane, E. P.: The Regional Anesthesia of Kulenkampff [Spanish]. Rev. med. latino-am. 25: 777-786, (April) 1940.

Wan, F. E.: The Use of Regional Anesthesia: an analysis of 2555 Cases. Nat. Med. J. of China 16: 730-738, (Dec) 1930.

Winnie, A. P. and Collins, V. J.: The Subclavian Perivascular Technique of Brachial Plexus Anesthesia. Anesthesiology 25: 353-363, 1964.

Winnie, A. P.: Brachial Plexus Block (Continuous). Correspondence. Anesthesiology 31: 195-196, 1969.

Wright, H. W. S.: Anesthesia of the Brachial Plexus. Brit. J. Surg. 14: 160-167, (July) 1926.

The evolution of interscalene brachial plexus block

Bahar, M., Magora, F., Rousso, M.: Observations on Interscalene Brachial Plexus. Anesthesia, 1977.

Etienne, J.: Regional Anesthesia: Its Application in the Surgical Treatment of Cancer of the Breast [French]. Doctoral Thesis, Faculté de Medecine de Paris, 1925.

Heffington, C. A., Thompson, R. C.: The Use of Interscalene Block Anesthesia for Manipulative Reduction of Fractures and Dislocations of the Upper Extremities. Journal of Bone and Joint Surgery 55-A: 83-86, 1973.

Hilarowicz, H.: The Technique of Conduction Anesthesia of the Brachial Plexus [German]. Zentralbl. f. Chir. 52: 2349-2351, (Oct 17) 1925.

Hilarowicz, H.: Anesthesia of the Brachial Plexus [German]. Zentralbl. f. Chir. 55: 2450. (Sept 29) 1928.

Kappis, M.: Conduction Anesthesia of the Abdomen, Breast, Arm, and Neck with Paravertebral Injection [German]. München. Med. Wochenschr. 59: 794-796, (April 9) 1912.

Mitchell, El., Murphy, FL., Wyche, MQ., and Torg, JS.: Interscalene Brachial Plexus Block Anesthesia for the Modified Bristow Procedure. Amer. J. of Sports Med. 2(10): 79-82. 1982.

Mulley, K.: A Modification of Kulenkampff's Brachial Block Technique in Order to Avoid Pleural Injury [German]. Beitr. z. klin. Chir. 114: 666-680, 1919.

Pauchet, V., Sourdat, P., Tabott, G., et al.: Regional Anesthesia, 4th Ed. [French]. Paris, Doin, 1928.

Pitkin, G. P.: Prolonged Local or Block Anesthesia with Regulated Cell Reception. Anesth. & Analg. 21: 1-12 and 83-95, 1942.

Santoni, A. D.: Regional Anesthesia of the Spinal Nerves [French]. Tosie de Paris, 1916.

Sharrock, N. E. and Bruce, G.: An Improved Technique for Locating the Interscalene Groove. In Clinical Reports. Brown, B. R. (Editor). Anesthesiology 44: 431-433, 1976.

Vidal-Lopez, F.: Brachial Plexus Anesthesia Using the Omotrapezoid Route. Anesth. & Analg. 56: 486-488, 1977.

Vongvises, P. and Panijayanond, T.: A Parascalene Technique of Brachial Plexus Anesthesia. Anesth. & Analg. 58: 267-273, 1979.

Ward, M. E.: The Interscalene Approach to the Brachial Plexus. Anesthesia 29: 147-157, 1974.

Winnie, A. P.: Interscalene Brachial Plexus Block. Anesth. & Analg. Current Researches 49: 455-466 (3), (May-June) 1970.

The evolution of infraclavicular brachial plexus block

Aillon, R.: Subcoracoid Technique for Brachial Plexus Block. (Personal Communication) (Aug) 1976.

Babitsky, P.: A New Way of Anesthetizing the Brachial Plexus [German]. Zentralbl. f. Chir. 45: 215-217, (Mar 30) 1918.

Balog, A.: Conduction Anesthesia of the Infraclavicular Portion of the Brachial Plexus [German]. Zentralbl. f. Chir. 51: 1563-64, (July 19) 1924.

Balog, A.: Brachial Plexus Anesthesia [German]. Zentralbl. f. Chir. 56: 1995-1996, 1929.

Bazy, L.: In Pauchet, V., Sourdat, P. and Labouré, J.: Regional Anesthesia, 2nd Ed., [French]. Doin, Paris, 1917.

Bazy, L. and Blondin, S.: Anesthesia of the Brachial Plexus [French]. Anesth. & Analg. 1: 190-198, (April) 1935.

Hilse, A.: Brachial Plexus Anesthesia [German]. Zentralbl. f. Chir. 56: 1348-1349, (June 1) 1929.

Kim, M. H.: Anesthesia of the Brachial Plexus via the Infraclavicular Groove [German]. Zentralbl. f. Chir. 55: 1423, (June 9) 1928.

Raj, P. P., Montgomery, S. J., Nettles, D., Jenkins M. T.: Infraclavicular Brachial Plexus Block – A New Approach. Anesth. & Analg. 52: 897-904, 1973.

Sims, J. K.: A Modification of Landmarks for Infraclavicular Approach to Brachial Plexus Block. Anesth. & Analg. 56: 554-555, 1977.

Whiffler, K.: Coracoid Block – A Safe and Easy Technique. British Journal of Anaesthesia 53: 845-848, 1981.

III. The Perivascular Techniques of Brachial Plexus Block

"Sooner or later some one will make a sufficiently close examination of the anatomy involved... so that an exact technique will be developed."   **Lundy**

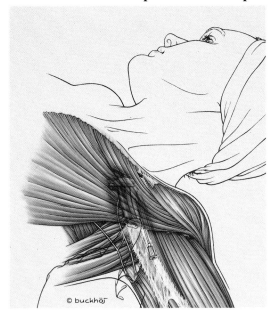

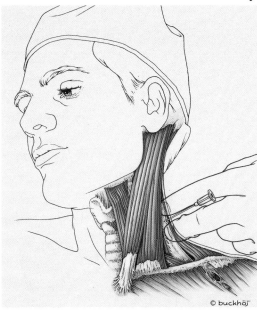

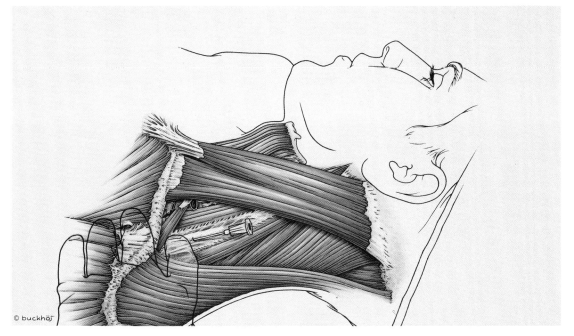

117

Clinical application of the anatomical concept of a continuous perineural and perivascular space surrounding the brachial plexus from roots to terminal nerves simplifies conduction anesthesia of the upper extremity and unites the several schools of brachial plexus block into a single school, that of perivascular (interfascial) plexus anesthesia. The continuity of this space was challenged briefly by Mathews, who, on the basis of roentgenographic studies using radiopaque dye in cadavers, felt that the supra- and infraclavicular portions of the space were separated by the coracoclavicular fascia. This hypothesis has been refuted by the author, both by roentgenographic studies using radiopaque dye in *living* subjects and by repeated clinical demonstration that high brachial and even cervical plexus anesthesia may be produced by injecting large volumes of anesthetic solution into the axillary sheath. Actually, this issue should never have become controversial, for it was stated almost as an axiom in the textbooks of surgery written in the "preantibiotic" era that a collection of pus under the prevertebral fascia would extend down this fascial tube and appear as a swelling on the medial aspect of the upper arm (the lateral wall of the axilla) along the course of the artery.

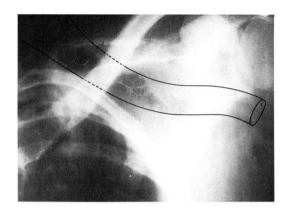

Interesting additional evidence is offered by an x-ray taken in a drugaddict who had run out of veins and injected his brachial artery with heroin. The perivascular tissues became infected with gasforming organisms, and this produced a "pneumogram" of the perivascular compartment.

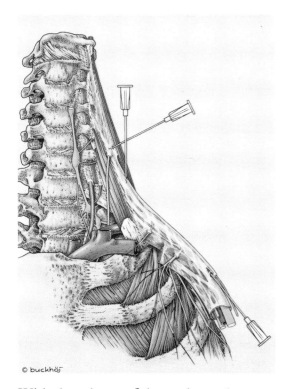

© buckhöj

With the advent of the perivascular concept, as stated earlier, brachial plexus anesthesia may be likened to peridural anesthesia, with the axillary technique of brachial plexus block being analogous to a caudal block, the subclavian perivascular technique being analogous to a lumbar epidural block, and the interscalene technique being analogous to a thoracic epidural block.

In other words, just as with peridural techniques, once the space surrounding the nerves has been entered, only a single injection is necessary, and the extent of anesthesia that results will depend upon the volume of local anesthetic utilized and the level at which it is injected. An advantage of the perivascular techniques of brachial plexus anesthesia over peridural techniques results from the fact that the perivascular space is surrounded throughout its course by soft tissue,

whereas the peridural compartment is encased in bone. The perivascular compartment can be deformed by extrinsic pressure to facilitate the flow and distribution of local anesthetics injected therein, whereas this is impossible with peridural techniques. As will be seen later on, properly applied digital pressure, variations in the needle direction, position of the arm, and even, to a lesser degree, the size of the patient, all can have a significant effect on the level of anesthesia resulting from a given volume of local anesthetic.

Axillary Perivascular Technique of Brachial Plexus Block

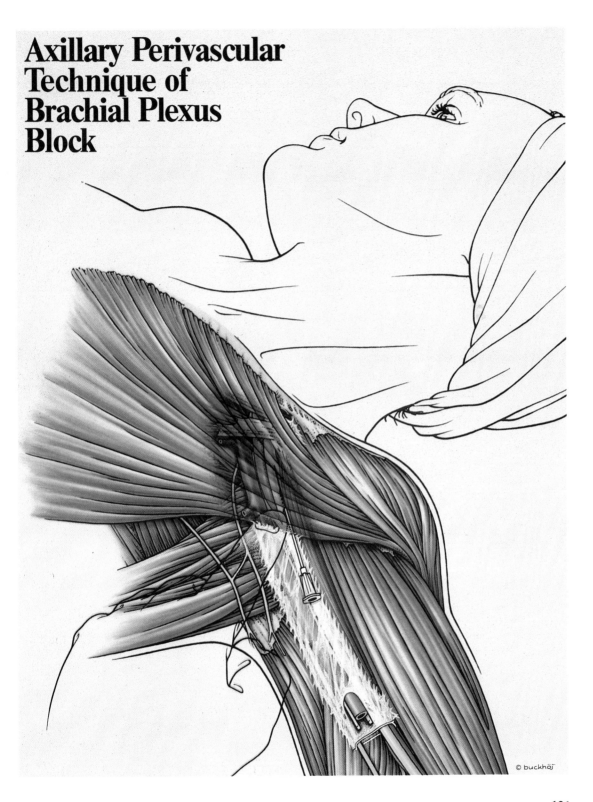

© buckhöj

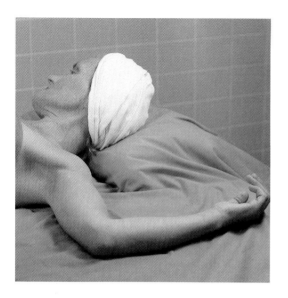 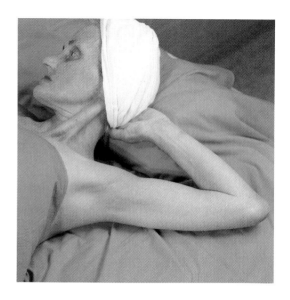

"Axillary block" is probably the most widely used technique of brachial plexus block in use today, most likely because the area in which the block is carried out is far removed from the dome of the lung and the phrenic nerve, so at the very least the likelihood of pulmonary complications is minimal. Furthermore, there are certainly more modifications and technical variations of axillary block than are associated with any other technique. And while some of these "tricks of the trade" can greatly enhance the effectiveness and extent of the anesthesia provided by axillary blocks, some actually decrease the effectiveness of the block.

The author carries out the axillary perivascular technique of brachial plexus block on the left as follows: the patient should be placed in the supine position with the arm abducted to approximately 90° and the forearm flexed to 90° and externally rotated so that the dorsum of the hand lies on the table and the forearm is parallel to the long axis of the patient's body.

It is tempting to both the patient and the anesthetist to have the patient's hand placed under the head. However, such a position actually makes performance of the technique more difficult, since the first step in carrying out an axillary block is identification of the axillary pulse, and it has been shown conclusively by Wright that hyperabduction of the arm will obliterate the brachial artery pulse in 83% of *normal* individuals.

This results from the fact that when the arm is hyperabducted there is stretching, torsion, and pinching of the subclavian-axillary vessels and of the plexus at three points: at the point where the subclavian vessels and the trunks of the plexus pass between the clavicle and the first rib; at the point where the axillary vessels and the cords pass around the tenderness attachment of the pectoralis minor muscle to the coracoid process; and at the point where they move around the head of the hyperabducted humerus. Obviously, then, hyperabduction should be avoided, since it makes identification of the pulse more difficult. As a matter of fact, in very muscular individuals if the degree of abduction of the arm is reduced to somewhat *less than* 90°, identification of the arterial pulse, occasionally difficult in these individuals, will be much easier.

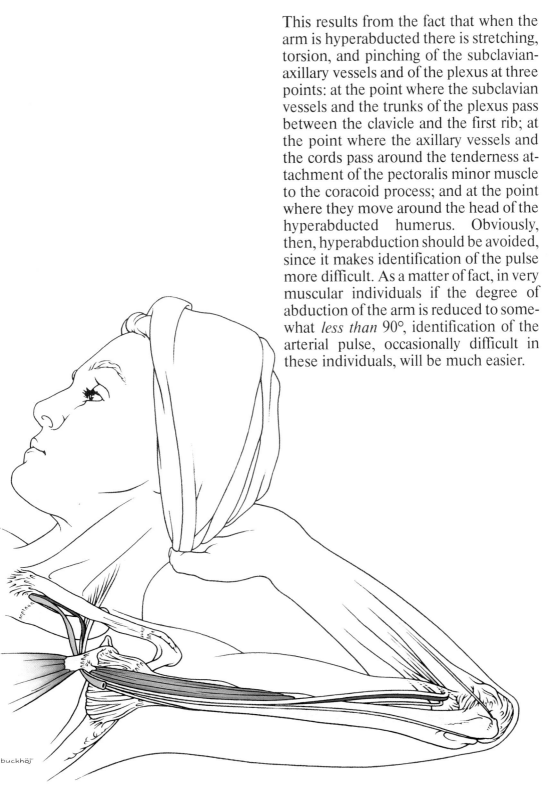

© buckhöj

123

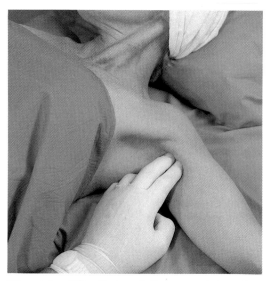

The identification of the arterial pulse should be carried out wherever the pulse is easiest to palpate. This may be at the level of the brachial artery in the upper arm, or it may be more proximal at the level of the axillary artery in the axilla.

In either case, having identified the artery, the pulse should be followed as far proximally as possible, ideally to the point where the pulse disappears under the pectoralis major muscle.

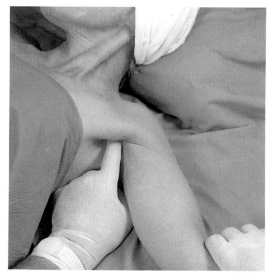

Again, it may be advantageous to have an assistant reduce the degree of abduction of the arm slightly to relax the pectoral muscles and allow palpation to proceed even further proximally. As will be seen later, this is important because if the needle can be inserted high enough in the axilla, the injection will be made above the level of the humeral head, which tends to obstruct the flow of anesthetic solution injected below it.

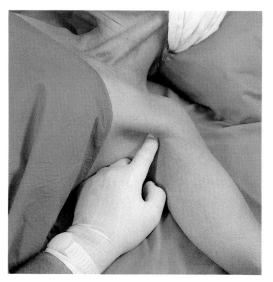

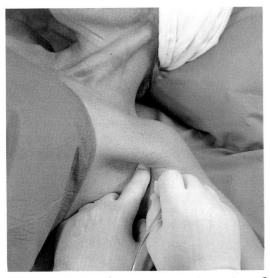

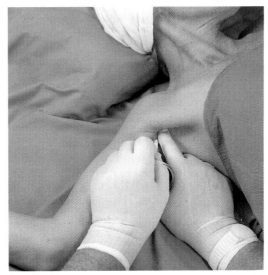

With the index finger still on the pulse of the axillary artery, a 1-1½ inch, 22-gauge, short bevel needle is inserted just superior to the finger tip, directing the needle toward the apex of the axilla so that the needle will be travelling in *almost* the same direction as the neurovascular bundle as it is advanced.

When performing a right axillary block, the same steps are followed but palpation is best carried out with the index finger of the right hand, using the left hand to manipulate the needle.

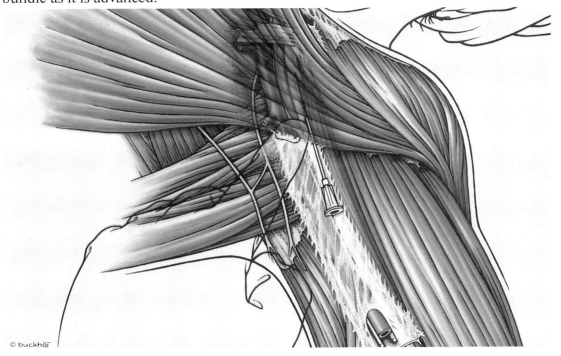

© buckhöj

The needle is advanced slowly, approaching the neurovascular bundle at a 10 to 20° angle, until one of three end-points indicates that the tip of the needle lies with the axillary perivascular space. (1) If a short bevel (45° angle) needle is utilized, *usually* a "fascial click" will be felt by the anesthetist as the tip of the needle penetrates the tough axillary sheath. If the anesthetist utilizes a conventional "A" bevel (17° angle) needle, there will be no audible "click", since this type of needle has a "cutting point" and incises the sheath with no click. The so-called "B" bevel needle, in common use today, the bevel of which is intermediate between a type "A" needle and a "true short bevel needle", will produce a "fascial click", but it takes more experience to appreciate the sound with this needle than with the short bevel needle. However, a "B" bevel needle is still far better in this respect than an "A" bevel needle. Furthermore, studies carried out by Selander in Sweden indicate that an added benefit of the short bevel needle is a significant reduction in the incidence of neural damage when a nerve is penetrated by this needle.

(2) The needle is advanced slowly until a paresthesia in the distribution of one of the nerves that lies within the sheath at this level indicates that the tip of the needle has encountered a nerve and hence lies in the axillary perivascular compartment. Some anesthetists insist on a paresthesia as an indication of sheath penetration, but recent studies carried out by Selander seem to indicate that this practice may carry an increased incidence of post-anesthetic neuropathy, and if so, the production of paresthesias probably should be avoided if possible. However, these same studies also indicated that even when an anesthetist attempts to carry out an axillary block *without* producing paresthesias, he will inadvertently encounter a nerve and produce a paresthesia 40% of the time. Clearly, even when paresthesias are not sought, if they are produced, the sheath has been penetrated, so the needle should be immobilized and the anesthetic injected. However, the practice of deliberately producing paresthesias of *more* than one nerve not only is unnecessary, but should be abandoned, since it may be associated with an even greater incidence of post-injection neuropathy.

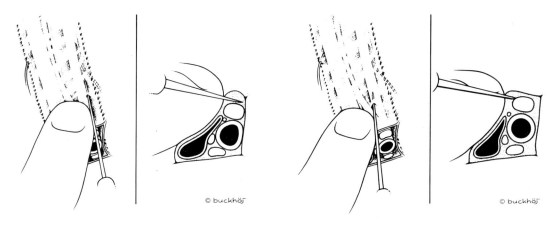

© buckhöj

(3) If bright red blood appears within the hub of the needle, the artery has been entered. When this occurs, the anesthetist should not withdraw the needle but he should advance it as quickly as possible through the posterior wall of the vessel, and inject the contents of the syringe. Advocates of the so-called "trans-arterial technique" immobilize the axillary artery between their index and middle fingers and *deliberately* penetrate both walls of the artery. They believe that penetration of the artery is the most certain and reproducible sign of entry into the axillary perivascular compartment. If this technique is utilized, whether intentionally or inadvertently, after penetration of the posterior wall of the artery, the entire volume of local anesthetic should be injected.

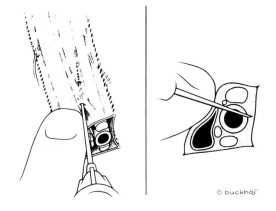

© buckhöj

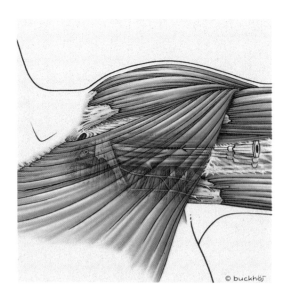

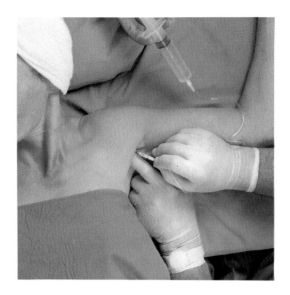

According to the technique of the author, when the axillary sheath has been penetrated, the tip of the needle should lie superiorly tangential to the arterial wall 1 to 1½ inches proximal to the most proximal palpable point of pulsation and probably proximal to the humeral head. If properly placed, the needle will clearly pulsate, a sign that *corroborates* proper placement of the needle but cannot be accepted as definitive.

Following aspiration in several quadrants, 20 to 40 ml of local anesthetic are injected, the actual volume depending on the patient's size, sex, and age and the desired level of anesthesia. Throughout the injection repeated aspiration for blood should be carried out intermittently.

Furthermore, firm digital pressure should be applied directly behind the needle during and immediately after the injection to prevent retrograde flow down the sheath.

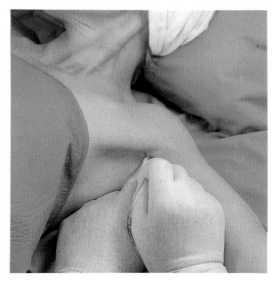

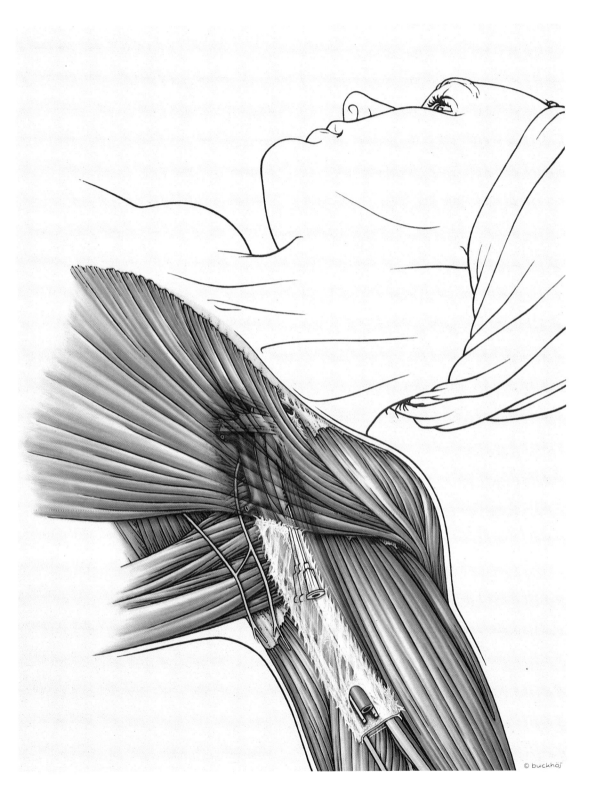

© buckhöj

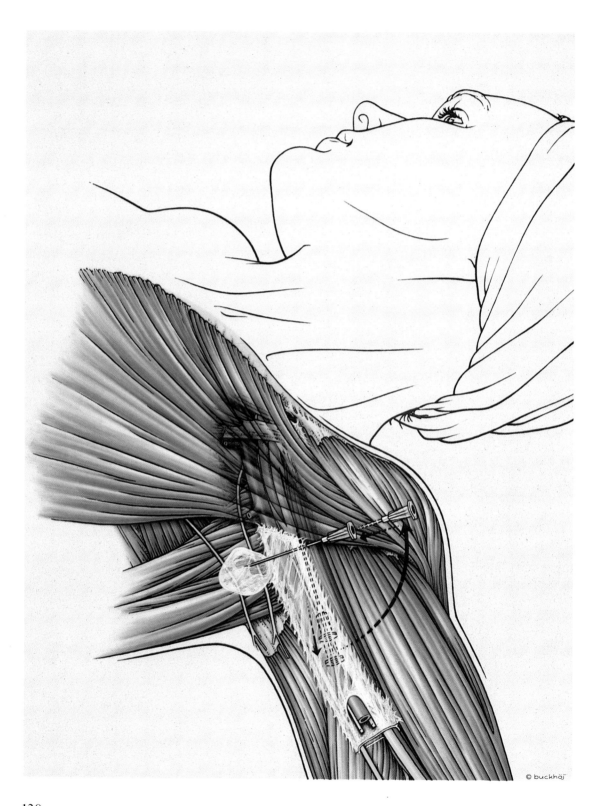

© buckhöj

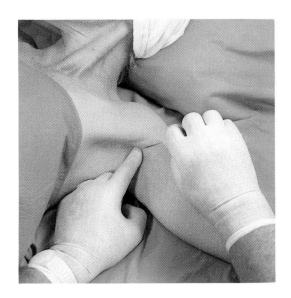 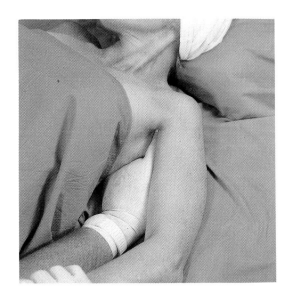

When the injection of the appropriate volume of local anesthetic has been completed, the needle is withdrawn until it lies in the subcutaneous tissue directly over the artery. At this point 3 to 5 ml of local anesthetic (which is usually the volume remaining in the tubing of an "immobile needle") are deposited, and this will effectively block the intercostobrachial nerve and the medial brachial cutaneous nerve, if it lies outside the sheath. Care should be taken not to withdraw the needle from the skin after blocking T_2, since to the patient this would require a "second stick", whereas injection of local anesthetic as the needle is withdrawn to a subcutaneous level is not considered to represent a "separate injection". Also, after withdrawing the needle to the level of the subcutaneous tissue, it is wise to change the direction so that inadvertent advancement of the needle during injection will not result in an intravascular injection.

As soon as the subcutaneous injection has been made, the needle should be quickly withdrawn and digital pressure maintained as the arm is brought down to the patient's side, a maneuver that removes the obstruction to central flow provided by the humeral head when the arm is abducted, as illustrated in the next section.

Axillary Perivascular Volume: Anesthesia Relationships

The relationship between the volume of anesthetic injected into the perivascular space and the extent of anesthesia it produces has been elucidated by the author by using local anesthetic solutions mixed with radiopaque dye. This tecnique allows us to compare x-rays showing a given volume of injected anesthetic with the level of anesthesia resulting from that injection.

20 ml injection

When 20 ml of radiopaque anesthetic solution are injected into the axillary sheath of an adult *without digital pressure,* it will not *consistently* reach the level of the cords of the plexus, a level indicated on x-ray by the coracoid process. Thus, with this volume the musculocutaneous and axillary nerves may *not* be blocked, and, as a result, sensation over the lateral aspect of the forearm and upper arm will remain intact and the powerful flexors of the forearm may remain active.

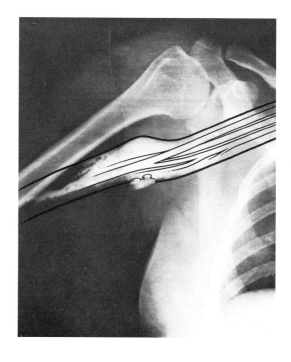

Anesthesia following the injection of such a low volume into the sheath will be adequate for hand surgery, but it must be remembered that the anesthetist cannot guarantee the surgeon a quiet field, since the block has not impaired the patient's ability to flex the forearm. This could be an important consideration in an un-cooperative or inebriated patient, who may move his arm, deliberately or inadvertently, during a surgical procedure and provide impossible working conditions for the surgeon.

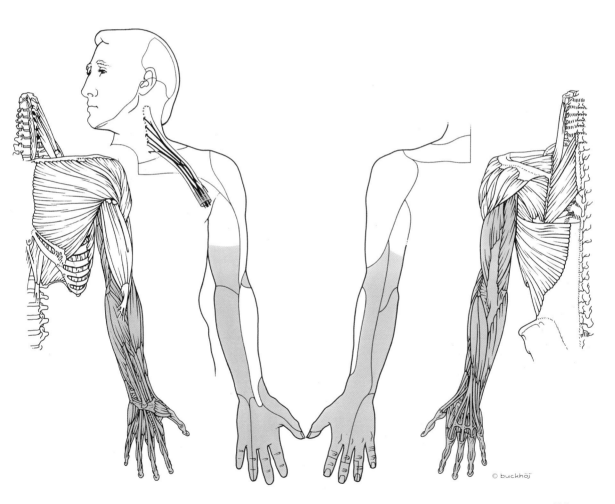

© buckhöj

40 ml injection

If the volume of anesthetic injected is increased to 40 ml, the most cephalad portion of the solution may be seen to reach the level of the first rib, and thus will ensure a complete sensory and motor block of the entire upper extremity. As mentioned earlier, by injecting even larger volumes (60 ml) into the axillary sheath (not shown here), the anesthetic can even be forced up into the cervical portion of the interscalene space and can therefore provide cervical as well as brachial plexus anesthesia. However, this technique is not recommended in clinical practice because of the inordinately large volumes of local anesthetic agents required.

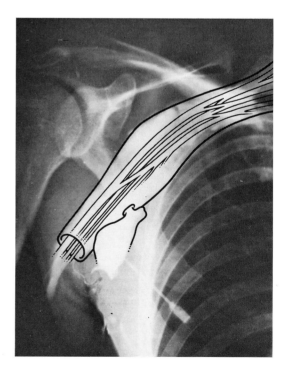

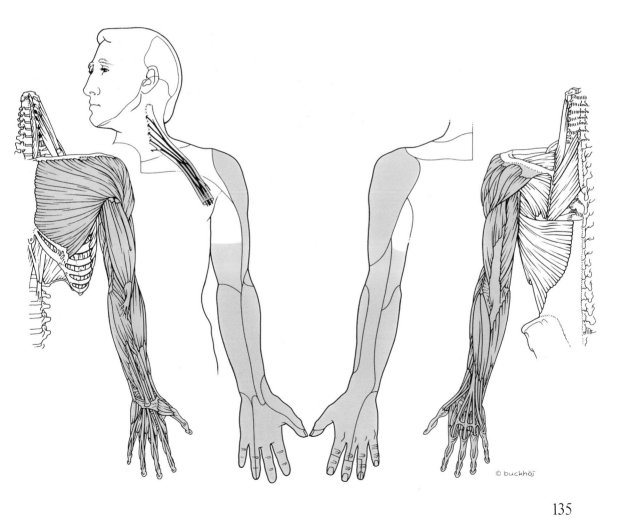

© buckhöj

135

Factors Influencing Axillary Perivascular Volume: Anesthesia Relationships

Most of the modifications of the axillary perivascular block technique have been introduced in an effort to promote the spread of the injected anesthetic solutions centrally and prevent their spread distally, but the efficacy of the various techniques advocated for doing this were never documented. In studies carried out recently by the author and his co-workers, two sequential 20 ml injections of a mixture of local anesthetic and radiopaque dye were made into the axillary sheaths of a series of healthy, adult, male patients to compare the influence of the level of needle insertion and injection and the direction of injection in promoting cephalad flow and to compare the efficacy of a tourniquet with that of digital pressure in preventing retrograde flow of the injected local anesthetic solution.

Level and direction of injection

As described in chapter II, Eriksson was one of the first to make a single injection into the axillary perivascular sheath. However, he advocated inserting the needle perpendicular to the axis of the neurovascular bundle and out in the distal axilla. In contrast to this, the author had always advocated inserting a single needle as high as possible in the axilla and as close to the same axis as that of the neurovascular bundle as possible. There were several reasons for advocating this level and direction of injection: first of all, inserting the needle as high as possible in the axilla and directing it cephalad placed the tip of the needle more than an inch

and a half (the length of the needle) closer to the level at which the musculocutaneous and axillary nerves leave the sheath.

Furthermore, since the direction of the needle was the same (or nearly the same) as the neurovascular bundle, then the thrust of the injected solution *should* tend to favor central spread and minimize distal or retrograde spread.

The first study was undertaken to determine the importance of the *level* and *direction* of the injection. The first pair of x-rays represent sequential injections of 20 and 40 ml at right angles to the neurovascular bundle at the level of insertion of the pectoralis major and latissimus dorsi muscles (Eriksson's technique).

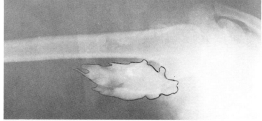

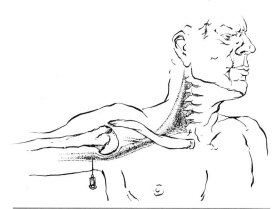

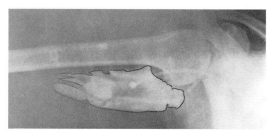

The level of injection is visible as the white dot (the hub) at the approximate midpoint of the radiopaque dye. It may be seen that while the solution injected in this manner moves both centrally and peripherally, proximal spread has been almost completely stopped by the head of the abducted humerus and, in fact, the extent of the distal spread exceeds the extent of the central spread considerably.

Contrast these x-rays with the next pair of x-rays taken after similar injections of 20 and 40 ml of radiopaque solution injected as high as possible in the axilla, the injection being made this time in a central direction.

It is evident that while there is some retrograde flow with this technique, too, the extent of central spread of the solution is much greater than the extent of peripheral spread. Furthermore, the most central portion of the solution not only has passed around the humeral head, it is actually medial to the coracoid process, the approximate level at which the musculocutaneous and axillary nerves leave the axillary sheath. Thus an additional reason for placing the needle as high as possible in the axilla and injecting in a central rather than perpendicular direction is to make the injection above the head of the abducted humerus, so that the latter cannot interfere with the central flow of the injected solution. Clearly, the preferable *level* of injection is as high as possible in the axilla and the preferable *direction* of injection is central.

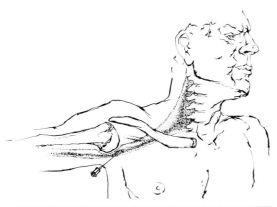

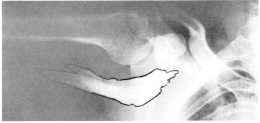

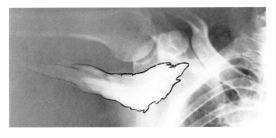

Tourniquet and digital pressure

In an attempt to minimize the required volume of local anesthetic solution, Eriksson and Skarby introduced the practice of placing a tourniquet tightly around the arm distal to the injection site assuming that the tourniquet would compress the axillary sheath and inhibit retrograde flow of local anesthetic.

As a means of documenting the efficacy of the tourniquet, Eriksson injected a mixture of local anesthetic and radiopaque dye into the axillary sheath, utilizing his technique, and he felt that the failure of the dye to reach and/or pass dis-

tal to the tourniquet indicated that the tourniquet did, indeed, prevent retrograde flow.

Actually, Eriksson utilized too small a volume to test the tourniquet's ability to prevent retrograde flow: because he injected only 10 ml of dye, the tourniquet *appeared* to be preventing retrograde flow, even though about one third of the injected volume moved distally toward the tourniquet. In reality this volume was simply not sufficient to reach the tourniquet and test its efficacy in preventing further retrograde flow.

Therefore, the author and his co-workers made two sequential 20 ml injections of local anesthetic mixed with radiopaque dye, according to the technique of Eriksson, i.e., with a tourniquet applied distally around the arm as close to the injection site as possible.

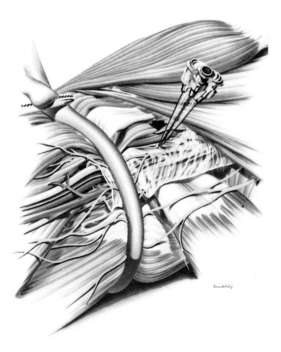

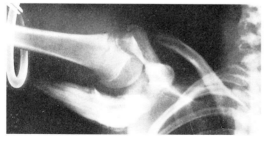

This pair of x-rays taken after these injections shows that, again, with the smaller volume the tourniquet *appears* to decrease the amount of solution that flows distally from the injection site, but as the volume increases, much of the dye passes through the barrier provided by the constricting tourniquet, without the tourniquet even making an indentation on the column of dye. In addition, it is apparent that even with the tourniquet applied, the dye is not able to ascend in the sheath beyond the obstruction provided by the humeral head.

Contrast these x-rays with the next pair of x-rays taken after two sequential 20 ml injections according to the technique of the author, that is, through a centrally directed needle placed as high in the axilla as possible, and with firm digital pressure applied immediately distal to the injection site.

Clearly, the digital pressure effectively prevents *any* significant retrograde flow whatsoever, and furthermore, the point of maximal central flow is medial to the head of the humerus and even medial to the level of the coracoid process, the level at which the musculocutaneous and axillary nerves leave the sheath.

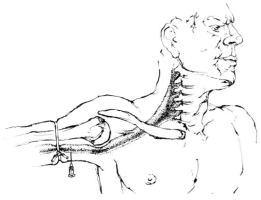

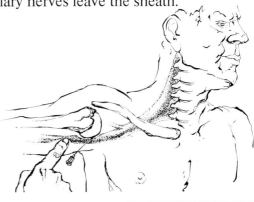

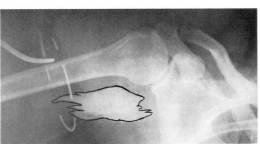

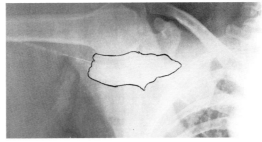

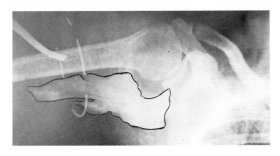

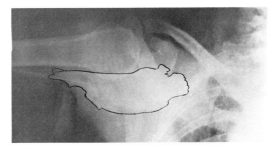

Position of the arm

From the foregoing studies it is apparent that the humeral head *may* significantly obstruct cephalad spread of injected local anesthetic. To test the efficacy of lowering the arm after the injection to remove this obstruction an additional x-ray was taken after the completion of two sequential 20 ml injections as in the previous pair of x-rays except that after the injection the arm was brought down to the side while digital pressure was continued.

It is obvious from this figure that lowering the arm to the side upon completion of the axillary block while maintaining firm digital pressure in the axilla *does* significantly enhance central flow of the injected solution by removing the barrier provided by the head of the abducted humerus.

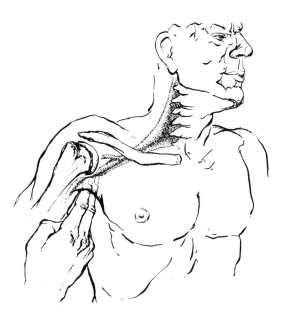

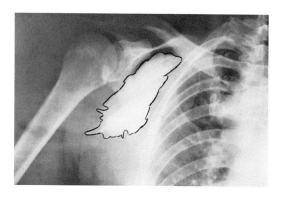

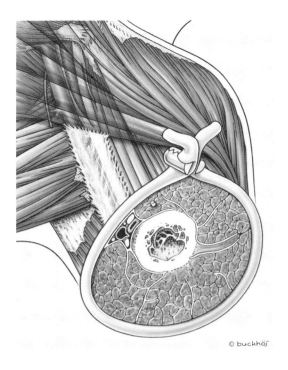

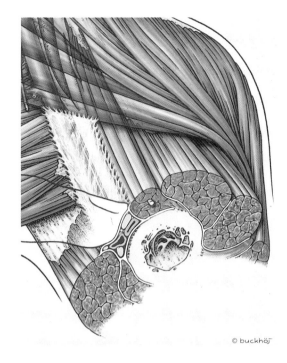

© buckhöj

© buckhöj

Conclusion

It would appear from these studies that digital pressure is preferable to a rubber tourniquet in preventing retrograde flow, undoubtedly because of two anatomical factors: (1) because of the bulky mass of the deltoid muscle, a tourniquet cannot be placed close enough to the site of injection to inhibit some retrograde flow, even if the tourniquet *were* effective in compressing the neurovascular bundle; and (2) because the neurovascular bundle is deeply situated in the groove between the coracobrachialis muscle and the long head of the triceps muscle, these two muscles actually protect the neurovascular bundle from the compressive force of the tourniquet.

However, when digital pressure is utilized distal to the needle to prevent retrograde flow, the compressing finger fits readily between these two muscles and completely occludes the perivascular space.

Lastly, these studies indicate that even if the injection is carried out through a needle directed centrally along the main axis of the neurovascular bundle, *if* it cannot be placed high enough in the axilla, the humeral head still *may* interfere with central spread of the local anesthetic. Therefore, following completion of the injection into the axillary sheath, and deposition of a small amount of local anesthetic subcutaneously to block the intercostobrachial nerve superficial to the sheath, bringing the arm down to the side while maintaining firm digital pressure will remove the obstruction to flow provided by the humeral head and will allow the anesthetic solution to reach a higher level with any given volume.

Low Volume Axillary Perivascular Technique

In certain patients who are critically ill, particularly those with cardiovascular disease, it may be necessary to use a low volume technique in order to minimize the number of milligrams of local anesthetic that will be absorbed systemically. Since the large volume utilized in an axillary block is *usually* necessary to assure blockade of the musculocutaneous nerve, a much smaller volume can be injected into the sheath if the musculocutaneous nerve is blocked separately. If this is the desired technique, then the axillary block is carried out as indicated before, but utilizing 10-15 ml injected into the sheath, with firm digital pressure just behind the needle.

After the injection into the axillary sheath is complete, the needle is withdrawn until the tip lies in the subcutaneous tissue; and then, with the finger still on the artery, the needle is redirected into the substance of the coracobrachialis muscle, just superior to the axillary artery and sheath, and 5-7 ml of local anesthetic are injected. It is not necessary to obtain a paresthesia of the musculocutaneous nerve, since the coracobrachialis muscle is a small muscle, and its fascia will confine the injected local anesthetic to the area of the nerve, facilitating the onset of anesthesia. The needle should then be withdrawn to the subcutaneous tissue again and several ml's injected superficial to the axillary artery in order to block the intercostobrachial and medial brachial cutaneous nerves. With this low volume axillary perivascular technique a total of 20-25 ml are utilized for the entire anesthetic procedure.

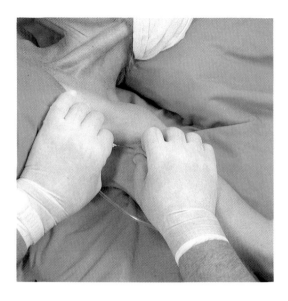

Of course, with this technique as with any other, T_2 must also be blocked if the tourniquet is to be utilized by the surgeon. Therefore, after completing the above two injections but *before* withdrawing the needle completely, the needle is redirected so as to deposit a few ml of local anesthetic superficial to the artery pulse.

An alternative is that of de Jong described in the preceeding chapter, but it must be remembered that with that technique only a sensory block of the musculocutaneous nerve will result, so a silent surgical field can not be guaranteed.

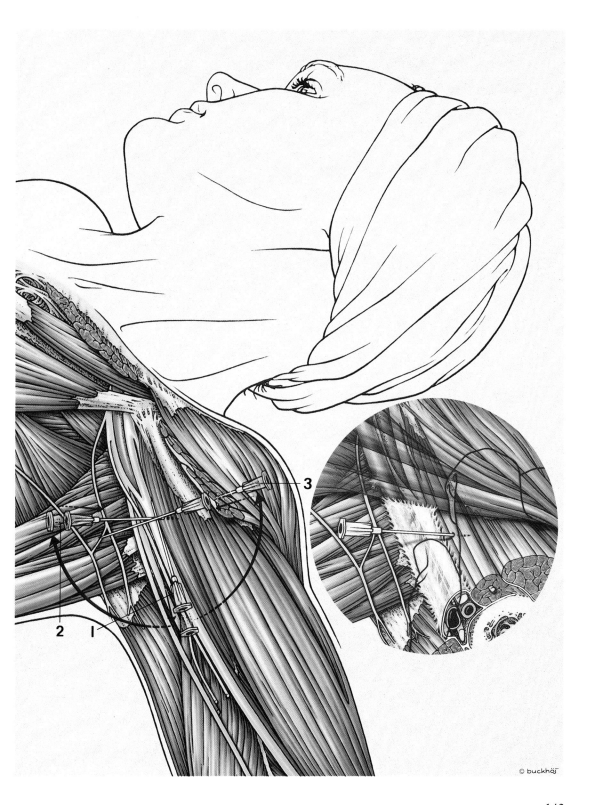

© buckhöj

143

Subclavian Perivascular Technique of Brachial Plexus Block

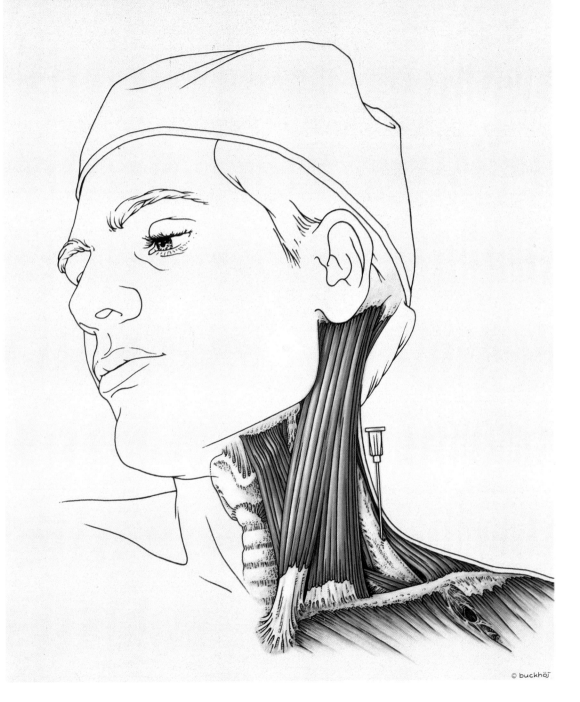

© buckhöj

The author carries out the subclavian perivascular technique of brachial plexus block on the left as follows: the patient is placed in the dorsal recumbent position with the head turned somewhat to the side opposite that to be injected. The head should not be turned too far to the opposite side, or the muscles to be palpated will be taut and more difficult to feel with the palpating finger. It may be convenient to tell the patient "to reach for his knee" to lower the clavicle, but if this maneuver is utilized, it is important that the patient then completely *relax* the arm and shoulder, again, so that the scalene muscles are relaxed and easily palpable.

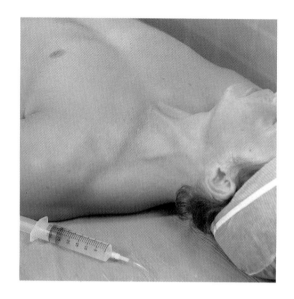

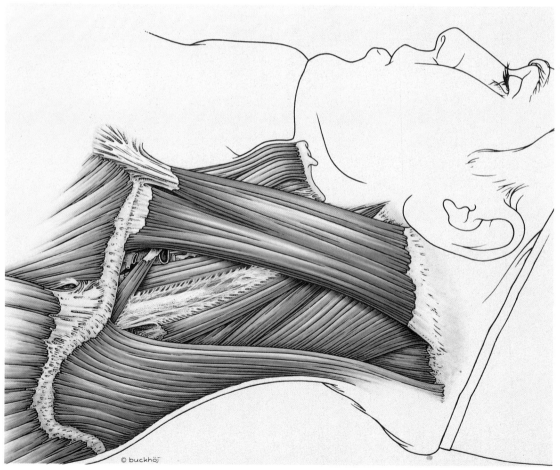

© buckhöj

The patient is asked to lift his head off the table slightly, in order to bring the *clavicular* head of the sternocleidomastoid muscle into prominence. In some patients only the sternal head is prominent, but even in such a patient, though the clavicular head may not be *visible,* it is almost invariably palpable.

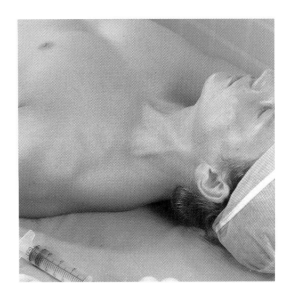

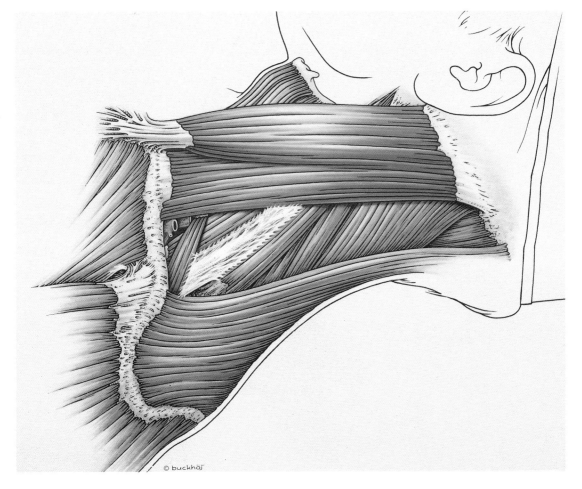

© buckhöj

The index finger is placed immediately behind (posterior to) the lateral border of the sternocleidomastoid muscle at the level of C_6, which is determined by dropping a line laterally from the cricoid cartilage.

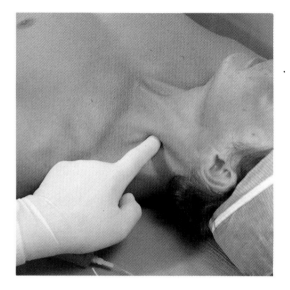

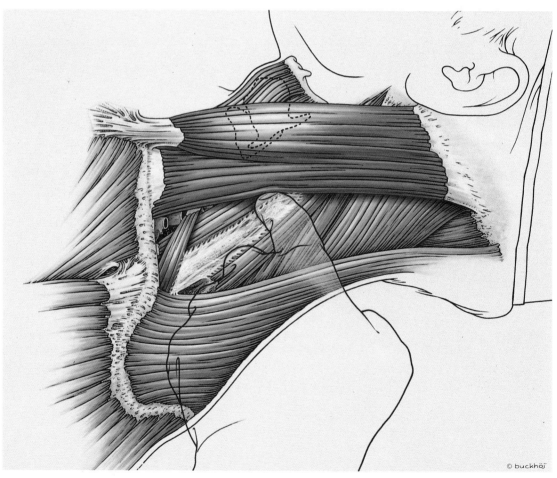

© buckhöj

Now, when the patient puts his head back on the table (and he must be *told* to do so) and the taut sternocleidomastoid muscle relaxes, the palpating finger actually moves medially and the fingernail on the palpating finger almost disappears behind the sternocleidomastoid muscle.

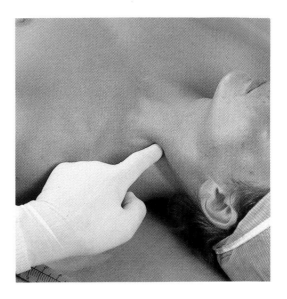

The index finger now lies on the belly of the anterior scalene muscle and under the lateral edge of the sternocleidomastoid muscle.

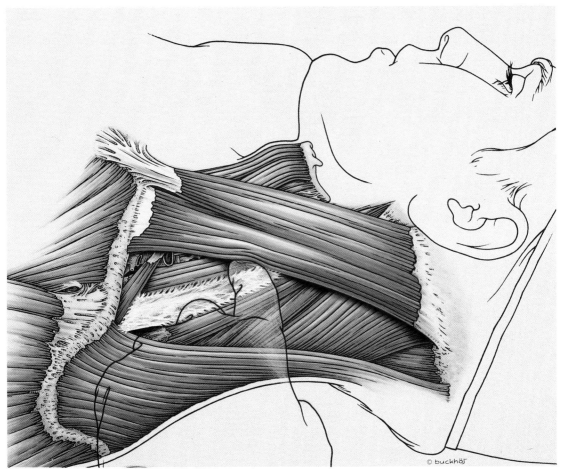

The palpating finger is now rolled laterally across the belly of the anterior scalene
muscle until it encounters the interscalene groove, the groove which separates
the middle and anterior scalene muscles.
It is important that identification of the
interscalene groove be carried out as indicated above at the approximate level of
C_6, since at a point lower than this the
groove may be obscured by the omohyoid muscle, which crosses the groove
in its inferior portion.

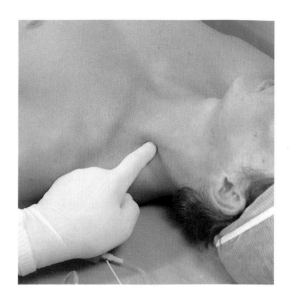

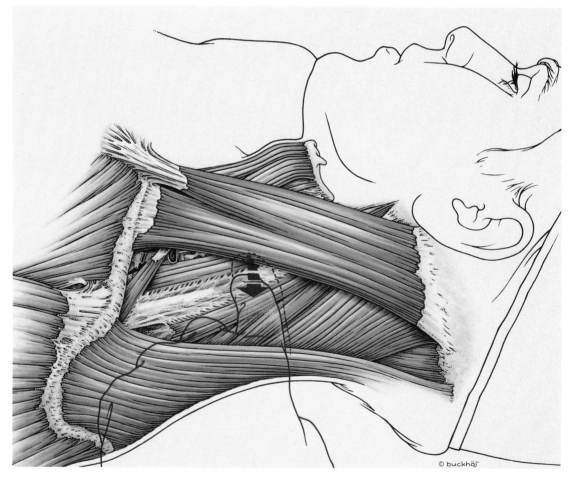

© buckhöj

When the interscalene groove has been identified, the finger is now moved inferiorly along this groove as far as it can *conveniently* be followed. In many cases, the groove can be followed inferiorly to the point where the pulse of the subclavian artery can be palpated as it emerges with the trunks of the plexus from between the anterior and middle scalene muscles.

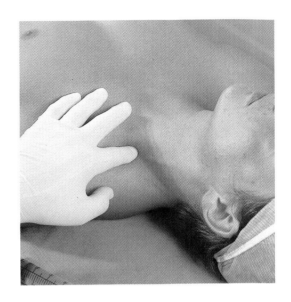

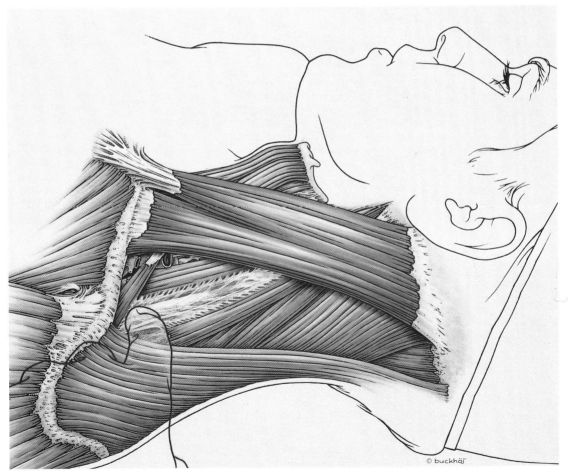

On the other hand, in some patients as the finger is moved inferiorly in the groove, the groove will be obscured by an unusually high omohyoid muscle. In most of these patients, the groove can again be picked up inferior to the omohyoid muscle, though in a few this is impossible. However, it is not critical that the groove is followed as far inferiorly as the artery, since it is just as effective to insert the needle higher in the neck and advance it inferiorly to the desired level of injection.

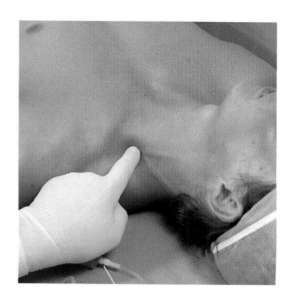

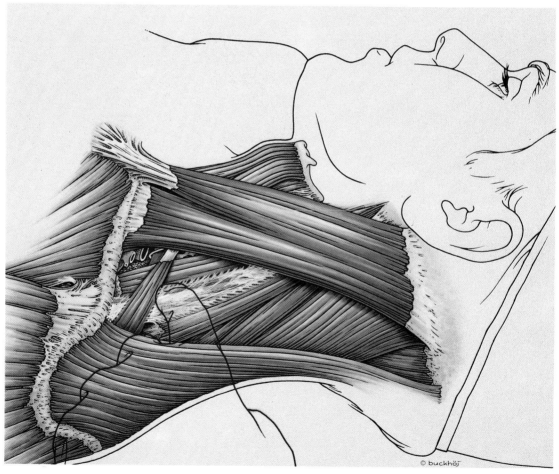

© buckhöj

When the interscalene groove has been identified and the palpating finger has been moved inferiorly along the groove as far as it can be palpated, with the finger still in the groove (and/or on the artery), a 1½ inch, 22-gauge, short-bevel needle should be inserted just above the palpating finger and advanced in a direction that is directly caudad, but not mesiad or dorsad.

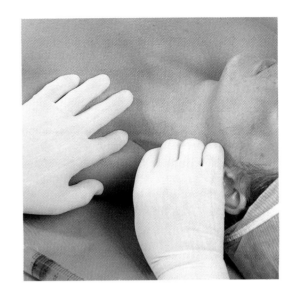

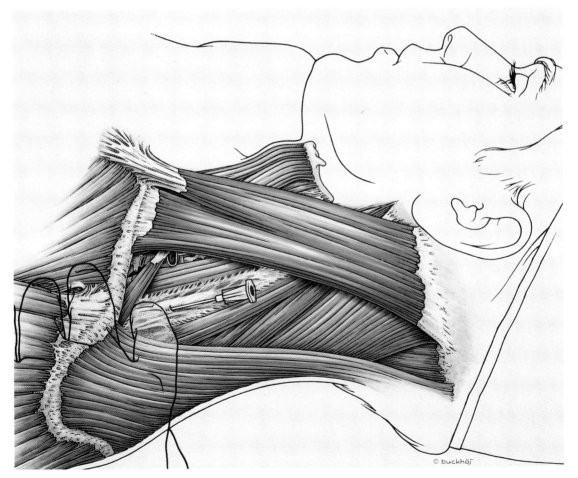

During its insertion and advancement, the hub of the properly directed needle should actually lie against the skin of the neck; so with this technique the needle must be held between the thumb and forefinger or forefingers, since there is no room between the hub of the needle and the neck for the anesthetist to use the traditional "pencil-grip". In carrying out the subclavian perivascular technique of brachial plexus block for surgery on the *left* arm, the anesthetist will find it most convenient to utilize his left index finger for palpation and to hold the needle in his right hand.

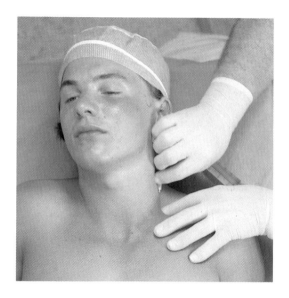

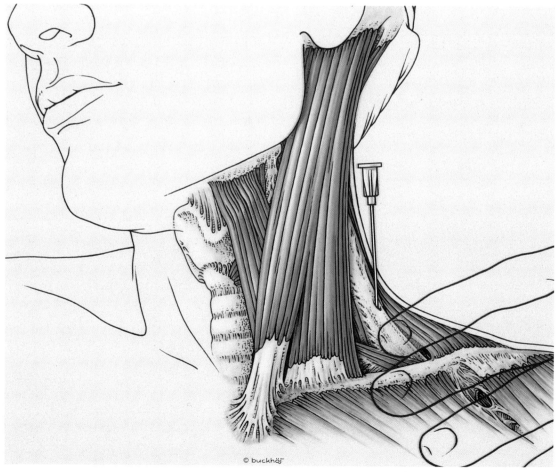

© buckhöj

In carrying out the block for surgery on the *right* extremity, the anesthetist will find it most convenient to utilize his right index finger for palpation and hold the needle in his left hand.

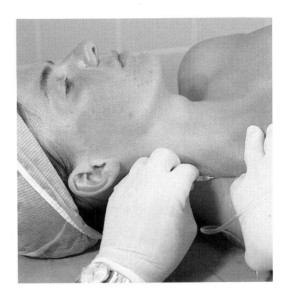

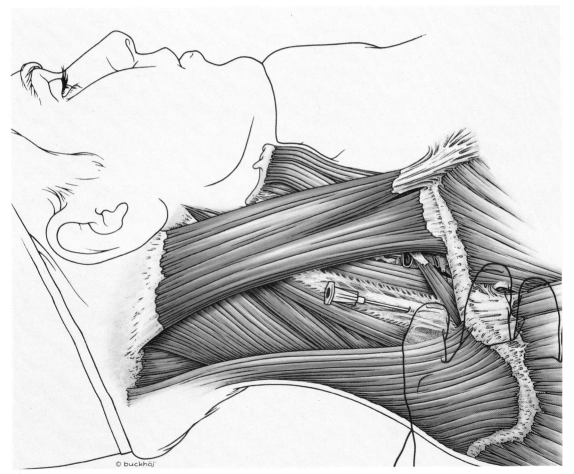

© buckhöj

It is critically important that the needle be advanced in a direction that is directly caudad, since this allows the needle to enter the subclavian perivascular space, the lower one-third of the interscalene space, in its longest dimension. The needle is advanced deep to the palpating finger until a paresthesia below the shoulder confirms the fact that the needle lies within the subclavian perivascular space.

If the needle is advanced slowly, the short bevel of the needle *may* produce a palpable "click" as the needle penetrates the scalene fascia, the "sheath of the brachial plexus", though this "click" is much less pronounced than that felt when a needle penetrates the axillary sheath. Finally, in carrying out this technique, one should remember that the trunks of the brachial plexus lie slightly closer to the middle scalene muscle than to the anterior, so the needle should be inserted slightly closer to the middle than to the anterior scalene muscle.

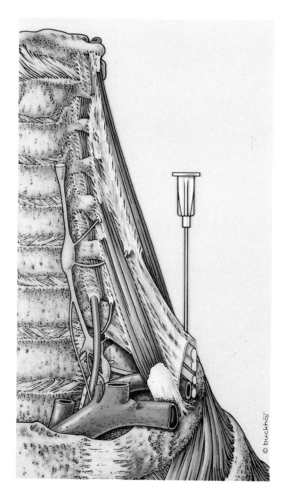

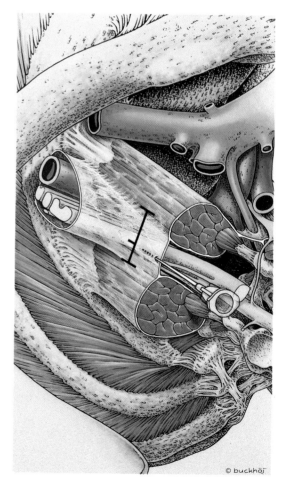

It is important before beginning a sub-clavian perivascular block to instruct the patient to say "stop" when he feels an "electric shock" to the arm and to tell the anesthetist *verbally* (not by pointing) *where* he feels it. The reason this is important is that a paresthesia to the shoulder is unacceptable, since it indicates that the needle has contacted the suprascapular nerve, and it is impossible then to tell whether this nerve has been contacted inside or outside the sheath of the brachial plexus. Therefore only a paresthesia that radiates to any point *below* the shoulder is acceptable.

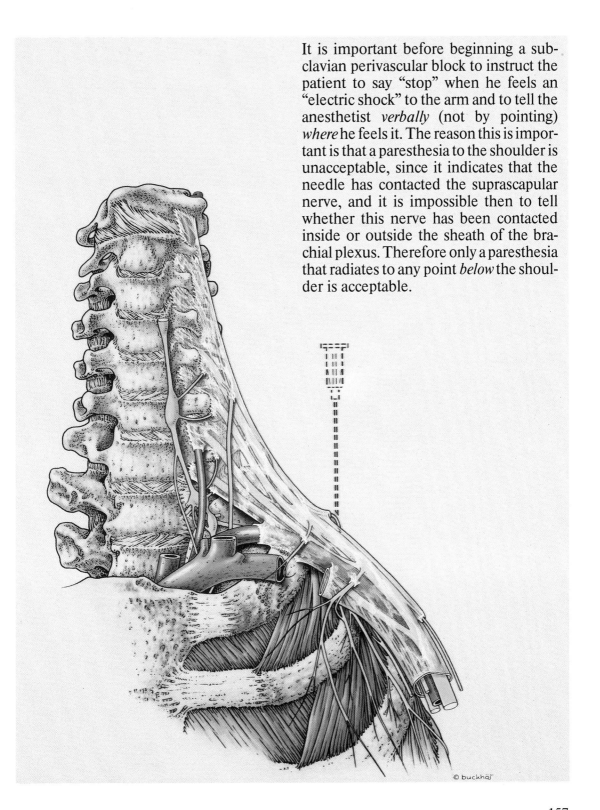

© buckhöj

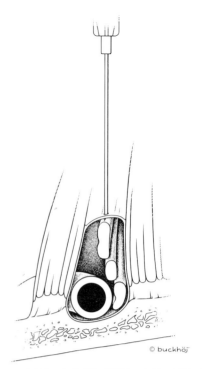

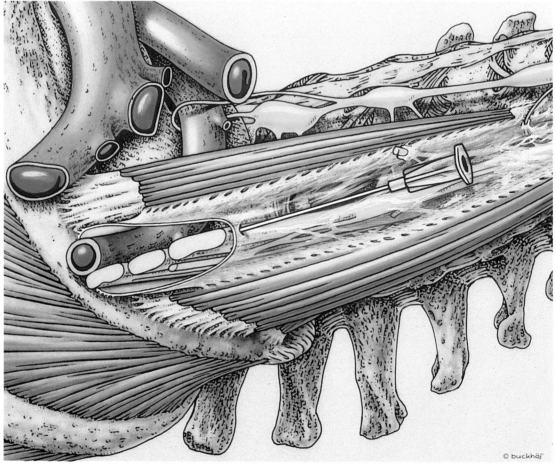

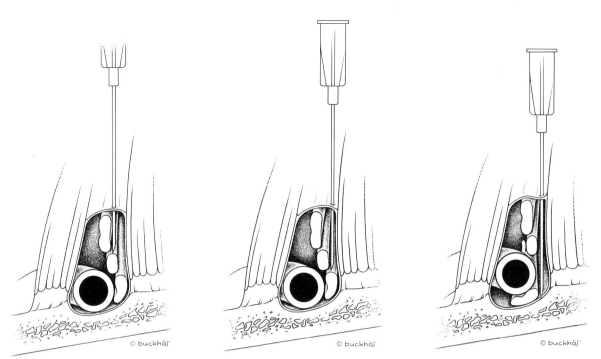

Again, recalling the anatomy at this level, the anesthetist really has three chances to produce a paresthesia as he advances the needle, for if the needle fails to contact the superior trunk, it may hit the middle trunk; if it misses the middle trunk, it may contact the inferior trunk, and of course, if the needle fails to make contact with any of the three trunks, it will "insert" on the first rib with the scalene muscles. So while contact with the first rib is *not* sought with this technique, the rib does provide a "backstop", which will prevent the properly directed needle from further advancement.

If the subclavian artery is penetrated by the advancing needle, it simply indicates that the needle is placed too far anteriorly, so when arterial blood is obtained, the needle should simply be withdrawn to the subcutaneous tissue and reinserted closer to the middle scalene muscle.

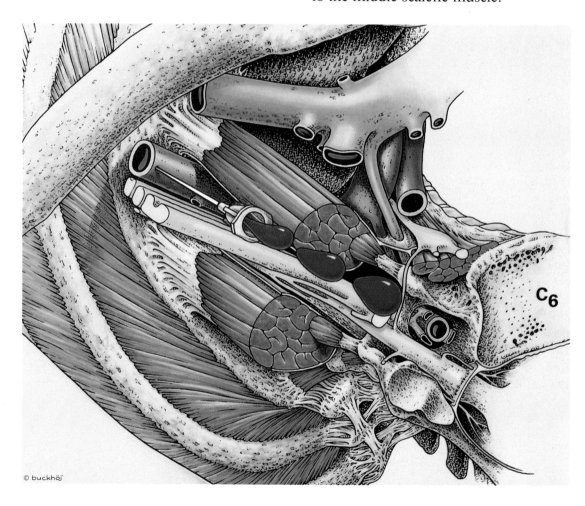

© buckhöj

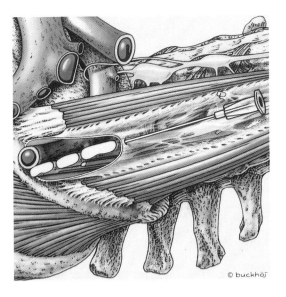

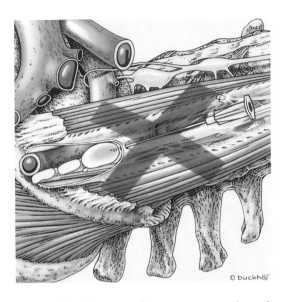

As soon as a paresthesia has been produced and the patient has indicated that it travels beyond the shoulder, the anesthetist attempts to aspirate in four quadrants and then injects 2 or 3 ml of the local anesthetic agent *rapidly*. Usually, this maneuver produces a "pressure paresthesia", a dull aching feeling in the same distribution as the "electrical" paresthesia, offering further proof that the tip of the needle is properly placed. Usually this "pressure paresthesia" elicits a slight grimace or "ooh" from the patient, which is quite different from the agonizing pain produced by an intraneural injection.

Obviously, if the injection of the first few ml's of local anesthetic produces such *severe* pain, it must be assumed that the needle is intraneural, and the injection must not be made without repositioning the needle. The "pressure paresthesia" that is being sought is undoubtedly due to the sudden increase in pressure produced as the solution is forced around the nerve into the subclavian perivascular space, which prior to the injection is simply a potential space. This is not unlike the "aching pain" experienced by a patient when local anesthetic is rapidly injected into the caudal canal. After the "pressure paresthesia" has been produced, the next few ml's of local anesthetic should be injected slowly, simply in an effort to minimize patient discomfort. However, after 8-10 ml of local anesthetic have been injected, the remainder may be injected as rapidly or as slowly as is desirable without producing discomfort to the patient. When the injection is complete and the needle withdrawn, the interscalene groove should be massaged vigoriously in a cephalad-caudad direction to enhance the distribution of the local anesthetic.

With this technique, as with any other, the intercostobrachial and medial brachial cutaneous nerves must be blocked separately by the subcutaneous injection of a few ml's of local anesthetic over the axillary artery pulse if a tourniquet is to be utilized during the surgical procedure.

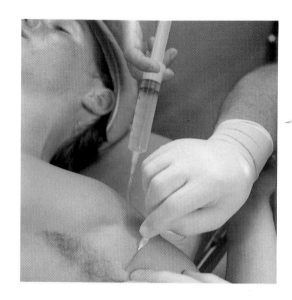

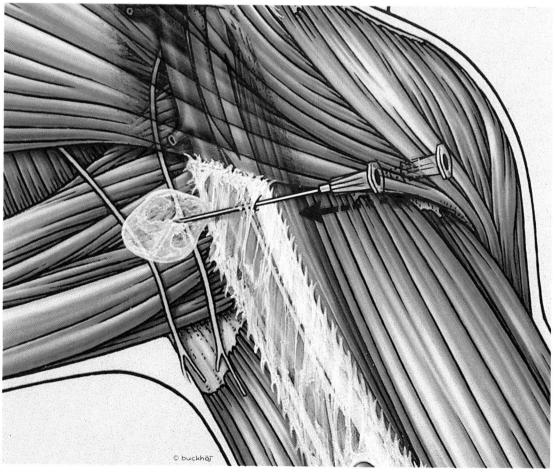

162

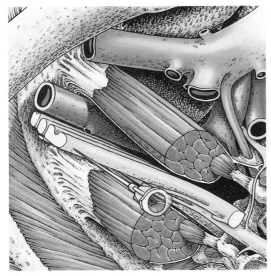

© buckhöj

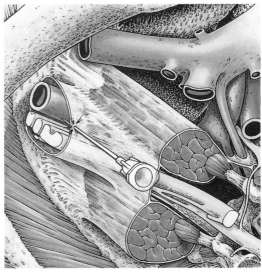

© buckhöj

In comparison with other supraclavicular techniques that attempt to block the brachial plexus by making multiple injections along the top of the first rib, the subclavian perivascular technique of brachial plexus block, because of the direction of needle insertion and advancement, the use of a short needle, and the use of a single injection, not only improves the incidence of satisfactory results but also minimizes the possibility of pneumothorax. Since the direction of needle insertion is parallel to the borders of the scalene muscles and since these muscles always insert on the first rib, the positions of the plexus, the subclavian artery, and the rib are located more precisely than with any other technique, even though with this technique contact with the rib is not sought, and usually paresthesias are obtained before such contact occurs.

It should be emphasized that with this technique, and with any technique carried out above the clavicle, the production of paresthesias is the most accurate indicator that the needle is properly placed within the sheath. The technique *can* be carried out without the production of paresthesias, relying on the perception of a "fascial click" as the needle enters the sheath, but in the hands of the author this has resulted in a 15% decrease in the incidence of success with the technique.

163

Subclavian Perivascular Volume: Anesthesia Relationships

Again, studies carried out by injecting local anesthetic agents mixed with radiopaque dye indicate the volume-anesthesia relationships obtained with this technique. Because the subclavian perivascular technique of brachial plexus block is carried out at a level where the entire plexus is contained in the fewest component parts, a smaller volume of local anesthetic is required than with any other technique.

20 ml injection

20 ml of local anesthetic are injected with this technique, when the entire brachial plexus is blocked and the extent of anesthesia is identical to that resulting from a 40 ml injection into the axillary perivascular space.

However, while the ultimate *extent* of anesthesia produced by the two injections is identical, the *onset* of motor blockade is quite different, due to the difference in the position of the needle with the two techniques: when asked to elevate the arm without bending the elbow 3-5 minutes post-injection, the patient having received the 20 ml subclavian perivascular block will be unable to do so, as the nerves supplying the flexors and abductors of the arm are the first to be bathed with local anesthetic, whereas the patient who has received the 40 ml axillary block *will* be able to elevate his arm, but as it approaches the vertical position, the hand will fall, since the extensors of the

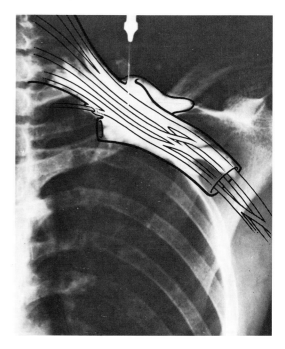

forearm are the first to be bathed with local anesthetic with this technique. In carrying out this test of early blockade with the axillary technique, the anesthetist must protect the patient so that the hand does not strike him in the face when it falls.

While 20 ml are, as indicated above, frequently sufficient to block the entire brachial plexus, if the injection is made fairly high in the subclavian perivascular space, as would be the case when a paresthesia is elicited by contacting the superior (or even middle) trunk, the onset of anesthesia may be delayed or even absent in the distribution of the inferior trunk, especially if that trunk is "trapped" between the subclavian artery and the upper surface of the first rib in the subclavian groove, so a larger volume is preferable, unless it is contraindicated.

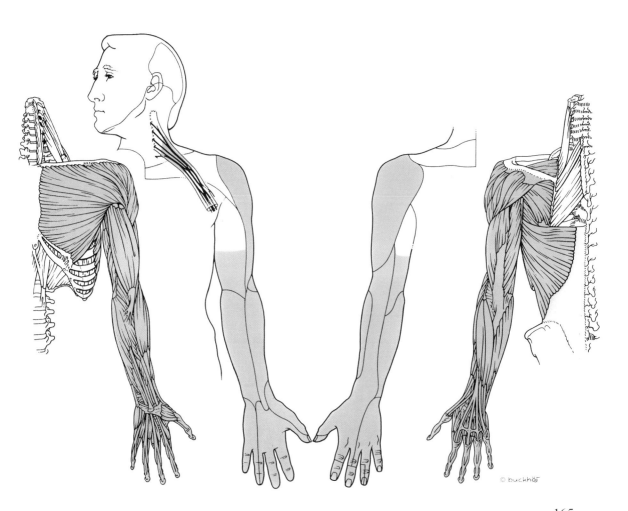

40 ml injection

An x-ray taken after an injection of 40 ml of the anesthetic-dye mixture into the subclavian perivascular space shows that with this volume the solution spreads proximally into the upper interscalene space and distally into the axillary perivascular space; so when this volume of anesthetic is used with the subclavian perivascular technique, anesthesia of the lower cervical plexus will result, in addition to anesthesia of the brachial plexus.

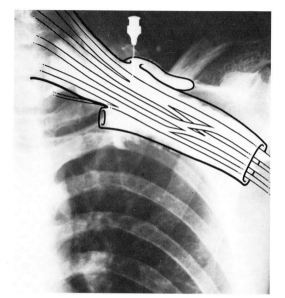

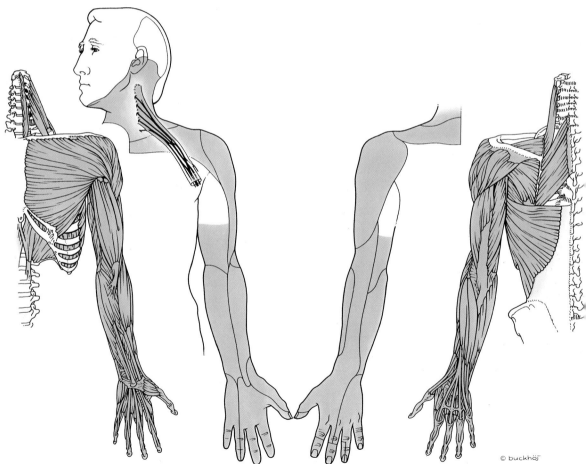

© buckhöj

Interscalene Perivascular Technique of Brachial Plexus Block

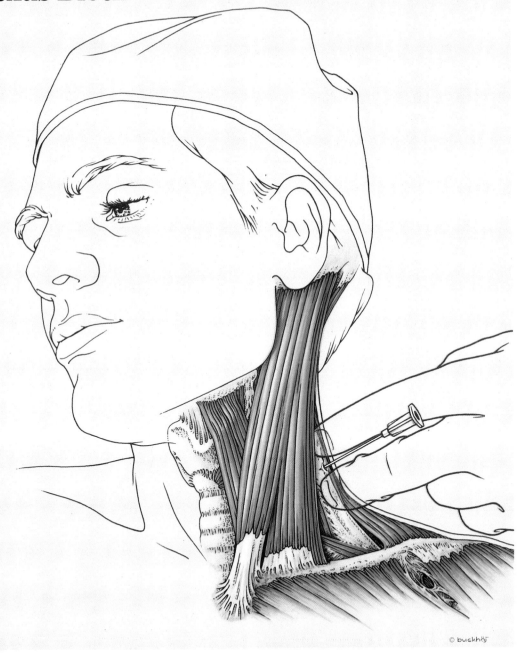

© buckhöj

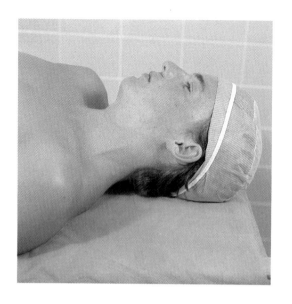

The author carries out the interscalene technique of brachial plexus block as follows: the patient is in the dorsal recumbent position with the head turned somewhat to the side opposite that to be blocked. The head should not be turned too far laterally, as doing so tends to stretch the scalene muscles, making palpation of the interscalene groove more difficult.

The block is carried out at the level of the sixth cervical vertebra, which is determined by extending a line laterally from the cricoid cartilage. The location of Chassaignac's tubercle, the prominent

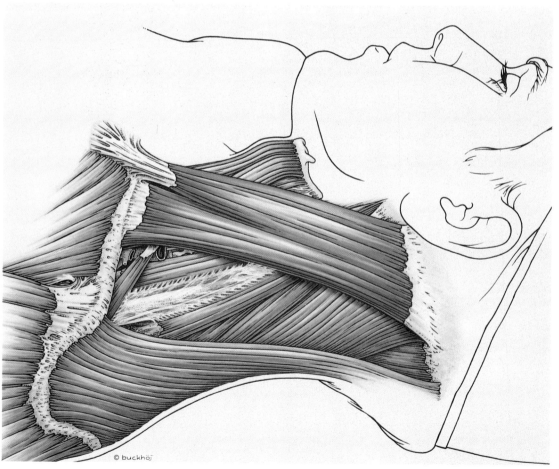

© buckhöj

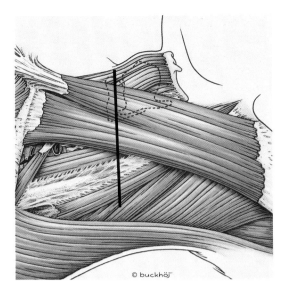

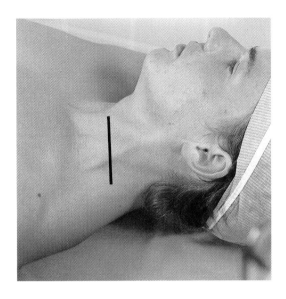

anterior tubercle of C_6, should *not* be sought as a landmark, since locating it usually causes considerable discomfort at a time that is psychologically disadvantageous in terms of patient cooperation.

An additional useful landmark is provided by the external jugular vein, when visible, for it crosses the interscalene groove at the level of C_6 virtually 100% of the time.

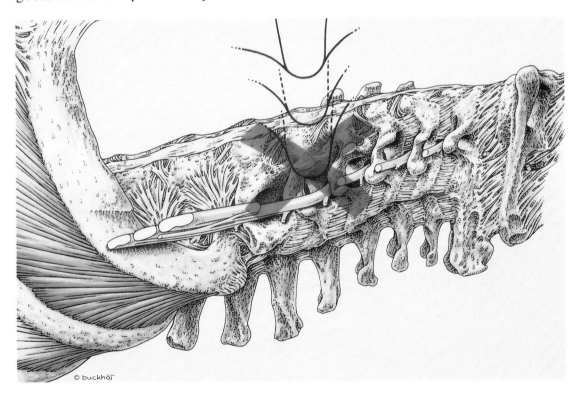

After explaining the procedure to the patient, he is asked to elevate his head slightly in order to bring the clavicular head of the sternocleidomastoid muscle into prominence. In some patients only the sternal head is prominent, but in virtually all patients, the clavicular head can be palpated, even when it is not visible.

A right-handed anesthetist should place the index and middle fingers of the left hand immediately behind (posterior to) the lateral edge of the sternocleidomastoid muscle and instruct the patient to relax; as the sternocleidomastoid muscle relaxes, the palpating fingers will actually move medially behind this muscle.

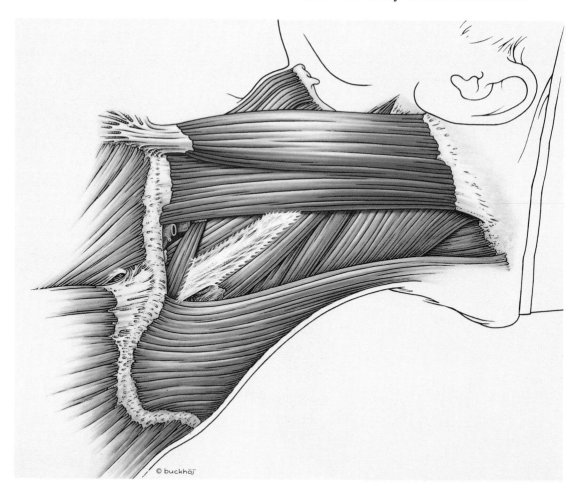

© buckhöj

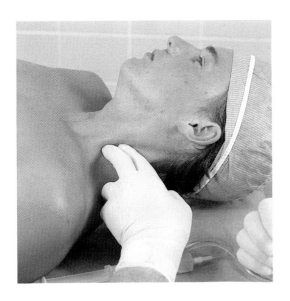
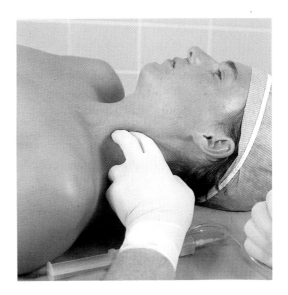

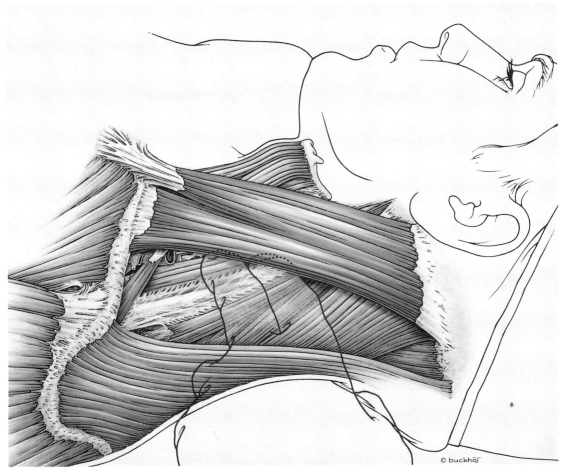

© buckhöj

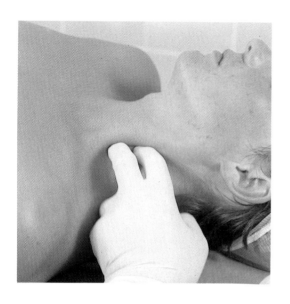

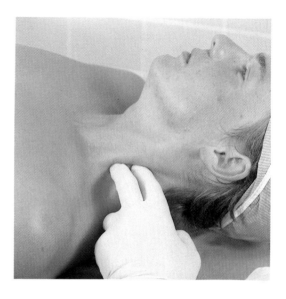

The palpating fingers now lie on the belly of the anterior scalene muscle.

They are rolled laterally across the belly of this muscle until the interscalene groove, the groove between the anterior and middle scalene muscles, is palpated.

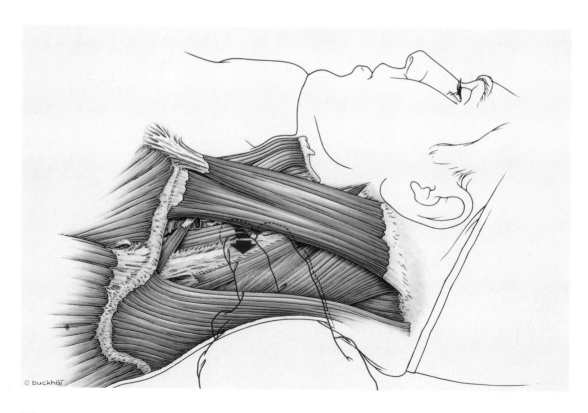

© buckhöj

The likelihood of eliciting paresthesias on the first insertion of the needle will be enhanced with this technique if it is remembered that the roots of the brachial plexus lie closer to the middle than to the anterior scalene muscle; obviously, then, when the needle is inserted between the palpating fingers in the interscalene groove, it should be inserted and advanced slightly closer to the middle than to the anterior scalene muscle.

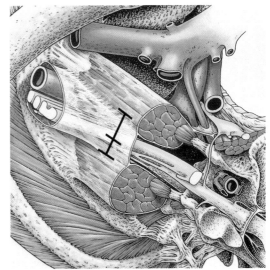

© buckhöj

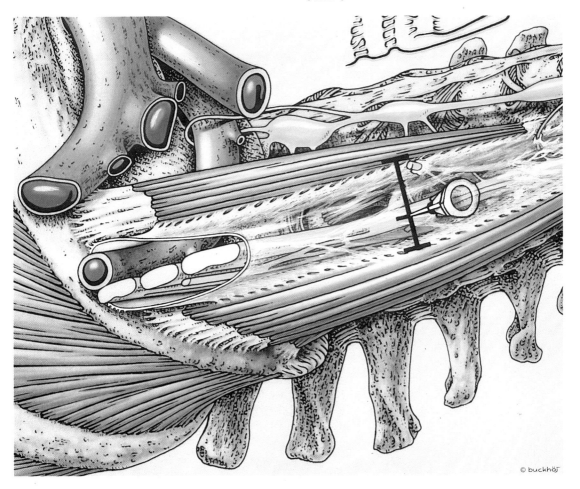

© buckhöj

With both the index and middle fingers in the interscalene groove, a 22-gauge, $1\frac{1}{2}$ inch short-bevel needle is inserted between them at the level of C_6, in a direction that is perpendicular to the skin in every plane, i.e., mostly mesiad, but slightly dorsad and slightly caudad. The injection site may have to be moved a millimeter or two superiorly to avoid the external jugular vein, if it is prominent, since the vein almost always crosses the interscalene groove at the level of C_6.

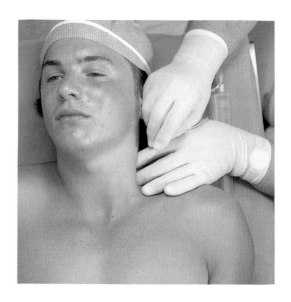

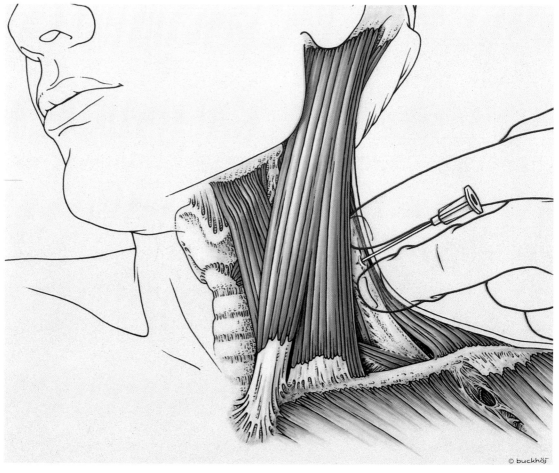

© buckhöj

The reason that the needle is inserted between the two palpating fingers with this technique, instead of above or below a single palpating finger as with other techniques, is that the two fingers depress the skin between them into the interscalene groove, decreasing the distance between skin and transverse process and thus decreasing the depth to which the needle must be inserted in order to obtain a paresthesia.

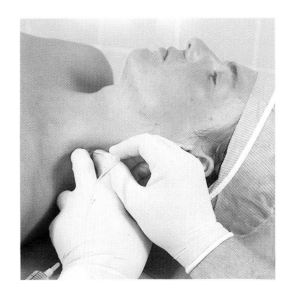

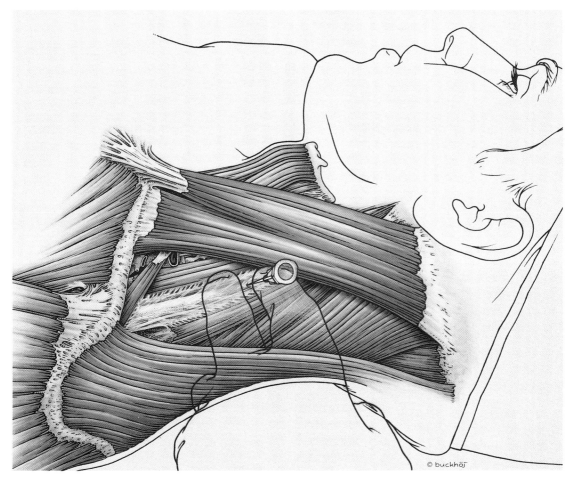

The needle is advanced slowly until a paresthesia is elicited or until a transverse process has been encountered. As with the subclavian perivascular technique, the patient must be instructed to say "stop" when he feels an "electric shock" to the arm and to tell the anesthetist verbally (not by pointing) where he feels it. Only a paresthesia *below* the level of the shoulder is acceptable, since a paresthesia to the shoulder could result from stimulation of the suprascapular nerve inside *or* outside the sheath.

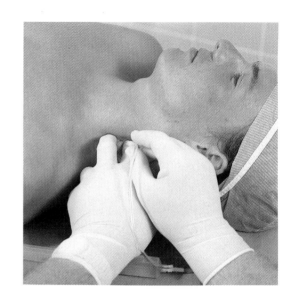

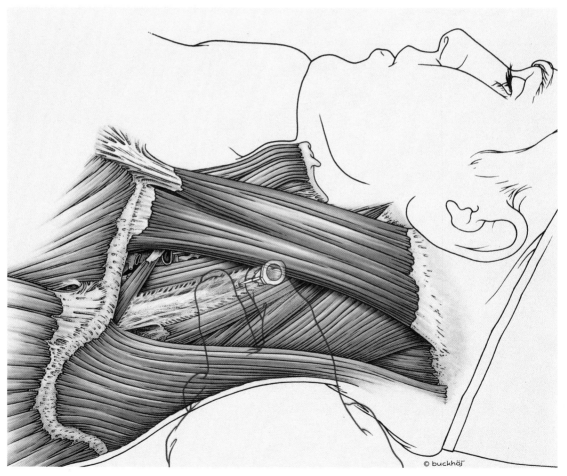

If bone is contacted without producing a paresthesia, the U-shaped end of the transverse process is "walked" millimeter by millimeter until a paresthesia is evoked.

Furthermore, the slightly caudad direction of the needle is absolutely essential to the safety of this technique, for it assures the anesthetist that if he misses the roots of the plexus with the needle, the needle will be stopped by bone (1). On the other hand, if the needle is inserted improperly in a directly mesiad direction, i.e., in a horizontal plane, and the roots of the plexus are not contacted, the advancing needle may penetrate the vertebral vessels (2) or may even enter the epidural space or spinal canal (3).

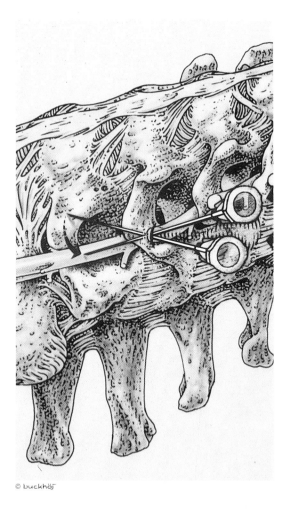

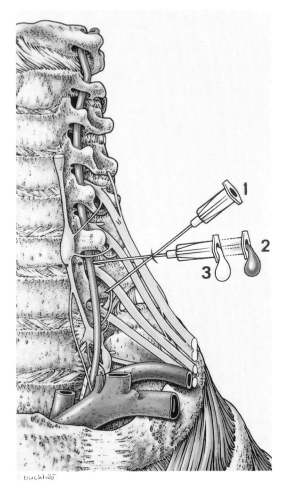

© buckhöj

buckhöj

Once a paresthesia has been obtained, and the patient has stated that it travels beyond the shoulder, aspiration is carried out in four quadrants and then, several ml's of local anesthetic are injected rapidly to elicit a "pressure paresthesia", a dull, aching feeling along the same distribution as the original "electrical paresthesias", probably due to the sudden increase in pressure in the interscalene space around the nerve roots. Following the production of the "pressure paresthesia", the next few ml's should be injected slowly to minimize discomfort to the patient, but after 8-10 ml of local anesthetic have been injected, the solution can be injected as rapidly as is desired without causing any discomfort to the patient; as always throughout the entire injection intermittent attempts to aspirate for blood should be made repeatedly.

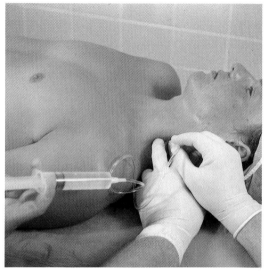

When the injection is completed and the needle withdrawn, the interscalene groove should be massaged vigorously in a cephalad-caudad direction to enhance the distribution of the local anesthetic.

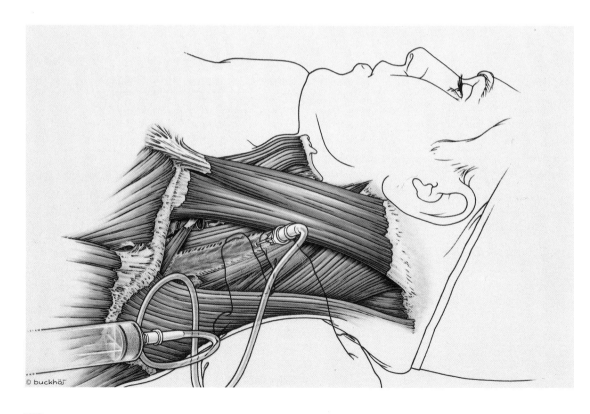

© buckhöj

Unlike other techniques, interscalene brachial block may be carried out with either hand on either side of the patient. While the right-handed anesthetist is usually more comfortable utilizing the left hand for palpation and the right hand for manipulating the needle on both sides, and the left-handed anesthetist the opposite, the ambidextrous anesthetist will find it more convenient to use the right hand for palpation and the left to manipulate the needle when performing an interscalene block on the right side.

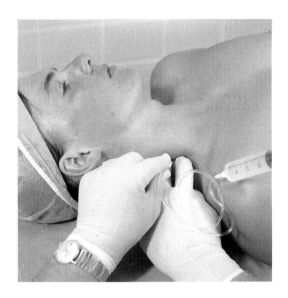

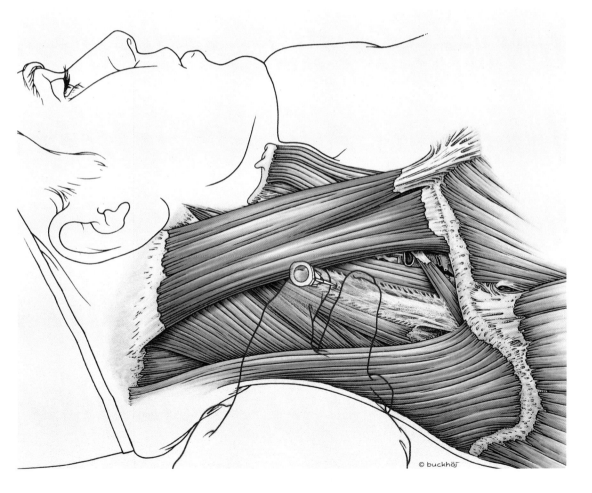

© buckhöj

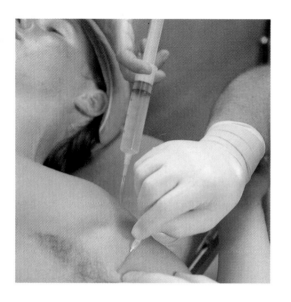

With this technique, as with any other, the intercostobrachial and medial brachial cutaneous nerves must be blocked separately by the subcutaneous injection of a few ml's of local anesthetic over the axillary artery pulse if a tourniquet is to be utilized during the surgical procedure.

Interscalene Perivascular Volume: Anesthesia Relationships

Again, the volume-anesthesia relationships of the interscalene technique of brachial plexus block are best illustrated by x-rays taken after the injection of a mixture of anesthetic agent and radiopaque dye.

20 ml injection

The first x-ray indicates that a 20 ml injection at the level of C_6 places the solution in the upper portion of the interscalene space, so such an injection results in anesthesia of the lower cervical plexus, which

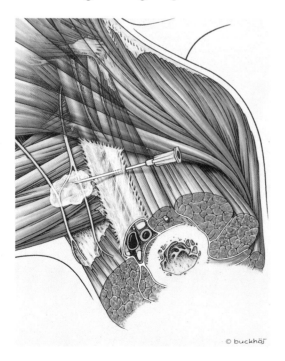

© buckhöj

also forms between the anterior and middle scalene muscles, as well as the brachial plexus. However, because the injection with this technique is made at such a high level, 20 ml are frequently inadequate to diffuse far enough inferiorly to reach the lower roots of the plexus, and as a result not infrequently anesthesia in the distribution of C_8 and T_1 is delayed and occasionally absent.

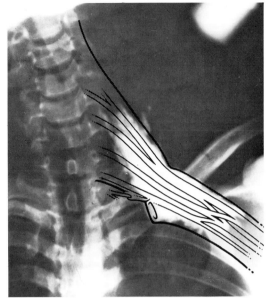

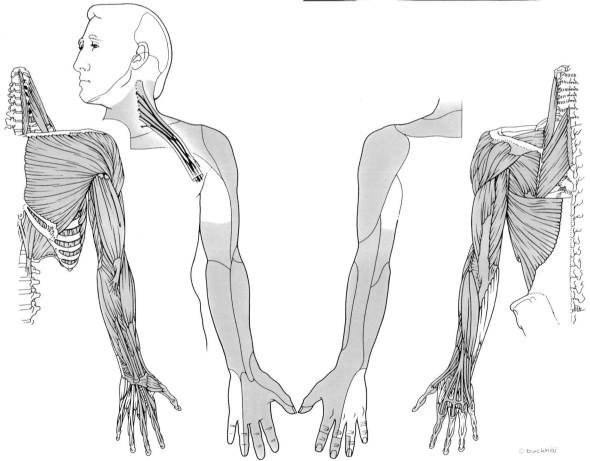

40 ml injection

The second x-ray shows that when the volume injected at this level is increased to 40 ml, the entire interscalene space is filled from the transverse processes of the upper cervical vertebrae all the way down to the cupola of the lung; therefore, while anesthesia in the distribution of C_8 and T_1 may be somewhat delayed as compared with other techniques, a 40 ml injection into the interscalene space will *usually* provide anesthesia of the entire cervical and brachial plexuses.

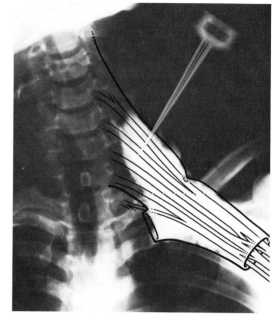

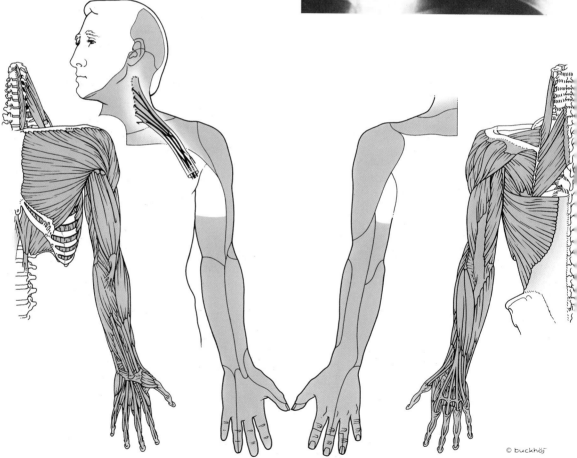

© buckhöj

Factors Influencing Interscalene Perivascular Volume: Anesthesia Relationships

Reference has been made repeatedly to the anatomical concept upon which the perivascular techniques of brachial plexus block are based, namely, that the brachial plexus is surrounded from the cervical vertebrae to the junction of the middle and upper thirds of the upper arm by a fascial envelope, which creates a continuous perineural and perivascular compartment. When an anesthetist is carrying out an axillary perivascular brachial block, he is injecting into the lower end of this continuous compartment; and in addition to the use of volume as indicated earlier, several technical maneuvers are utilized to increase the extent of spread up the sheath in order to block those elements which leave the sheath at a high level, i.e., the axillary and musculocutaneous nerves.

With an interscalene brachial block, the situation is somewhat reversed in that the injection is made high in this continuous space, and the elusive components of the plexus are the eighth cervical and first thoracic roots, which lie a considerable distance *below* the site of injection. As has already been described, the use of a large volume injection increases the incidence of successful blockade of these roots; but just as with an axillary block, when performing an interscalene block, the local anesthetic solution both ascends and descends within the interscalene space, which is the reason that following the injection of a large volume, part or all of the cervical plexus is blocked in addition to the brachial plexus. Because of proven efficacy of digital pressure in controlling the distribution of local anesthetics in carrying out an axillary block, the author has advocated digital pressure just *above* the site of injection in carrying out an interscalene brachial block, to inhibit the cephalad spread of the solution and to enhance the caudad spread, increasing the likelihood of blocking the lower roots of the plexus, whatever volume is injected. To document the efficacy of this maneuver the author and his co-workers compared sequential injections of 20 and 40 ml of a mixture of local anesthetic and radiopaque dye into the interscalene space with and without digital pressure above the site of injection.

Injection without digital pressure

The first pair of x-rays represents sequential injections of 20 and 40 ml of local anesthetic mixed with radiopaque dye into the interscalene space at the level of C_6 without digital pressure: the upper x-ray depicts the injection of 20 ml. The injected solution may be seen to move both up and down the interscalene compartment. The lower x-ray, taken after the volume has been increased to 40 ml, demonstrates extensive spread of the solution cephalad into the cervical portion of the interscalene compartment and caudally and laterally over the first rib and under the clavicle into the axillary portion of the sheath.

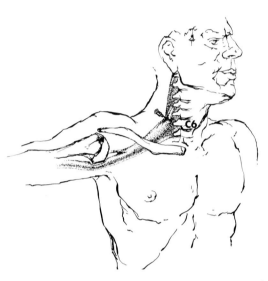

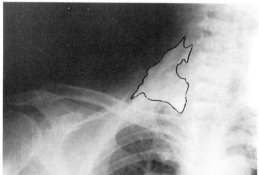

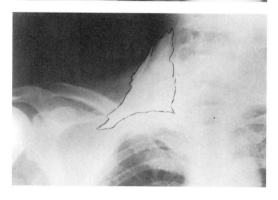

Injection with digital pressure

The second pair of x-rays represents identical injections, but made with firm digital pressure above the needle throughout the injection. Both x-rays show vividly how the digital pressure almost completely prevents the cephalad migration of the solution, with virtually all of the solution being forced caudally and laterally into the axillary portion of the sheath. The lower x-ray simply indicates that even after the injection of 40 ml into the interscalene space at C_6, continued, firm, digital pressure prevents any cephalad spread of the solution, with virtually all of the additional solution moving down to the cupola of the lung and out along the axillary sheath.

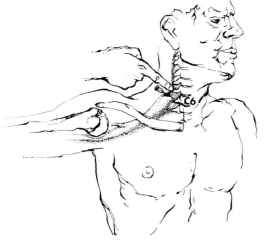

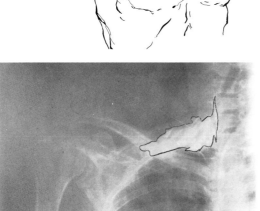

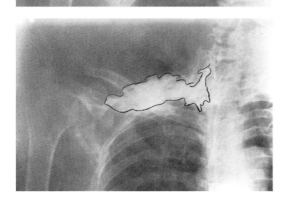

Conclusion

In short, these studies document the efficacy of digital pressure applied just above the needle during the performance of an interscalene block in inhibiting cephalad flow and promoting caudad flow, thus reducing the volume of anesthetic necessary with this technique to provide complete anesthesia of the entire brachial plexus.

Obviously, then, this is an important maneuver in carrying out interscalene brachial block, *provided* that anesthesia in the distribution of the cervical plexus is not necessary for the surgical procedure.

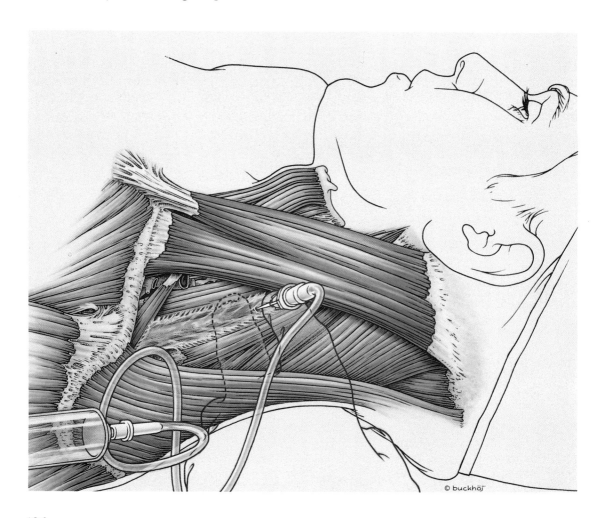

© buckhöj

186

Low Volume Interscalene Perivascular Brachial Plexus Block

In the occasional patient in whom the total dose of local anesthetic agent must be minimal for medical reasons, the volume of local anesthetic injected into the interscalene space can be reduced to 10-15 ml provided firm digital pressure is applied during the injection and the area is massaged vigorously afterward. Ordinarily with this volume and digital pressure, all of the plexus except C_8 and T_1 will be blocked. If surgery is confined to the hand, then, the ulnar nerve may be blocked quite painlessly at the elbow and anesthesia of the hand will be complete. However, if the surgery involves the forearm, and the medial antebrachial cutaneous nerve is not blocked, injection into the axillary perivascular space *below*

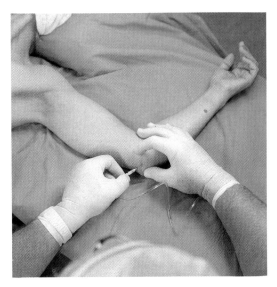

the artery will be necessary to block both of these derivatives of the lower roots of the plexus. Such a combination of axillary and interscalene injections has been proposed by Reese as a routine method of providing brachial plexus anesthesia.

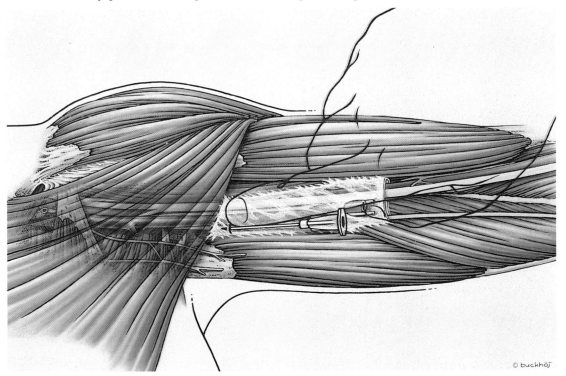

© buckhöj

187

References & Bibliography

Clausen, E. G.: Postoperative ("Anesthetic") Paralysis of the Brachial Plexus. Surgery 12: 933-942, 1942.

Eriksson, E. and Skarby, H.: A Simplified Method of Axillary Block. [Swedish]. Nord. Med. 68: 1325, 1962.

Selander, D., Dhunér, K. -G., and Lundborg, G.: Peripheral Nerve Injury Due to Injection Needles Used for Regional Anesthesia. Acta Anaesth Scan 21: 182-188, 1977.

Selander, D., Edshage, S., and Wolff, T.: Paresthesiae or No Parasthesiae? Nerve Lesions After Axillary Blocks. Acta Anaesth Scand 23: 277-33, 1979.

Winnie, A. P. and Collins, V. J.: The Perivascular Techniques of Brachial Plexus Anesthesia. Scientific Exhibit, ASA Annual Meeting, Denver, (Oct 23-27) 1965.

Winnie, A. P. and Collins, V. J.: The Subclavian Perivascular Technique of Brachial Plexus Anesthesia. Anesthesiology 25: 353-363, 1964.

Winnie, A. P.: Interscalene Brachial Plexus Block. Anesth. & Analg... Current Researches 49: 455-466 (3), (May-June) 1970.

Winnie, A. P.: Regional Anesthesia. Surgical Clinics of North America 54: 861-892, 1975.

Winnie, A. P., Radonjic, R., Akkineni, SR., and Durrani, Z.: Factors Influencing Distribution of Local Anesthetic Injected into the Brachial Plexus Sheath. Anesth. & Analg. 58: 225-234. 1979.

IV. Clinical Considerations

"The technique to be used in any given case should be determined on the basis of the surgical site, the required level of anesthesia, and the physical status and habitus of the patient, not on the basis of the anesthetist's bias for training."
Winnie

Primary Consideration: The Patient

As with any anesthetic technique, the choice of brachial plexus anesthesia must be made with the patient's welfare, both physiological and psychological, as the primary consideration. Since consciousness or loss of consciousness is optional with brachial plexus anesthesia, a preoperative visit, if possible, is even more important with this form of anesthesia than with general anesthesia, not only to evaluate the physical, psychological, and emotional status, but also to explain the anesthetic technique and the various options so that the surgical experience need not be a frightening or painful one. It is human nature to "want to be asleep" during an unpleasant or painful experience, because to most patients sleep is equated with freedom from pain. However, when properly informed that brachial plexus block is the safest form of anesthesia in a particular case, most patients readily agree to "whatever the anesthetist thinks is best". Furthermore once they are convinced that they will feel no discomfort other than that of the initial injection, many patients actually enjoy being awake and being an active participant in the surgical experience. On the other hand, some patients fear is "being awake", and these individuals almost invariably agree to a block when they learn that they will be given drugs preoperatively to sedate them and to minimize the discomfort of the block and intraoperatively to allow them to sleep and to be unaware of the surgical proceedings. Obviously, if a patient still prefers a general anesthetic after the merits of regional anesthesia and the possible risks of general have been explained, the anesthetist *must* comply.

While many anesthetists do not even consider regional anesthesia in infants and children, in many situations the pediatric patient is a better candidate for regional anesthesia than his adult counterpart, *provided* that the anesthetist is willing to spend the time necessary to establish rapport and gain the child's confidence. After the age of 3 or 4, or when the child can really understand the anesthetist's explanation, most children will cooperate *if* the anesthetist promises "just one pinch". The secret to fulfilling such a seemingly dangerous promise is that the "pinch" is the needle stick to raise a skin wheal, a practice that I feel is worthwhile *only* in infants and children. If the youngster is unable or unwilling to cooperate, we have found that "permissive" doses of ketamine 1 mg/kg administered intramuscularly will readily render the patient passively permissive but awake. In any case, when contemplating a brachial block to a minor, the procedure should be explained *first* to the parents and *then* with their concurrence to the child himself.

In any case, whether the patient is an adult or child, the surgeon must also agree that brachial plexus anesthesia is appropriate for the anticipated surgical procedure. If the surgeon has counseled the patient as to the advantages of this form of anesthesia *prior* to the patient's admission or, at least, prior to the anesthetist's preanesthetic visit, it is a rare patient who will not readily agree to its use. However, once the patient has been told that brachial plexus block is "the best anesthetic", it is unwise, if the block is partially or even totally unsuccessful, to abandon the technique and administer a general anesthetic, when to everybody's understanding a general anesthetic is *not* "the best anesthetic for this procedure". It is far better to repeat the block if there is no anesthesia or block the missed nerves if there is only partial anesthesia. Obviously, if there are medical reasons why this becomes impossible, they should be explained to the patient and entered into the patient's chart before beginning a general anesthetic under these circumstances.

Pharmacologic Considerations
Perioperative Medication

Never in the history of our specialty has there been available to the anesthesiologist such a wide variety of drugs that can be utilized to alter consciousness and enhance the anesthetic experience, and nowhere can these drugs be used more effectively than in the patient undergoing regional anesthesia. By combining ataractics, sedatives, and narcotics the anesthetist can, to a large degree, control the emotional and mental status of the patient. The decision as to the need for such pharmacological control is made on the basis of the degree of apprehension and anxiety exhibited by the patient and his desire to be asleep or awake, the degree of pain that will be produced by the particular technique selected, and upon the anesthetist's need for the patient's cooperation in performing that technique. For example if the block is to be carried out with the use of a nerve stimulator, the technique will require little patient cooperation and will produce minimal, if any pain, so the anesthetist is free to utilize very heavy sedation, if desirable, and can use sedatives and/or ataractics without narcotics. On the other hand, if one is going to utilize a technique that relies on the production of paresthesias, since the technique is painful *and* requires patient cooperation, the anesthetist might in this case rely more heavily on narcotics and/or ataractics. An additional advantage of narcotics is obvious if the surgery is for a painful and/or traumatic injury, in which case the analgesia provided by narcotics will be welcome even while the patient is awaiting surgery.

Clearly, with the multitude of drugs

available, there is no one correct way to premedicate a patient, particularly since each preanesthetic prescription should be individualized for the particular patient to be anesthetized. However, over the past twenty years the author has tried many combinations of drugs and feels that for the average, healthy, adult male about to undergo a brachial plexus block the following regimen provides, in the vast majority of cases, an optimal preoperative and intraoperative course: our regimen calls for premedication with morphine sulfate 0.2 mg/kg intramuscularly one hour prior to the anticipated time of the regional procedure. The morphine produces an excellent state of euphoric tranquility, and provides sufficient analgesia to minimize the discomfort of the nerve block procedure without interfering with the patient's perception of paresthesias. Following the performance of the block and after the *onset* of anesthesia, incremental doses of diazepam are given intravenously, titrating the patient to the point where he will sleep if allowed to but can be aroused and cooperate if and when the need arises.

Usually this endpoint is achieved after the administration of 0.1 to 0.15 mg/kg. If it is anticipated that the surgical procedure will last more than an hour to an hour and a half, hydroxyzine, in a dose that is ten times the dose of diazepam just administered, is injected intramuscularly into the anesthetized area, since this agent can be painful when administered intramuscularly. The sequential use of these two agents is based upon the fact that diazepam has a rapid onset but very short clinical duration, while hydroxyzine, which cannot be administered intravenously, has a slow onset but a prolonged duration of action; so the two drugs together, particularly with morphine as a "background", provide effects that have an immediate onset of action and a prolonged duration. Both drugs contribute to the sedation and in most cases to a high degree of retrograde amnesia; and in addition, diazepam elevates the convulsant threshold of the patient to local anesthetics and hence enhances the safety of the anesthetic, while hydroxyzine has analgesic effects of its own, which are additive with the effects of morphine. It is important to note that in our experience the occasional idiosyncratic, dysphoric responses attributed to morphine simply have not been apparent, though when the morphine has been omitted and diazepam has been utilized alone, such reactions have occurred. It is our opinion, therefore, that these ataractic drugs provide optimal effects when they are administered *after* morphine premedication.

Clinical pharmacokinetics of local anesthetics during brachial plexus blocks

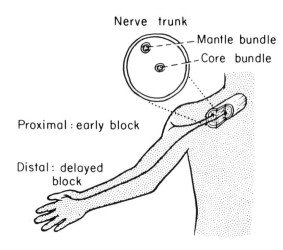

de Jong, R. H.: Local Anesthetics, pp. 65-71. Charles C. Thomas, Springfield, Illinois, 1977.
Reprinted by permission from Charles C. Thomas.

In order to offer a patient the maximal benefit of brachial plexus anesthesia it is essential for the anesthetist to be intimately familiar with the pattern and sequence of onset and recovery of the sensory and motor blockade which results when a local anesthetic is injected into the brachial plexus sheath. In other words, one must understand the clinical pharmacokinetics of local anesthetics in order to understand the clinical course of brachial plexus anesthesia, and in order to select the agent which will provide the optimal onset and duration of sensory block along with an appropriate degree of muscular relaxation.

The traditional concept concerning the pattern and sequence of the blocking process was synthesized in 1963 by de Jong, who described a theoretical model on the basis of physiological data obtained in the laboratory up to that time: he conceived of a nerve trunk as composed of many fascicles or bundles of nerve fibers, each tightly packed with hundreds of axons and encased in perineurium, all surrounded by the thick, fibrous epineurium. Within each fascicle, individual nerve fibers are surrounded and separated from one another by the thin, membraneous endoneurium. De Jong referred to those bundles that are close to the surface of the nerve as mantle bundles and to those situated deep within the nerve as *core bundles,* and pointed out that axons in the mantle bundles innervate the proximal portions of the arm, whereas axons in the core bundles innervate the more distal portions.

Critical to de Jong's concept is the assumption that the vascular supply of the nerve trunk is predominantly extraneural, with only minimal distribution intraneurally, so that perfusion is greatest in the periphery and poorest in the core. Thus the vascular uptake of an injected local anesthetic (the mechanism controlling its concentration gradient and hence its diffusion) was considered to occur predominantly at the periphery of the nerve trunk.

On the basis of this *theoretical* model de Jong predicted the following sequence of events after the performance of a brachial plexus block:

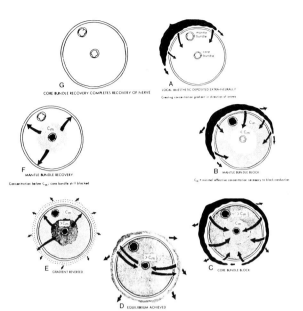

Theory of De Jong

Schematic drawing of diffusion-distribution sequences of a local anesthetic during nerve block according to De Jong. Arrows indicate the direction of the concentration gradient; the relative density of the stippling represents the relative concentration. The C_m density is the minimal effective concentration necessary to block conduction. (A) After perineural injection of a local anesthetic at a concentration well above C_m, the solution diffuses from the exterior of the nerve inward to the center with a steep diffusion gradient. (B) The mantle fibers of the nerve trunk are exposed to the local anesthetic before the core fibers, so these fibers are blocked while fibers in the core still conduct normally. (C) As diffusion continues inward, the concentration at the core reaches the C_m. The entire nerve is now blocked. (D) During the induction period the perineural concentration of local anesthetic has gradually been reduced by dilution, spread, and vascular absorption, while the core concentration has increased progressively until the external and internal concentrations are about equal and equilibrium is achieved. (E) With continued vascular absorption of the perineural pool of local anesthetic, the direction of diffusion is reversed so that the gradient is now from the core outward. As a result the concentration in mantle fibers has just fallen to C_m; conduction will soon be reestablished in these fibers while the core fibers are still solidly blocked. (F) The function of the mantle fibers has recovered, while the core fibers are still blocked, since the concentration in the core is at C_m. (G) With continued diffusion from the core outward, the concentration of all fibers falls below C_m so normal nerve conduction will be resumed throughout the entire nerve trunk.

de Jong, R. H.: Local Anesthetics, p. 66. Charles C. Thomas, Springfield, Illinois, 1977.
Reprinted by permission from Charles C. Thomas.

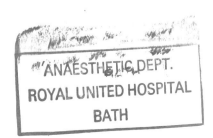

"Analgesia becomes evident first in the upper arm, then spreads towards the fingers until the entire arm is numb. While the analgesic front sweeps down the limb, weakness of the muscles of the upper arm begins to appear, becoming more pronounced until motor block ensues. Paresis, superseded by paralysis, now extends down the limb and eventually the entire arm is rendered numb and powerless. Recovery takes place in the reverse order. The C_m of motor fibers being greater than that of pain fibers, motor function returns before pain perception, both spreading in a proximal to distal direction." Therefore, de Jong concluded, "in as much as motor nerves are blocked last and recover first, the duration of motor block is shorter than that of sensory block, and seeing that outward diffusion during recovery is much slower than inward diffusion during induction, sensory block persists long after motor function has recovered."

Data obtained by the author and his colleagues at the University of Illinois Medical Center using the subclavian perivascular technique of brachial plexus block as a *clinical* model is in disagreement with de Jong's theoretical model. The results of our studies indicate that in man, provided the concentration of the local anesthetic injected is greater than the critical concentration of that agent needed to block motor nerves, the onset of motor blockade precedes or, at least, occurs simultaneously with the onset of sensory blockade, first in the mantle bundles and then in the core bundles.

Since the minimal effective concentration (C_m) of motor fibers is approximately twice that of sensory fibers, how can one explain the fact that analgesia does *not* precede paresis as predicted by de Jong?

193

In discussing the somatotopic representation of fasciculi within a nerve, de Jong accurately pointed out that fibers to or from the proximal regions of the arm travel in the mantle bundles, while those to or from the distal regions travel in the core bundles. However, within a given mantle bundle, there is similar organization of the nerve fibers, with the fibers nearest the surface of the nerve innervating the most proximal portions of the nerve distribution and fibers innervating a slightly more distal distribution farther from the surface, or deeper within the mantle bundle. It is axiomatic that the muscles controlling any segment of an extremity do so from the segment immediately proximal to the segment being controlled. In other words, the muscles controlling movements of the hand (other than the intrinsic muscles of the hand) are in the forearm; the muscles controlling movement of the forearm are in the arm; and the muscles controlling the arm are in the shoulder girdle and chest wall. Therefore, the motor nerves to muscles controlling the movement of any given segment will come off before sensory fibers innervating that segment, so the more peripheral fibers in any given bundle of fibers will be motor and the more deeply located fibers will be sensory.

In our studies using the subclavian perivascular technique of brachial plexus block, the local anesthetic was deposited at the level of the trunks, but it also bathed the roots, divisions, and upper cords. Since, with the exception of the suprascapular nerve, there are no cutaneous sensory branches derived from the brachial plexus proximal to the distal portion of the cords, it is obvious that the more peripheral fibers of a mantle bundle in the trunk are motor, and only the deepest fibers are sensory. Therefore, as a local anesthetic penetrates the epineurial barrier, the first fibers encountered are motor, and hence the blocking process *begins* in motor fibers before the local anesthetic has even reached the sensory fibers. Thus, if the molecules of the local anesthetic agent arrive at a mantle bundle in a concentration significantly above the critical motor concentration, the geographical arrangement of the nerve fibers, not size, determines the sequence of blockade. It follows then, that the earliest sign of success following either the subclavian perivascular or interscalene techniques of brachial plexus block is the inability of the patient to lift his arm off the table due to blockade of the fibers innervating the potent flexors of the arm. With the axillary perivascular technique the

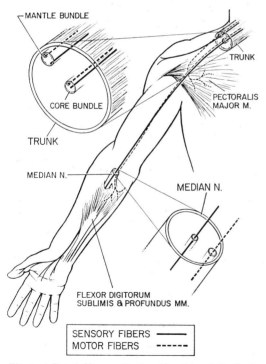

MANTLE BUNDLE
TRUNK
CORE BUNDLE
PECTORALIS MAJOR M.
TRUNK
MEDIAN N.
MEDIAN N.
FLEXOR DIGITORUM SUBLIMIS & PROFUNDUS MM.

SENSORY FIBERS ———
MOTOR FIBERS - - - - - -

Winnie, A. P. et al: Pharmacokinetics of Local Anesthetics During Plexus Blocks. Anesth. & Analg. 56: 852-861, 1977.
Reprinted by permission from International Anesthesia Research Society.

local anesthetic is injected at the level of the terminal nerves, below the level at which the nerves to the flexors of the arm leave the cords; so the earliest evidence of blockade is the inability of the patient to maintain the forearm in extension when asked to "point to the ceiling", due to blockade of the extensors of the forearm, which occurs prior to blockade of the flexors of the arm when the local is injected at this level. Furthermore as long as the appropriate musculature is tested, the onset of motor block will be found to occur 1-3 minutes after an injection into the perivascular compartment with any technique.

The other major difference between data obtained in our clinical studies and that proposed in de Jong's theoretical model is the sequence and pattern of recovery. According to de Jong, motor recovery precedes sensory recovery in both mantle and core fibers, and recovery of both modalities proceeds in a proximal to distal direction. Our studies have shown a sequence and pattern of recovery which are quite the opposite: first of all, recovery takes place in a distal to proximal direction, so that the hand recovers before the upper arm. Furthermore, sensory fibers do *not* remain blocked long after motor fibers have recovered, as postulated by de Jong; as a matter of fact, a significant degree of paresis usually persists after pain perception has returned.

What is the explanation for the difference between these theoretical and clinical models? De Jong assumed that recovery from nerve block follows the same *diffusional pattern* as that responsible for the induction of nerve block, but in reverse order. Hence, he hypothesized that after complete blockade, the extraneural anesthetic reservoir is steadily depleted by dif-

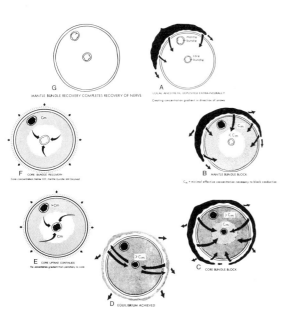

Theory of Winnie

Schematic drawing of diffusion-distribution sequences of a local anesthetic during nerve block according to the present author. The difference from De Jong's sequence may be seen in (E) and (F). Because of the internal circulation of the nerve, the concentration does not reverse as indicated by de Jong, so recovery takes place first in core fibers. Thus the sequence is as follows: (A) After perineural injection of a local anesthetic at a concentration well above C_m, the solution diffuses from the exterior of the nerve inward to the center with a steep diffusion gradient. (B) The mantle fibers of the nerve trunk are exposed to the local anesthetic before the core fibers, so these fibers are blocked while fibers in the core still conduct normally. C) As diffusion continues inward, the concentration at the core reaches the C_m. The entire nerve is now blocked. (D) During the induction period, the perineural concentration of local anesthetic has gradually been reduced by dilution, spread, and vascular absorption, while the core concentration has increased progressively until the external and internal concentrations are about equal and equilibrium is achieved. (E) Because of the intraneural vascular network, vascular absorption continues to be greater in the core than in the periphery, so the concentration gradient continues to be from mantle to core. (F) As core uptake continues to predominate, the concentration falls below the C_m in the core fibers and the core fibers recover while the mantle fibers are still blocked. (G) As uptake continues from mantle to core, the mantle bundles finally recover and full recovery of the entire nervetrunk is completed.

Winnie, A. P. et al: Pharmacokinetics of Local Anesthetics During Plexus Blocks. Anesth. & Analg. 56: 852-861, 1977.
Reprinted by permission from International Anesthesia Research Society.

fusion, dispersion, and vascular absorption, until the concentration of anesthetic drops below C_m. Thus, *if* the concentration gradient is reversed, then diffusion should proceed from the intraneural to extraneural space; and since the fibers in the mantle bundle are nearest the surface of the nerve, they should be subjected sooner to the "anesthetic exodus" than those in the nerve core. Therefore, de Jong theorized that the anesthetic concentration in the mantle drops below the C_m, first of motor fibers and then of sensory fibers, with recovery occurring first in the upper arm, recovery of the core fibers being delayed until peripheral diffusion decreases the concentration sequentially below the C_m of motor and then sensory fibers.

Since the data obtained in our clinical studies clearly indicate that this is *not* the sequence of events in recovery, then the diffusional pattern must be quite different. The sequence and pattern of recovery described by de Jong have as their basis the assumption that reversal of the local anesthetic gradient occurs primarily due to *extraneural* vascular absorption of the drug. However, this assumption fails to consider the *intraneural* vascular supply, which we feel has a dramatic impact on the intraneural concentration of local anesthetic and the resulting gradient. It is well established, yet not widely appreciated, that each peripheral nerve is abundantly vascularized throughout its entire length by a succession of vessels, the vasa nervorum, which by their repeated division and anastomosis within the nerve form an unbroken intraneural vascular net. This network of vessels is supported by the nutrient arteries and veins, which arise either from a main arterial trunk or from one of its branches.

All nutrient arteries, before breaking up into finer branches, divide at least once inside or outside the nerve into ascending and descending branches, which travel in the epineurium of the nerves supplied. From these epineurial arteries or arterioles, penetrating arterioles arise at irregular intervals, and from these penetrating arterioles are derived the intraneural arterioles, precapillaries, and capillaries, which by their repeated division and anastomosis, form the continuous, longitudinal, intravascular net which extends the length of the nerve. So extensive is this intraneural vascular network that many surgeons consider the intraneural blood supply to be sufficient to maintain full nutrition of the nerve trunk after obliteration of large segments of its perineural supply. The significance of this intraneural vascular architecture in regional anesthesia relates to the fact that as the vessels move from periphery to core, continuously branching and rebranching, the interface between blood vessels and nerve fibrils increases progressively. Thus, following the establishment of blockade of mantle and core fibers, in

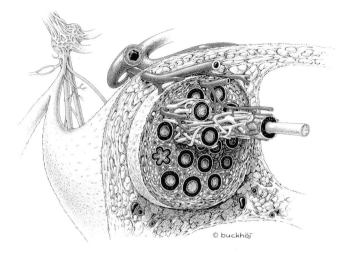

© buckhöj

addition to the process of extraneural uptake of local anesthetic, there is an even greater intraneural removal of the drug, which on the basis of the density of the capillary network, should be greatest in the core of the nerve. As a result the gradient of local anesthesia will *not* reverse with the passage of time, but will continue from mantle to core. Consequently, sensory fibers, which are the most centrally located, will recover first as the concentration of local anesthetic decreases in the core until it is below C_m, after which time the motor fibers in the core which are somewhat more peripherially placed will recover. As the process continues, the sensory fibers in the mantle should recover next, since they are more central than their motor counterparts; and finally the motor fibers in the mantle, by virtue of their being closest to the periphery, should recover last. Such a diffusional pattern explains precisely the sequence and pattern of recovery observed in our clinical studies.

This information complex though it may seem, is of more than academic interest; for it is only with a complete understanding of these pharmacokinetic principles that the anesthetist can assess the progress of anesthesia after performing a brachial plexus block, advise the surgeon of the adequacy of the anesthesia, and respond intelligently to the patient's questions concerning the anesthetic experience.

Choice of local anesthetic agents

It is, in large part, the current availability of local anesthetic agents having a wide spectrum of activity, particularly in terms of duration of action, that has expanded the usefulness of brachial plexus anesthesia to include surgery for which this type of anesthesia was previously unacceptable or undesirable. Until recently, in choosing a local lanesthetic agent capable of providing appropriate anesthesia, the limiting factor has been duration of action. Today regional anesthetists have available to them anesthetic agents, the duration of action of which range from about 20 minutes to 12-24 hours, depending on the concentration and volume of the agent and the presence or absence of vasocontrictors. It is beyond the scope of this book to provide a comprehensive discussion of the pharmacology of local anesthetic agents, for this will be provided in a subsequent volume of the same series; but it is important to appreciate that there is currently available a sufficient variety of local anesthetics that the duration of anesthesia can be tailored to the individual surgical procedure.

Thus for example, if one wishes to provide anesthesia for a short procedure of 20-30 minutes one can utilize 2% procaine, while for a procedure lasting 30-60 minutes one could add epinephrine 1:200,000 to procaine, or give plain 2% chloroprocaine. Similarly for a procedure anticipated to last 1-1½ hours, the anesthetist may utilize 2% chloroprocaine with epinephrine 1:200,000 or 1% lidocaine without epinephrine, whereas if the anticipated duration is 2½-3 hours he may elect to add epinephrine 1:200,000 to 1% lidocaine or to utilize mepivacaine 1% without epinephrine. If the desired duration of anesthesia is 3-4 hours, one may elect to utilize prilocaine 1%, and if the duration of anesthesia desired is 5-6 hours tetracaine 0.15-0.2% with 1:200,000 will be the agent of choice. For prolonged anesthesia of 10-12 hours bupivacaine 0.5% or etidocaine 0.5-1.0% are both effective, though both have a very wide *range* of duration and can on occasion result in anesthesia lasting well over 24 hours. Like tetracaine, bupivacaine has a very slow onset of action, whereas etidocaine has an onset of action even faster than that of lidocaine, but the latter agent has the disadvantage of providing motor blockade that long outlasts sensory blockade, an experience which is frightening to most surgical patients, since they fear that, with the return of sensation, the block has worn off and the arm is paralyzed!

In an effort to overcome the disadvantage of slow onset shared by tetracaine and bupivacaine, many anesthetists have mixed them with short-acting agents in an effort to provide a mixture that would provide both a rapid onset and a prolonged duration. Thus, Moore introduced the very effective mixture consisting of mepivacaine 1% and tetracaine 0.2% with epinephrine 1:200,000; in almost 500 brachial blocks carried out with this mixture, utilizing both the axillary and supraclavicular approaches, Moore reported an onset time of 5-8 minutes, the establishment of surgical anesthesia within 12-25 minutes (compared to 20-40 minutes when tetracaine was utilized alone), and a duration of anesthesia of 4-5½ hours and longer. The author and his colleagues have had similar success with this mixture, which is prepared by dissolving 40 mg of tetracaine crystals (Niphanoid®) in 20 ml of 1% mepivacaine, to which is added 0.1 ml of 1:1000 epinephrine, giving a solution that contains 1% mepivacaine, 0.2% tetracaine, and epinephrine 1:200,000. Other short-acting agents have been added to tetracaine in an effort to provide the "ideal" mixture, and these have included the amides lidocaine and prilocaine and the esters procaine and 2-chloroprocaine,

but none were found to have any advantage over mepivacaine, so their use with tetracaine has never become popular.

Early studies in animals *appeared* to indicate that the toxicity of a solution resulting from the mixture of two local anesthetics was greater than the sum of the toxicities of the two agents, i.e., that the toxicity was synergistic rather than additive. These studies indicated that the compounding of local anesthetics increased the severity of systemic toxic reactions and even the incidence of death in certain laboratory animals, implying that the use of such mixtures in humans might be dangerous. Fortunately, the extrapolation of such data from animals to humans is invalid for several reasons: first of all, animals catabolize ester derivatives quite slowly, while humans metabolize them rapidly; so when a mixture of an ester and an amide is utilized in man, because of the rapid metabolism of the ester, the peak blood levels of the two drugs occur at different times, with the peak blood level of the ester occurring very rapidly and the blood level of the amide rising much more slowly. Secondly, the animal studies utilized intravenous injections of the two local anesthetics, which would obviously result in simultaneous peak levels, whereas following the injection of a mixture of local anesthetics clinically in man, the achievement of peak blood levels will be delayed by the time required for vascular uptake of the agents. Furthermore, the use of epinephrine in mixtures of local anesthetics in man markedly decreases the magnitude of the peak levels of both local anesthetics, but without changing the time differential of the two peaks, thus enhancing further the safety of using such mixtures in man.

Efforts to compound bupivacaine to shorten the time of onset have been less successful than with tetracaine. One of the reasons is that when two *solutions* of a local anesthetic are mixed, both solutions are diluted to concentrations lower than those considered optimal when either agent is utilized alone. Nonetheless, the early report of Cunningham and Kaplan indicated excellent results with a solution containing 1% chloroprocaine and 0.33% bupivacaine, compounded by mixing 20 ml of bupivacaine 0.5% and 10 ml of chloroprocaine 3%. They compared the results achieved with this mixture with the results obtained using bupivacaine 0.5% alone, both solutions being injected into the axillary perivascular compartment. As expected, the time of onset was reduced significantly by the use of the mixture, but more important, the time to surgical anesthesia was reduced by slightly more than 50%. Furthermore, the compounded drug appeared to spread faster than bupivacaine alone; and the duration of the block was not affected whatsoever, since both solutions provided 19 hours of sensory blockade, and this without the addition of epinephrine to either solution! They also noted that bupivacaine appeared to provide a prolonged period of analgesia that lasted long after normal sensory function had returned in both groups.

Unfortunately, although this is the only report of this combination of agents used for brachial plexus block, other investigators utilizing the mixture for epidural anesthesia have been unable to reproduce their results. An early report by Villa and Marx appeared to indicate that the combination of these two agents resulted in a mixture having the best characteristic of each, namely rapid onset and prolonged duration; but subsequent studies carried out by investigators at several institutions indicate that for epidural anesthesia the mixture of chloroprocaine and bupivacaine has the same onset and duration as chloroprocaine utilized alone! In other words, when chloroprocaine is mixed with bupivacaine for epidural anesthesia, the chloroprocaine enhances the rate of *onset* over bupivacaine alone, but bupivacaine does *not* enhance the duration of chloroprocaine. Galindo has postulated that the reason the addition of bupivacaine fails to prolong the duration of chloroprocaine is that the pH of the mixture of bupivacaine and chloroprocaine (3.60) is so far from the pKa of bupivacaine (8.1) that only 1% of the free base of bupivacaine available at the pH of the commercial solution of bupivacaine (5.60) is available in the mixture. The pKa, of course, is that pH at which the anesthetic in solution is 50% base and 50% cation; and the clinical significance of this results from the fact that the amount of free base available determines the rate of diffusion of a local anesthetic. Since the pH of commercial chloroprocaine (3.56) is so similar to the pH of the mixture (3.60), the available base of chloroprocaine remains about the same, and the mixture behaves virtually as though it was chloroprocaine alone. Galindo confirmed his hypothesis by demonstrating, at least in the laboratory, that the addition of bicarbonate to the mixture to raise the pH to 5.56 (close to the pH of the commercial solution of bupivacaine) caused the mixture to retain the rapid onset of chloroprocaine and to provide the prolonged duration of bupivacaine. The importance of the pH of a local anesthetic and its dissociation constant (pKa) on the activity of local anesthetic agents has been reemphasized by Galindo, who showed both in laboratory studies and in clinical studies utilizing brachial plexus block that adjusting the pH of virtually all commercially available local anesthetic agents to about 7.0 significantly reduces the onset time and prolongs the duration of a nerve block. Even more recently the importance of alkalinization of local anesthetics was demonstrated clinically by Hilgier of Poland who compared bupivacaine alkalinized to a pH of 6.4 with commercial bupivacaine in fifty patients, in whom anesthesia was provided by the subclavian perivascular technique of brachial plexus block, twenty-five patients receiving each solution. The data obtained in his study indicated that the alkalinization of bupivacaine reduces the onset time from 20-30 minutes to 7-14 minutes, provides a greater *intensity* of motor block, and increases the duration of sensory block from 5-10 hours. It would appear, in view of reports such as this, that alkalinization of slow onset, long-acting local anesthetics just prior to their use should obviate the necessity of compounding local anesthetics altogether. Thus, Galindo has advocated the addition of 0.1 ml of sodium bicarbonate to each 10 ml of commercially available solutions of bupivacaine or etidocaine to bring the pH to approximately 7.0 just before the agents are injected, and similarly, the addition of 1.0 ml for each 10 ml of chloroprocaine, lidocaine, and mepivacaine.

Another mechanism by which the effect of pH has been utilized to hasten the onset of blockade with local anesthetics is that of carbonation. In theory, when a carbonated local anesthetic is injected, the free base is liberated quickly due to rapid buffering, and the liberated carbon dioxide diffuses very rapidly across cell membranes, causing a fall in the intracellular pH. Thus the analgesic base is brought closer to the nerve more rapidly and in a higher concentration, decreasing the time required for penetration of the nerve; and then because of the lower intracellular pH, ionization takes place rapidly after penetration, enhancing the quality and duration of the block. Carbonated lidocaine was first introduced by Bromage almost twenty years ago, and he demonstrated that when utilized for epidural anesthesia, the carbonated lidocaine reduces the latency of onset by one-third as compared to the hydrochloride solution. Several years later Schulte-Steinberg in Germany, and after him Bromage in Canada, demonstrated that when utilized for brachial plexus block the carbonated solution of lidocaine had an even greater effect, reducing the latency to full analgesia by two-thirds as compared to the hydrochloride solution. Schulte-Steinberg also pointed out that while duration was unaffected by the carbonate, perhaps the most important impact of carbonation was on the *spread* of the solution, to such an extent that he was able to reduce the volume required for a supraclavicular brachial block by 30-50%! Bromage, on the other hand, noted that in addition to the remarkable improvement in onset provided by carbonated lidocaine, there was a 12% reduction in duration, a phenomenon not seen when the carbonate was utilized for epidural analgesia. In his subsequent studies, however, Bromage also demonstrated that a *mixture* of 1% carbonated lidocaine and 0.25% bupivacaine resulted in a combination which masked the disadvantage of each drug by the advantage of the other, for this combination provided an onset time of less than 7 minutes and a mean duration of more than 7 hours.

Because of the clinical advantages of carbonated lidocaine, Bromage proposed the carbonation of other slow-onset, long-acting agents; but when McClure and Scott compared carbonated bupivacaine and bupivacaine hydrochloride for interscalene brachial plexus block, there was little difference between the time taken by each agent to achieve its maximal spread. However, the real advantage of the carbonated bupivacaine over the hydrochloride was indicated by the fact that even with a volume of 40 ml, none of the patients receiving bupivacaine hydrochloride had anesthesia of the 8th cervical or 1st thoracic dermatome at the end of 30 minutes, while all of the patients receiving carbonated bupivacaine did! Furthermore, these investigators felt that the carbonated solution of bupivacaine produced, not only a more widespread block, but also a more intense block. Unfortunately, the advantages of carbonated lidocaine are only available in Canada, and similarly, the advantages of carbonated bupivacaine only in Germany.

It is obvious from all of the foregoing discussion that the choice of a local anesthetic for a brachial plexus block is made *primarily* on the basis of the duration of anesthesia desired: thus for procedures where full and immediate return of function is desirable, as in ambulatory surgery or diagnostic blocks in a Pain Clinic, the objective is to match the duration of anesthesia with the anticipated duration of surgery as closely as possible. On the other hand, when prolonged postoperative pain relief, immobilization, and sympathetic blockade are desirable, as after reimplantation and other vascular procedures, then the longest acting agents available should be selected. The concentration of an agent should be selected *primarily* on the basis of the degree of motor blockade required. While the author disagrees with several eminent authorities (see Chapter V) that concentrations of lidocaine and mepivacaine greater than 1% are neurotoxic, rarely is a concentration greater than 1% necessary, since both of these agents produce adequate relaxation of all of the muscles except those controlling the fingers of the hand in the vast majority of cases. Increasing the concentration of most agents will speed the onset and prolong the duration of the agent somewhat, but this should only be a secondary concern, since choice of a particular agent (or mixture) should be made on the basis of these characteristics.

It is common clinical practice to add epinephrine to a local anesthetic for one of two reasons (or both): first of all, epinephrine delays vascular uptake of the local anesthetic from the site of injection, thus shortening slightly the time of onset and prolonging the duration of action. Secondly, the reduction in vascular uptake will decrease the peak blood level of the local anesthetic and hence reduce the possibility of systemic toxicity. However, the decision to utilize epinephrine with a given local anesthetic should be based on several considerations: first of all epinephrine alters the absorption of different local anesthetics to differing degrees: for example, the addition of epinephrine markedly prolongs the duration of some local anesthetic agents and has little effect on others. Similarly, epinephrine significantly reduces the peak blood levels of some agents and has only a minimal influence on others. In general, the shorter the duration of a local anesthetic when administered alone, the greater will be the impact of epinephrine, both in increasing duration and in reducing peak blood levels. Thus, epinephrine markedly increases the duration of chloroprocaine, procaine, and lidocaine, and has *much* less effect on mepivacaine, prilocaine, bupivacaine, and etidocaine. Similarly, epinephrine produces significant reductions in peak blood levels of chloroprocaine, lidicaine, and mepivacaine, but effects only minimal reductions in the peak levels of prilocaine, bupivacaine, and etidocaine. The glaring exception to this general inverse relationship between duration and the effectiveness of epinephrine is tetracaine, for though it is considered to be a long-acting agent, the addition of epinephrine markedly prolongs its action *and* enhances its safety. As a matter of fact, it is almost an absolute rule at the author's institution that for reasons of safety neither lidocaine nor tetracaine should be utilized without epinephrine.

Another important consideration when one is contemplating the addition of epinephrine to a local anesthetic is the systemic effect of the epinephrine itself. Even when utilized in its optimal concentration, the epinephrine will enter the circulation and produce significant hemodynamic effects. Obviously, the optimal dose of epinephrine is that which would produce maximal increase in the duration of a local anesthetic agent and minimal hemodynamic effects. Kennedy and his co-workers have demonstrated that a supraclavicular brachial block carried out with 30 ml of 1.6% lidocaine has virtually no hemodynamic effects, while the same agent with epinephrine produces a dose-related increase in cardiac rate, cardiac output, and stroke volume that persists for 90 minutes, and decreases in peri-

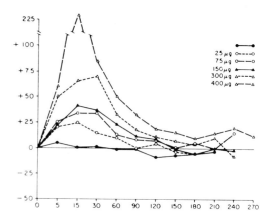

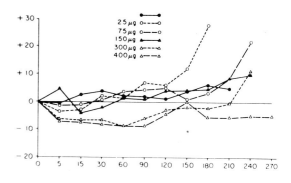

The effect of epinephrine on the duration of a brachial plexus with 30 ml of 1.5% Lidocaine			
Epinephrine		Mean Duration (min)	Range
ug	Concentration		
0	–	186.00	150-210
25	1:1.200.000	195.00	180-210
75	1:400.000	240.00	210-270
150	1:200.000	264.00	210-300
300	1:100.000	247.50	240-270
400	1:75.000	255.00	240-270

Kennedy Jr., W. F., Bonica, J. J. et al: Cardiorespiratory Effects of Epinephrine when Used in Regional Anesthesia.
Acta Anaest. Scand. (Suppl. XXIII, Proceedings I of the 2nd European Congress of Anaesthesiology). pp. 320-333, 1966.

pheral resistance and concomitant changes in mean arterial pressure that persist for 120 minutes.

Further, they showed that epinephrine produces a dose-related increase in the mean duration of anesthesia but only *up to* a concentration of 1:200,000, above which, the cardiocirculatory changes continued to increase *without* any further increase in the duration of anesthesia.

Obviously, then if epinephrine is utilized to prolong the duration of anesthesia provided by a local anesthetic, it is pointless to exceed the concentration of 1:200,000, a concentration which virtually all clinicians accept as optimal. Furthermore in patients whose cardiac status is such that these cardiocirculatory changes are undesirable and in patients whose medical problems render them sensitive to catecholamines (i.e., hypertension, hyperthyroidism, etc.), epinephrine should be omitted. In those patients, as in patients where blockade may be desirable for several days, a continuous technique may be preferable.

And finally, if epinephrine *is* desirable, ideally it should be added to the local anesthetic just before the local anesthetic is utilized. The reason for this is that commercial local anesthetic solutions containing epinephrine are buffered to a lower pH than the standard solution of that agent in an effort to minimize the oxidation of the epinephrine; such acidification clearly moves the pH even farther from the pKa of that solution, reducing the availability of the free base, the rate of diffusion of the local anesthetic, and ultimately delaying the onset of surgical anesthesia. When epinephrine is added to a local anesthetic, it should be carefully measured utilizing a tuberculin syringe, and this is most conveniently accomplished by simply adding 0.1 ml of epinephrine to 20 ml of the local anesthetic agent to give a final concentration of 1:200,000. Since the size of a "drop" of a solution varies with the size of the apperture in the dropper, the practice of measuring epinephrine by drops should be considered archaic and is to be condemned.

Surgical Considerations

The important concept developed in the first chapter of this book is that of a continuous fascia-enclosed space surrounding the brachial plexus from the cervical transverse processes to several centimeters beyond the distal axilla. And in the third chapter techniques have been described whereby this space can be entered at any level; and, just as with peridural techniques, the extent of anesthesia that will result following the injection of a local anesthetic into this space will depend on the volume of anesthetic utilized and the level at which it is injected. Extending the analogy between the perivascular and peridural compartments, the axillary perivascular technique of brachial plexus block has been compared to a caudal block in that the injection is made into the lowermost portion of the space, the subclavian perivascular technique has been compared to a lumbar epidural, in that the injection is made into the midportion of the space, and the interscalene technique has been compared with a thoracic epidural, in that the injection is made into the upper portion of the space. And finally, to continue the analogy one step further, just as with peridural anesthesia, the choice of a particular perivascular technique will depend *primarily* on the site of surgery. Frequently, clinical studies have been carried out to compare the efficacy of brachial plexus block by various techniques *without* respect to the site of surgery, and this simply leads to erroneous conclusions. One would never compare the relative efficacy of epidural and caudal anesthesia in a heterogenous group of patients, some of whom are undergoing rectal surgery while others are undergoing lower abdominal surgery. Caudal, is ordinarily better for rectal surgery, and lumbar epidural is usually better for lower abdominal surgery. However, it is common to find such comparisons of the efficacy of the various techniques of brachial plexus block for "upper extremity surgery", without respect to the level at which the operation is carried out!

Obviously, the axillary perivascular technique of brachial plexus block is most suitable for surgery involving the distal part of the upper extremity, hand, wrist, and lower forearm; the subclavian perivascular technique is most suitable for surgery involving the mid-portion of the upper extremity, the upper forearm, elbow, and lower part of the upper arm; and finally, the interscalene techniques most appropriate for surgery and manipulations involving the more proximal portion of the upper extremity, the upper arm, shoulder, and shoulder girdle. Thus it follows that to provide *optimal* anesthesia for upper extremity surgery, an anesthetist must be equally competent with all three techniques. Each has its advantages and each its disadvantages. On the other hand, while the surgical site is *usually* the primary consideration in selecting one technique over another, if other considerations are more important in a particular case, anesthesia of the entire extremity

can be achieved by an alternate technique simply by increasing the volume of the local anesthetic and/or by adding a supplemental block. For example, while axillary block is ideal for surgery on the hand, if the hand is infected and enlarged axillary nodes make an injection into the axilla undesirable, anesthesia can be provided by the subclavian perivascular technique, or even by an interscalene technique, provided a large volume is utilized and firm digital pressure is provided above the needle during the injection. Similarly, while interscalene block is ideal for surgery on the upper arm and shoulder girdle, enlarged scalene lymph nodes or a localized skin infection might make insertion of a needle at this level unwise, in which case a subclavian perivascular technique or even an axillary technique with a large volume of local anesthetic and firm digital pressure distal to the injection site can provide adequate anesthesia.

In selecting the appropriate technique of brachial plexus block for a particular surgical procedure, it is important to consider the level at which the injection is made with that technique and the components of the brachial plexus which will be bathed with the injected solution: for example, interscalene brachial plexus block is a block at the level of the *roots* of the brachial plexus; and since the injection is made at C_6, the level of the *upper* roots, if one fails to block all of the components of the plexus with this technique, the distribution of anesthesia and the distribution of the area that has been missed will be the distrubition of one or more roots. It has often been said that with interscalene brachial block, anesthesia in the distribution of the ulnar nerve may be delayed or absent, but it must be remembered that it is actually anesthesia in the distribution of C_8 and T_1 that is delayed or absent. Therefore, if surgery is to be carried out in the hand in this situation (though interscalene block is ordinarily a poor third choice for hand surgery), then blockade of the ulnar nerve at the elbow will be sufficient to complete the anesthesia *of the hand.* However, if surgery will be carried out on the forearm, blockade of the ulnar nerve at the elbow will be inadequate, since it is the medial antebrachial cutaneous nerve, also derived from C_8 and T_1, which supplies the medial aspect *of the forearm,* not the ulnar nerve. Thus when charting the extent of anesthesia following an interscalene brachial block, it is more appropriate to do so utilizing a dermatome chart rather than a peripheral nerve chart.

When the subclavian perivascular technique is utilized to provide brachial plexus anesthesia, the distribution of anesthesia that results and the distribution of an area which is missed, will be in the distribution of the three trunks of the plexus, since with this technique the local anesthetic solution is injected at the trunk level. Therefore, if the inferior trunk is missed, then anesthesia will usually be lacking in the distribution of C_8 and T_1, since those two roots together comprise the inferior trunk. Similarly, if only the superior trunk is bathed with local anesthetic solution, then the anesthesia that results will be in the distribution of C_5 and C_6, the two roots that together comprise the superior trunk; and anesthesia will be lacking in the distribution of C_7, C_8, and T_1, since the middle trunk is composed exclusively of fibers from C_7. However, because the subclavian perivascular technique deposits the local anesthetic at a point where the plexus has contracted into the fewest component parts, incomplete anesthesia is less frequent with this technique than with any other.

Finally, because the injection of local anesthetic with the axillary perivascular technique is carried out at a level where all of the peripheral nerves have formed, anesthesia and inadequate anesthesia, will be in the distribution of the various peripheral nerves. Since the axillary and musculocutaneous nerves leave the axillary sheath at a higher level than any of the other terminal nerves, these are the nerves most commonly missed following an axillary perivascular block, although the use of a sufficient volume injected high in the axilla with firm digital pressure *should* reach the nerves in the vast majority of cases. Actually, the axillary nerve is probably missed more frequently than the musculocutaneous, but usually when one chooses an axillary block appropriately, the site of surgery is such that missing the axillary nerve is not important. The musculocutaneous nerve, on the other hand, innervates the extensive lateral portion of the forearm from the wrist to the elbow, so it is extremely important to block this nerve for wrist and forearm surgery. If the musculocutaneous nerve has been missed, it can be blocked at either of two levels: it can be blocked an inch or two above the elbow, where it emerges from between the biceps and brachialis muscles to become subcutaneous (Chapter II, de Jong's technique); but it must be remembered that when the nerve is blocked at this level, it has already given off its muscular branches to the powerful flexors of the forearm, so blockade at this level will not provide relaxation of these muscles. If one needs to block both the muscular and cutaneous portions of the musculocutaneous nerve, this can be done by injecting 5-7 ml superior to the axillary artery into the substance of the coracobrachialis muscle (Chapter III); for as soon as the musculocutaneous nerve leaves the axillary sheath, it immediately penetrates the substance of the coracobrachialis muscle and runs the entire length of that muscle giving off its muscular branches to the coracobrachialis, brachialis, and biceps muscles (Chapter I). A single injection of 5-8 ml into the coracobrachialis muscle is sufficient to block the musculocutaneous nerve, since the fascia investing this small cylindrical muscle will confine the local anesthetic to the muscle around the nerve.

Medical problems of the surgical patient, though unrelated to the surgery, may also affect the anesthetist's choice of technique: for example, in the patient with severe bronchial asthma or advanced pulmonary disease of any sort, techniques carried out above the clavicle are best avoided, because of the fact that phrenic block, or pneumothorax, no matter how unlikely, could be disastrous, and in the asthmatic even sympathetic block could produce adverse results (Chapter V). As a matter of fact, if bilateral blockade is required for surgery in any patient, while the interscalene or subclavian perivascular technique can be sequentially administered, it is perhaps wisest to utilize an axillary block on one side and either of the supraclavicular techniques on the other.

Another factor that affects the choice of a particular technique of brachial plexus block is the ability of the patient to cooperate: the axillary and subclavian perivascular techniques of brachial block require a considerable degree of patient cooperation, because very slight movement can make it extremely difficult and potentially dangerous to carry out the technique. On the other hand, the interscalene technique is particularly useful in patients who are unwilling or unable to cooperate due to inebriation, disorientation, or the extremes of age. Infants and small children, for example, may be simply but effectively immobilized by applying firm pressure on both shoulders and on the forehead, which is held turned to the opposite side. In such patients, it is particularly important that the needle be inserted with the syringe attached by a length of tubing, so that when contact with the transverse process is made or a paresthesia is elicited, aspiration and injection can be accomplished quickly. If the needle has been properly directed with special care being taken to assure the slight caudad direction, there are no vital structures at this level that could cause complications, should the patient move suddenly.

Choice of technique in infants and children

As stated earlier, in the hands of a competent and empathetic anesthetist, brachial plexus anesthesia can be utilized most effectively in infants and children, not only for surgery, but also as a means of providing a sympathetic block or even as a means of providing postoperative pain relief after painful surgery carried out under general anesthesia. Whatever the indication, in infants little cooperation is required; the infant is simply immobilized and the block carried out as quickly as possible. In older children capable of communication and understanding, a sympathetic but straightforward approach with strong parental support can usually convince the child to cooperate, *provided* he understands exactly what is going to happen to him, and most importantly, how much it will hurt. It may help, where the parent is not too anxious, to have the father and/or mother present during the performance of the block to enlist the cooperation of the child. On the other hand, if the parents are anxious and nervous about the procedure, it is better to deal with the child on a one-to-one basis.

As stated earlier, children are the only patients in whom the author utilizes a skin wheal, so that the patient can be promised that he or she will only experience one "stick" or "pinch". Frequently it is helpful for the anesthetist to demonstrate to the patient that he can stick himself with the small 25 or 26-gauge needle used to raise a skin wheal without any apparent pain. Obviously, if the patient is unable or unwilling to cooperate, even after sincere and sympathetic attempts to gain his or her cooperation, "permissive" doses of ketamine (1-2 mg/kg) may be administered intramuscularly to render the patient passively permissive but able to cooperate. However, ketamine should be a last resort, and should not be used as a "crutch" routinely to obviate the need for establishing rapport with the child.

While the author has utilized all three approaches to the brachial plexus in infants and children, the axillary and subclavian perivascular techniques have been abandoned, except in special cases, in favor of the interscalene technique, which can be used almost *routinely* in infants and children. The reason for this is the fact that in infants and children the anterior and middle scalene muscles are not yet fully developed and hence are not in contact with one another. As a result, the interscalene groove is truly an inter-scalene space, and the palpating fingers of the anesthetist can easily discern, in most cases, the tips of the cervical transverse processes. Therefore, having raised a skin wheal at the level of C_6, a short, 25-gauge needle is simply inserted and advanced until contact with the transverse process is made, after which aspiration and injection are carried out very quickly. In this age group, paresthesias are *not* sought, and because the space between the scalenes is so wide, most of the time it is possible to contact the transverse process without encountering a nerve root. It is important that, as the block is being carried out, the anesthetist keep constant verbal contact with the patient, explaining precisely what is going on and assuring him that "we're almost through".

In assessing the onset and progression of a block in children, it is necessary to rely heavily on the signs of motor block-ade, saving sensory testing with a needle until anesthesia is complete. In an infant one can readily demonstrate the onset of flaccid paralysis in the extremity and then much later, demonstrate lack of a response to pinprick. Most children, after they are convinced that they will be pain free, completely relax and become fascinated with their surroundings and eager to talk to the anesthetist, who now has demonstrated his "magic" and made him a good friend. Because the interscalene space is "wide open" in infants and children, and because the artery is still small, provided the volume is adequate; the anesthetic solution has ready access to *all* of the roots of the plexus, and unlike the situation in adults, it is the exception rather than the rule to have inadequate anesthesia in the distribution of C_8 and T_1.

Schulte-Steinberg feels regional anesthesia in the awake pediatric patient should be reserved for children with full stomachs whose surgery cannot await gastric emptying and for those with such severe systemic disease that general anesthesia would, be life threatening, but even in these situations, only if the child is amenable and the surgeon is accustomed to working under regional anesthesia. He prefers to induce basal anesthesia with nitrous oxide and oxygen, ketamine, or barbiturates and utilize the technique described by Aizenberg, who utilizes a nerve stimulator to carry out brachial plexus anesthesia in children so that he does not require their cooperation. Like Eriksson and Nielsel, Schulte-Steinberg prefers the axillary approach in children, and all three agree with Aizenberg that muscle contractions evoked by a nerve stimulator provide a better index of proper needle placement than pulsation, though Nielsel only achieved a 60% success rate using a nerve stimulator to carry out axillary block. Interestingly enough, the table developed by Nielsel indicating appropriate volumes of prilocaine for axillary block in children gives volumes very similar to those advocated by the author.

Axillary Brachial Plexus Block Volumes Equipotent to One Per Cent Prilocaine

Age (years)	Volume (ml)
1-3	6-9
4-6	9-11
7-9	14-20
10-12	21-25
13-15	28-35

After Eriksson and Nielsel.

Data from Eriksson, E.: Axillary Brachial Plexus Anesthesia in Children with Citanest. Acta Anaesthesiol. Scand., 16:291, 1965; and Nielsel, H.C., Rodrigues, P., and Wilsmann, I.: Regional Anaesthesie der oberen Extremität bei Kindern, Anaesthetist., 23:178, 1974.

Determination of volume of local anesthetic

The volume-anesthesia relationships described in Chapter III are the result of studies carried out on healthy adult males. As with peridural anesthesia, the appropriate volume of anesthetic required to produce a given level of anesthesia will vary somewhat with size, and to a lesser extent, with age and sex. Our experience has shown *height* to be the single most important factor in determing the correct volume for either sex at any age. In infants and children, of course, sex and age become operative only because they have a direct bearing on height.

That height is the most important determinant of volume is not surprising, since it is well known that the distance from fingertip to fingertip closely approximates the height; so it follows that, since the fingertip to fingertip distance will be related to the length of the brachial plexus "sheath", the height can be utilized as an index of this length. If an individual patient is fully grown, i.e., if he has achieved "adulthood", then in the vast majority of cases the appropriate volume can be determined by dividing the height in inches by 2, with the understanding that if *extensive* anesthesia is required in the areas missed most frequently by that technique, the volume should be increased 5–10 ml, whereas if only limited anesthesia is required, the volume may be reduced by 5–10 ml. In infants and children determination of the appropriate volume is more complicated, and a table has been developed empirically to facilitate calculation of the proper volume and concentration in the pediatric age group. Again, the calculated volume must be increased or decreased slightly if "extensive" or "limited" anesthesia is desired,

Guide to Determination of Volume in Perivascular Anesthesia

Age, years	Sex – Height in inches				Formula to determine volume, ml.	Concentration
	Male	Volume, ml.	Female,	Volume, ml.		
Birth	21	4	20	4		
1	30	6	30	6		
2	36	7	36	7	Height / 5	0.7 to 0.8
3	40	8	40	8		
4	43	9	43	9		
5	46	12	45	11		
6	49	12.5	48	12	Height / 4	0.8 to 0.9
7	52	13	51	12.5		
8	54	14	53	13		
9	56	18.5	55	18		
10	58	19	57.5	19		
11	60	20	60	20		
12	62	21	63	21	Height / 3	0.9 to 1.0
13	65	22	65	22		
14	68	23	66	22		
15	70	23	66	22		
16	71	25	66	22.5		
After maximum growth	70 and above	Use formula	66 and above	Use formula	Height / 2	1.0 to 1.5

and the concentration may be decreased somewhat in patients of poor physical status.

It is to be emphasized that this table, like tables for determining the proper size of an endotracheal tube, is provided as a rough guide for the beginner. The anesthesiologist experienced in perivascular brachial plexus techniques in children does not require such a table, any more than one experienced in pediatric endotracheal anesthesia needs a table to determine the proper size of a tube. Certainly, no table replaces the clinical judgment obtained through experience, but one may be useful until such experience has been gained.

In adults many anesthetists simply "flood" the brachial plexus, using 40 ml of local anesthetic routinely, regardless of technique. Since this large volume will increase the chances that all of the components of the plexus will be bathed at any given level and because the "excess" local anesthetic will ascend and descend in the perivascular compartment bathing a greater *length* of the component parts, the chances of a complete successful block are enhanced. With this approach, however, it is important to make certain that the maximum dosage for that agent is not exceeded.

Two injection techniques

As stated in Chapter III, one of the more common techniques of performing axillary block is to make two injections into the axillary sheath, one superior to and the other inferior to the axillary artery. To the author this practice seems illogical, since the axillary perivascular space com-

209

14

pletely surrounds the vessels and nerves of the plexus and a single injection of an adequate volume is sufficient to bathe all of the contents of that space. Furthermore, in making a separate injection above and below the vessels, into the perivascular compartment, one is really carrying out two separate axillary blocks in the same patient; and since every technique has a finite failure rate, performing the technique twice is going to enhance the likelihood of missing the sheath at least once. In this situation only half of the calculated volume of local anesthetic will be in the sheath, minimizing the extent of the block and maximizing the possibility that several nerves will be missed.

This two-injection technique *appeared* to become more logical when Rorie and Thompson demonstrated the presence of septa which they feel divides the perivascular space into several compartments, so that more than one injection would be required in order to fill each of the compartments. However, the high success rate achieved with single injections into the perivascular compartment would seem to indicate that these septa, undoubtedly present, must be porous membranes incapable of altering the flow of injected local anesthetic solutions within the perivascular space.

However, since with any of the perivascular techniques success depends not only on bathing all of the component parts of the plexus but also on bathing these components for an adequate distance, it was logical for someone to consider two injections, one into the upper part and one into the lower part of the perivascular compartment. And indeed, several years ago Reese, and more recently Galindo, described a technique consisting of two injections, one made above the clavicle to block the upper components of the plexus and the other in the axilla to block the lower components, with half the calculated volume being deposited at each location. The only criticism the author has of this approach is that it makes a simple technique more complex, and in the vast majority of cases, it is simply unnecessary. Continuing the analogy with peridural techniques, this practice is similar to the combination, popular in some institutions, of lumbar epidural anesthesia for labor and caudal for delivery: it seems anatomically and physiologically logical, but complicates a simple technique and in the vast majority of cases is unnecessary. However, if an interscalene or subclavian block fails to provide *complete* anesthesia of the brachial plexus, a supplemental axillary block is most appropriate since paresthesias are unnecessary.

Technical Considerations

Sterile technique

The same antiseptic preparation of the skin should be carried out prior to the performance of a brachial plexus block as is carried out with a spinal or epidural block. Thus, after palpating the landmarks of a patient, the skin is prepared carefully with alcohol, betadine, or both. In preparing the skin for an axillary block, it is important that, unless the patient routinely shaves the axilla, the axilla should *not* be shaved. While there are no studies concerning a causal relationship between the shaving of axillary hair and infection, one can extrapolate the studies carried out concerning such a relationship between the shaving of pubic hair and infection: in a five-year prospective study of 23,649 surgical wounds, Cruse and Foord found that in patients who were shaved, the surgical infection rate was 2.3%; in patients who had no shave, but only had their hair clipped, the infection rate fell to 1.7%; and in patients who had no shave or clipping the infection rate was only 0.9%. Obviously, the irritation and the minor trauma produced by shaving or clipping must actually *contribute* to infection, rather than preventing it. This finding is in agreement with another study published by Seropian and Reynolds who reported that in 406 patients undergoing lower abdominal surgery, the infection rate was 5.6% after razor preparation, 0.6% after depilatory preparation, and 0.6% after no preparation whatsoever. Furthermore, they also showed that the *time* of razor preparation had a dramatic effect of infection rate: when the patient was shaved just prior to surgery, the infection rate was 3.1%; when the patient was shaved up to 24 hours prior to surgery, the infection rate was 7.1%; and when the shave was carried out over 24 hours before surgery, the infection rate was 20%! It is clear from these studies that bacterial liberation and growth after razor preparation injury actually enhances the possibility of infection, and therefore it would seem that shaving the axilla, especially just prior to the administration of an axillary block, would only serve to increase, rather than decrease, the likelihood of infection. The author and his colleagues have utilized aseptic preparation of the skin in several thousands of patients without shaving the axilla, and not a single case of infection has been encountered. It is possible that the antimicrobial activity of all of the presently available local anesthetics plays more of a role in infection control than the antiseptic preparation of the skin. (See chapter V). Nonetheless, sterile preparation of the skin provides the first line of defense against infection.

Following preparation of the skin, the author does not ordinarily drape off the area of the block, as is done with spinal or epidural anesthesia, since such draping masks or obscures many important landmarks. Needless to say, sterile gloves are worn during the performance of the block, and care is taken that all of the equipment utilized in the performance of the block by the anesthestist is sterile. An exception is occasionally made in patients whose landmarks are difficult to palpate: in such a case, if it is anticipated that the use of rubber gloves will jeopardize the possibility of locating landmarks that might be difficult to palpate, the hands of the anesthetist may be scrubbed and prepared just as the neck is prepared. If the antiseptic solution can, indeed, control or eliminate the bacterial flora of the patient on contact, it should logically do likewise on the hands of the anesthetist. Nonetheless, when working without gloves, the anesthetist should attempt to avoid touching the shaft of the needle and should penetrate the skin of the patient at a site untouched by the palpating fingers.

The Immobile Needle

Success with any nerve block depends not only on the initial, precise placement of the needle, but also on subsequent stabilization of that needle during aspiration and injection of the local anesthetic solution. Attaching and detaching a syringe directly to a needle may dislodge the tip of the needle from its original desired position and result in incomplete or inadequate anesthesia. To avoid this possibility, about 15 years ago the author began to utilize a simple and inexpensive technique which allows complete immobilization of the needle throughout the entire performance of the block: a small-bore disposable, intravenous extension tubing is interposed between the needle and the syringe containing the anesthetic solution.

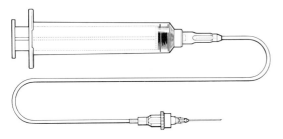

After the entire system has been filled with anesthetic solution, the needle is properly placed for the desired nerve block procedure. After obtaining an appropriate paresthesia or after entering the proper fascial plane, aspiration is carried out and the anesthetic is injected, with repeated, intermittent aspiration throughout the injection. The important feature of this system is that, because of the interposition of the flexible plastic tubing between the needle and the syringe, movement of the syringe does not produce movement of the needle. Many anesthetists find it more convenient to utilize two 20 ml syringes instead of a single 50 ml syringe. This, of course, requires that after the first 20 ml syringe is empty, that syringe must be detached and another full syringe attached. With this system, such activity can be carried out without the possibility of dislodging the needle by moving it. The use of the "immobile needle" has unquestionably avoided many failures or partial blocks, particularly in cases where removal and attach-

ment of the syringe to the needle would have proven to be mechanically difficult or awkward. Furthermore, the use of the immobile needle is the only way that the hub of the needle can lie in its proper position against the skin of the neck in carrying out the subclavian perivascular technique of brachial block, since connection of a large syringe for injection of the local anesthetic directly to the needle would require that the hub of the needle be tilted away from the neck. Again, such movement of the proximal end of the needle would undoubtedly alter the position of the tip of the needle and jeopardize the success of the block. Worthy of mention is the fact that if care is not taken to fill the extension tubing completely with local anesthetic agent, several ml's of air may be injected during performance of the block. This is not a serious occurrence, assuming the injection is not intravascular, but it could give rise to needless alarm on the part of the anesthetist that this "subcutaneous emphysema" represents a developing pneumothorax!

There are two other characteristics of the immobile needle that are important, both for success and for safety: the first is a short-bevel needle, and the second is a translucent (or preferably, transparent) plastic hub.

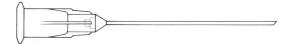

Originally, the author advocated the use of a short-bevel needle because such a bevel allows better perception of the "click" produced when the needle penetrates fascial planes; and indeed, this is still a valuable feature provided by the short-bevel needle. However, more recently Selander has demonstrated that short-bevel needles produce significantly less nerve damage when they contact nerves, particularly if the needle is inserted such that the tip enters the nerve with the bevel in the long axis of the nerve fibers (see Chapter V). As a matter of fact, Selander, like many before him, has questioned the possibility of making an intraneural injection when a short-bevel needle is utilized, except under extremely unusual circumstances.

The reason a *translucent,* plastic hub is desirable is that it allows slightly earlier recognition of the intravascular placement of a needle during brachial plexus block: if the hub of the needle is translucent, then blood will become visible as soon as the shaft of the needle is filled, whereas if the hub of the needle is opaque, the entire shaft *and hub* must be filled before blood becomes visible to the anesthetist. While this may seem to be a minute detail, if the use of a translucent hub can prevent even the rare occurrence of an intravascular injection, then it assumes a much greater importance.

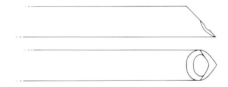

Unfortunately, the ideal block needle is not available in the United States. Selander's studies indicate that to minimize trauma to the nerves, the ideal bevel angle is 45°, a bevel that is available in the United States only on a Crawford point epidural needle, a needle having an opaque, metal hub and having a shaft that is simply too long.

However, the major needle manufacturers in the United States all make a "B-bevel" needle, which has a bevel of 19°, intermediate between the usual A-bevel (12°) and Selander's 45° bevel, and it is available with a translucent hub, 1½ inch length, and 22-gauge shaft.

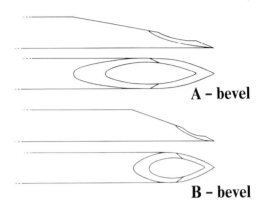

A – bevel

B – bevel

The immobile needle concept was recently adopted in Great Britain by Hillman and in Germany by Zenz and Glocker, and as a result a German manufacturer has made a unit consisting of a 24-gauge needle, having a 45° bevel and an opaque hub (unfortunately) connected to a small-bore extension tube with Luer-Lok fittings. The only disadvantages of this system, in the opinion of the author, are that the hub is not translucent, the 24-gauge needle limits the rate of injection, and the extension tubing is so short that it restricts somewhat the ability of the anesthetist to move the needle without "tugging" on the syringe. Nonetheless, at the present time this is the closest thing to an ideal needle currently available anywhere.

Continuous techniques

If sensory, motor, and/or sympathetic blockade are desirable for a longer duration than that provided by the long acting local anesthetics, as with peridural techniques a catheter may be inserted into the perivascular compartment to allow intermittent injections of local anesthetics over a period of many hours or days.

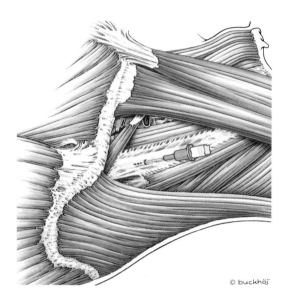

© buckhöj

Early experience with catheters inserted through a needle ("Intra-caths") were far from ideal, since the needle made a hole in the sheath which was larger than the catheter, and this resulted in excessive leakage of local anesthetic after removal of the needle. However, the advent of "around the needle" catheters ("Extra-caths"), particularly the more recently introduced small-bore versions, has rendered continuous brachial plexus anesthesia technically very simple. The author has utilized continuous brachial plexus block by all three approaches, and it is his belief that technically the subclavian perivascular technique provides the best results. When the axillary approach is utilized, movement of the upper extremity, whether active or passive, raises and lowers the apex of the axilla and thus tends to

move the indwelling catheter in and/or out of the perivascular compartment. With the interscalene technique, the catheter is at right angles to the sheath and skin, so that movement of the head or shoulders tends to advance or withdraw the catheter. When a catheter has been inserted utilizing the subclavian perivascular technique, the external part of the catheter lies flat against the neck and movement of the head and neck simply bends the catheter without the tendency to advance or withdraw it.

The continuous technique is carried out exactly like the single-injection technique, except that it may be advisable to raise a skin wheal and "nick" the skin with a large needle to prevent the catheter from "puckering" on the shaft as it penetrates the skin. Once a paresthesia has been obtained, the first injection is made through the needle to expand the perivascular compartment and ascertain (through the development of anesthesia) that the needle is properly placed. Then as the needle is withdrawn, the catheter is advanced *slightly* to prevent its leaving the sheath, after which it is "capped" with a rubber injection site and taped to the neck. Some authors have attached the catheter to a continuous-infusion pump to maintain anesthesia indefinitely, but it has been more desirable in our practice to make injections intermittently, allowing transient recovery from the block to allow assessment of function.

While continuous techniques of brachial plexus block were introduced even before the availability of plastic catheters to provide prolonged anesthesia of the brachial plexus, the development of longer-acting local anesthetics has reduced the necessity of continuous techniques for most surgical cases, though the introduction of sophisticated microvascular and reconstructive surgical techniques may reverse this trend. Nonetheless, Selander in Sweden has advocated the *routine* use of a catheter technique for axillary blocks to avoid the need for vasoconstrictors to prolong anesthesia, to allow supplemental injections of local anesthetic to be made when insufficient volume has resulted in an incomplete block, and of course, to allow for prolonged anesthesia, if such becomes desirable. Hemple in Germany has described a similiar *routine* catheter technique above the clavicle, similar in that the direction of needle insertion is identical to that utilized with the axillary technique but above the clavicle. From an anatomical standpoint it would appear that the risk of pleural puncture would be increased with this technique, but the results achieved by Hemple and his co-workers with this "longitudinal supraclavicular technique" were excellent, and the incidence of serious complications was nil. Again, this group felt that the catheter allowed supplemental injections to be made when the volume utilized for the first injection proved to be inadequate, and that their experience indicated that repeated injections of short-acting local anesthetics are superior to a single-injection of a long-acting agent.

Finally, Rosenblatt has demonstrated that a brachial plexus catheter can be inserted by a modified Seldinger technique, but this technique requires the introduction of an 18-gauge epidural needle into the interscalene space, and should nerve contact be made, the *potential* for nerve damage would seem to be excessive. Nonetheless, in the one case reported by Rosenblatt, this technique was used safely and effectively.

The nerve stimulator

Throughout this book, and particularly in Chapter III, little has been said concerning the use of a nerve stimulator in properly placing the needle with any of the techniques described. That is because the author firmly believes that there is no indicator which demonstrates more precisely that the needle is in close proximity to a nerve than the production of a paresthesia. The response to a nerve stimulator depends not only on the distance between the needle and the nerve but also on the magnitude of the stimulus producing the response. And finally, the perivascular techniques were developed in an effort to *simplify* conduction anesthesia of the upper extremity, and the use of a nerve stimulator would seem to complicate these techniques. But every technique has advantages and disadvantages, and the use of a nerve stimulator is no exception: the nerve stimulator provides an excellent teaching tool in that the student can visually determine which component of the plexus is being stimulated by noting the muscular response to that stimulation. When a nerve stimulator is used, there is no need to produce a paresthesia, an unpleasant, if not painful experience for the patient, although paresthesias may inadvertently be produced while using a nerve stimulator. Patient cooperation is unnecessary, which allows the technique to be utilized in patients who are heavily sedated, depressed, or semicomatose; and if contact with the nerve is not made, then the possibility of nerve damage from such contact is ruled out. A major disadvantage, other than the initial objection mentioned above, is the fact that it is possible to stimulate the various components of the plexus *through* the sheath and hence make an injection outside the sheath, resulting in complete or partial failure.

The use of electrical stimulation to carry out a brachial plexus block is not new: Perthes utilized electrical stimulation to locate the brachial plexus just one year after Kulenkampff first described his technique, but Perthes' equipment was cumbersome and his needles crudely insulated with lacquer, so the technique was readily forgotten. In 1955 Pearson demonstrated that motor nerves could be located by electrical stimulation with an insulated needle, but it was not until 1962, when Greenblatt and Denson reported a portable, transistorized nerve stimulator, that the use of electrical stimulation in regional anesthesia became practical and feasible. Using needles insulated except at the tip with plastic paint, these investigators demonstrated that because sensory stimulation requires a higher voltage than motor stimulation, nerves can be located using voltages high enough to stimulate motor fibers without causing any discomfort to the patient; and in fact, they demonstrated the quantitative relationship between the voltage required for motor stimulation and the distance of the needle from the nerve.

Nonetheless, even the equipment utilized by Greenblatt and Denson was expensive and, more important, was not readily available; so further reports concerning the use of electrical stimulation for regional anesthesia were not forthcoming until 1969, when Wright indicated the feasibility of utilizing a "Block-Aid Monitor" for nerve blocks and Koons reported the utility of the "Rochester" needle, the first "extra-cath", as an insulated needle. Now the tools required were readily available to all anesthetists; and yet it was the demonstration by Montgomery and Raj that standard, uninsulated needles could be utilized to stimulate nerves that gave the greatest impetus to the use of electrical stimulation in regional anesthesia. These investigators pointed out that, while some of the current applied to an unshielded needle leaves all along the shaft, the greatest density of current is at the tip.

The technique developed and popularized by Raj is as follows: the ground electrode is attached to an EKG pad which is placed on the opposite shoulder. The exploring electrode is connected to the hub or shaft (if the hub is plastic) of a 22-gauge, $1\frac{1}{2}$ inch needle connected to the syringe containing the anesthetic solution by an extension set. The voltage control is turned to the fourth marking, with a switch frequency of 1 pulse per second on the stimulator. The needle is advanced slowly while the forearm and hand are observed carefully for muscle movement. Flexion or extension of the elbow, wrist, or digits confirms that the needle is in close proximity to the nerve fibers of the brachial plexus. The best results will be obtained if movements of the hand or fingers are produced. When such movements have been produced, the voltage is reduced and the needle moved deeper and more superficially to find maximum contraction at the same stimulation. After careful aspiration, 1–2 ml of local anesthetic are injected through the needle, and this should result in reduced muscle movements at that voltage. If a reduction in muscle movement does not occur, stimulation may be coming from the side of the needle, in which case the needle should be repositioned and the procedure repeated. When muscle movements are reduced by several ml's of local anesthetic, the remaining anesthetic solution should be injected through the needle. One or two minutes later, further testing should show no muscle movement except at very high voltages.

The technique of electrical stimulation described by Raj has become quite popular, particularly at teaching institutions. Its major appeal, contrary to previous techniques, is that equipment readily available to all anesthetists is utilized. However, several controlled studies comparing nerve blocks carried out using a nerve stimulator with nerve blocks carried out using paresthesias showed no advantage of the nerve stimulator over paresthesias. Recently Galindo has stated that the failure of the nerve stimulator in such studies to provide results superior to those achieved with paresthesias is due to the equipment utilized: first of all, he points out it is the current, not the voltage, that causes a nerve to depolarize, and since the stimulators utilized by Raj and others control only the voltage, the current flowing from the needle at any voltage will depend upon the resistance between the two electrodes. Since this resistance is unknown but certainly variable, the flow of current from the needle will be completely unpredictable. Furthermore, since the needle is not insulated except at the tip, "false" localization of nerves because of current leakage from the shaft of the needle can lead to misplacement of the needle and anesthetic failure.

Since the minimal stimulating current or threshold current is constant for peripheral nerves from patient to patient, electrical stimulation should be carried out, according to Galindo, with an instrument that generates a "constant current" and with needles insulated by teflon except at the tip, so that the response to stimulation can *only* result from current flowing from the tip of the needle.

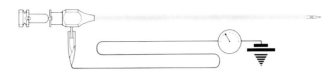

Galindo, A.: Special Needle for Nerve Blocks. Regional Anesthesia 5: 12-13, 1980.
Reprinted by permission from J. B. Lippencott Company.

Therefore, Galindo has designed an instrument that delivers a constant current and monitors the current dilivered continuously, and has also designed 22-gauge and 25-gauge $1\frac{1}{2}$ inch needles which are coated with teflon except at the tip. Using this equipment the technique is carried out in a manner similar to that described by Raj, but starting with a current of 3 milliamps. As the needle approaches a nerve, the current is reduced as the response increases. Galindo's experience indicates that if the current requried for a response is below 1 mA (ideally below 0.5 mA), there is contact between the uninsulated tip of the needle and the nerve. Conversely, if a current above 1 mA is required, there is some distance between the tip of the needle and the nerve. Thus, when stimulation has been produced by a current below 1 mA, after aspirating, two-thirds of the calculated volume is injected. If a motor response persists, the current is turned to the maximum setting, and the remainder of the anesthetic solution is injected until there is no motor response, even at maximal stimulation.

While evaluation of this refined technique awaits more widespread use, the fact that it requires "special equipment" not readily available may discourage such use. Furthermore, the needles are expensive and are only available with a "pencil point" (see Chapter V), which may discourage many anesthetists from using them. These needles, designed to minimize nerve trauma, have an apperture quite proximal to the true tip of the needle, so it is possible that the needle tip might have penetrated the sheath of the brachial plexus while the opening of the

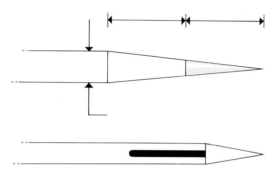

needle is still proximal to it. Again, further evaluation is necessary before the utility of these needles can be judged.

References & Bibliography

Pharmacological considerations

Akamatsu, J. T.: The Synergistic Toxicity of Local Anesthetics. Anesthesiology 28: 238, 1967.

Bieter, R. N.: Applied Pharmacology of Local Anesthetics. Am. J. Surg. 34: 500-510, 1934.

Bonica, J. J., More, D. C., and Orlov, M.: Brachial Plexus Block Anesthesia. Am. J. Surg. 98: 65-79, 1949.

Bonica, J. J.: Regional Anesthesia With Tetracaine. Anesthesiology 11: 606-622, 1950.

Bonica, J. J.: Regional Anesthesia With Tetracaine: Clinical Investigation of the Pharmacologic Properties of Tetracaine. Anesthesiology 11: 716-729, 1950.

Bromage, P. R., Gertel, M.: An Evaluation of Two New Local Anesthetics for Major Conduction Blockade. Can. Anaes. Soc. J. 17: 557-564, 1970.

Bromage, P. R., and Gertel, M.: Brachial Plexus Anesthesia in Chronic Renal Failure. Anesthesiology 36 (5): 448-493, (May) 1972.

Bromage, P. R., Gertel, M.: Improved Brachial Plexus Blockade with Bupivacaine. Hydrochloride and Carbonated Lidocaine. Anesthesiology 36: 479-487, 1972.

Büchi J. and Perlia X.: Structure-activity Relations and Physico-chemical properties of Local Anesthetics, Ch 2 in Lechat P. (Ed.): Local Anesthetics, Sect 8, Vol. 1, Intern Encycl Pharmacol Therap. Pergamon, Oxford, 1971.

Cohen, S. E.: The Rational Use of Local Anesthetic Mixtures. Regional Anesthesia 4: 11-12, 1979.

Cohen, S. E.: and Thurlow, A.: Comparison of a Chloroprocaine-Bupivacaine Mixture with Chloroprocaine and Bupivacaine Used Individually for Obstetric Epidural Analgesia. Anesthesiology 51:228-292, 1979.

Corke, B. C., Carlson, G., and Dettbarn, W-D.: The Intereaction of 2-Chloroprocaine and Bupivacaine. (Abstract) Anesthesiology 55: A162, 1981.

Cousins, M. J. and Bridenbaugh, P. O.: Neural Blockade in Clinical Anesthesia. J. P. Lippencot and Co. Philadelphia p. 49, 1980.

Covino, B. G., Vassalo, H. G.: Local Anesthetics, Mechanisms of Action and Clinical Use, p. 49, Grune & Stratton, 1976.

Covino, B. G., Marx, G. F., Finster, M. and Zsigmond, E. K.: (Editorial) Prolonged Sensory/Motor Deficits Following Inadvertent Spinal Anesthesia. Anesth. and Analg. 59: 399-400, 1980.

Cunningham, N. L., and Kaplan, J. A.: A Rapid-onset, Long-acting Regional Anesthetic Technique. Anesthesiology 41: 509-511, 1974.

Daos, F. G., Lopez, L., and Virtue, R. W.: Local Anesthetic Modified by Oxygen and by Combination of Agents. Anesthesiology 23: 755-761, 1962.

Defalque, R. J., and Stoelting, V. K.: Latency and Duration of Action of Some Local Anesthetic Mixtures. Anesth. & Analg. 45: 106-116, 1966.

Galindo, A., and Witcher, T.: Critical Blocking Length as Related to Conduction Velocity. (ASA Abstracts) Anesthesiology 51: S218, 1979.

Galindo, A., and Witcher, T.: Mixtures of Local Anesthetics: Bupivacaine- Chloroprocaine. Anesth. & Analg. 59: 683-685, 1980.

Galindo, A., Schou, M., and Witcher, T.: pH Adjusted Local Anesthetics. (Abstract) 6th Annual Meeting of the American Society of Regional Anesthesia, March-pages 12-15, 1979.

Galindo, A.: pH-Adjusted Local Anesthetics: Clinical Experience. (Meeting Abstracts) Regional Anesthesia 8:35-36, 1983.

Hilgier, M.: Alkalinization of Marcaine for Prolongation of Brachial Block. Regional Anesthesia 8: 1983.

Hodgkinson, R., Husain, F. J., and Bluhm, C.: Reduced Effectiveness of Bupivacaine 0.5% to Relieve Labor Pain After Prior Injection of Chloroprocaine 2%. (Abstract) Anesthesiology 57: A201, 1982.

Hollmen, A.: Axillary Plexus Block: A Double-Blind Study of 59 Cases Using Mepivacaine and LAC-43. Acta Anaesth. Scandinav. (Supplementum XXI): 53-65, 1966.

Hudgins P. M. and Putney J. W.: Distribution of Local Anesthetics and the Intracellular pH in Vascular Smooth Muscle. J. Pharmacol Exp. Ther. 181:538-546, 1972.

Kennedy, W. F. Jr., Ward, R. J., Tolas, A. G., Martin, W. E. and Grinstein, A.: Cardiorespiratory Effects of Epinephrine When Used in Regional Anesthesia. Acta Anaesth. Scandinav. 10 (Supp. 23) 320, 1966.

Kennedy Jr., W. F., Bonica. J. J., Ward, R. J., Tolas, C. G., Martin, W. E., and Grinstein, A.: Cardiorespiratory Effects of Epinephrine When Used in Regional Anesthesia. Acta Anaesthesiologica Scandinavica (Supplementum XXIII, Proceedings I of the 2nd European Congress of Anaesthesiology), pp. 320-333, 1966.

Kim, J-M., Goto, H., and Arakawa, K.: Duration of Bupivacaine Intradermal Anesthesia When The Bupivacaine is Mixed with Chloroprocaine. Anesth. & Analg. 58: 364-366, 1979.

Lalka, D., Vicuna, N., Burrow, S. R., Jones, D. J., Ludden, T. M., Haegele, K. D., and McNay, J. L.: Bupivacaine and Other Amide Local Anesthetics Inhibit the Hydrolysis of Chloroprocaine by Human Serum. Anesth. & Analg. 57: 534-539, 1978.

Leser, A. J.: Duration of Local Anesthesia in Relation to Concentrations of Procaine and Epinephrine. Anesthesiology 1: 205-207, 1940.

Lund, P. C., Cwik, J. C., Vallesteros, F.: Bupivacaine - A New Long-Acting Local Anesthetic Agent: A Preliminary Clinical and Laboratory Report. Anesth. & Analg. 49:103-112, 1970.

Lund, P. C., Cwik, J. C. and Pagdanganan, R. T.: Etidocaine – A New Long-Acting Local Anesthetic Agent: A Clinical Evaluation. Anesth. & Analg. 52: 482-494, 1973.

Löfström, B.: Clinical Evaluation of Local Anesthetics. Clin. Anesth. 2/ 1969:20-43, 1971.

Martin, W. E., Kennedy, W. F. Jr., Bonica, J. J., Stegall, F., and Ward, R. J.: Effect of Epinephrine on Arteriolar Vasodilation Produced by Brachial Plexus Block. Acta Anaesth. Scandinav. 10: Supp. 23, 313, 1966.

Mazze, R. I. and Dunbar, R. W.: Plasma Lidocaine Concentrations After Caudal, Lumbar Epidural, Axillary Block, and Intravenous Regional Anesthesia. Anesthesiology 27: 574-579, 1966.

McClure, J. H. and Scott, D. B.: Comparison of Bupivacaine Hydrochloride and Carbonated Bupivacaine in Brachial Plexus Block by the Interscalene Technique. Br. J. Anaesth. 53: 523-526, 1981.

Meffin, P., Long G. J., and Thomas, J.: Clearance and Metabolism of Mepivacaine in the Human Neonate. Clin. Pharmacol Ther. 14:218-225, 1973.

Moore, D. C.: Pontocaine Hydrochloride for Brachial Block Analgesia: One Hundred and Fifty Cases. Anesthesiology 9: 281-284, 1948.

Moore, D. C.: An Evaluation of Hyaluronidase in Local and Nerve Block Analgesia: A Review of 519 Cases. Anesthesiology 11: 470-484, 1950.

Moore, D. C.: The Use of Pontocaine Hydrochloride for Nerve Block and Infiltration Analgesia, Therapeutic, and Diagnostic Blocks: 1004 Cases. Anesthesiology 11: 65-75, 1950.

Moore, D. C., Bridenbaugh, L. D., Bridenbaugh, P. O. and Tucker, G. T.: Bupivacaine for Peripheral Nerve Block: A Comparison with Mepivacaine, Lidocaine, and Tetracaine. Anesthesiology 32: 460-463, 1970.

Moore, D. C., Bridenbaugh, L. D., Bridenbaugh, P. O., and Thompson, G. E.: Bupivacaine Hydrochloride: A Summary of Investigational Use in 3274 Cases. Anesth. & Analg. 50: 856-869, 1971.

Moore, D. C., Bridenbaugh, L. D., and Thompson, G. R., and Tucker, G. T.: Does Compounding of Local Anesthetic Agents Increase Their Toxicity in Humans? Anesth. & Analg. 51: 579-585, 1972.

Moore, D. C., Bridenbaugh, L. D., Thompson, G. E., Balfour, R. I. and Horton, W. G.: Factors Determining Dosages of Amide-Type Local Anesthetic Drugs. Anesthesiology 47: 263-268, 1977.

Moore, D. C., Bridenbaugh, L. D., Thompson, G. E., Balfour, G. E. and Horton, W. G.: Bupivacaine: A Review of 11,080 Cases. Anesth. & Analg. 57: 42-53, 1978.

Moore, D. C: "Toxic Effects of Local Anesthetics": JAMA 240: 434, 1978 (Letters)).

Moore, D. C.: The pH of Local Anesthetic Solutions. Anesth. & Analg. 60: 833-834, 1981.

Munson, E. S., Paul, W. L., and Embro, W. J.: Central-Nervous-System Toxicity of Local Anesthetic Mixtures in Monkeys. Anesthesiology 46: 179-183, 1977.

Poppers, P. J.: Evaluation of Local Anesthetic Agents for Regional Anaesthesia in Obstetrics. Br. J. Anaesth. 47:322-327, 1975.

Raj, P. P., Rosenblatt, R., Miller, J., Katz, R. L., and Garden, E.: Dynamics of Local-Anesthetic Compounds in Regional Anesthesia. Anesth. & Analg. 56: 110-117, 1977.

Rud, J.: Local Anesthetics. An Electrophysiological Investigation of Local Anesthesia of Peripheral Nerves, with Special Reference to Xylocaine. Acta Physiol Scand. (Suppl.) 178:1-171, 1961.

Selander, D.: Supraclavicular Brachial Plexus Block with Etidocaine without Vasoconstrictor. Acta Anesth. Scand. 60: 29-32, 1975.

Seow, L. T., Lips, F. J., Cousins, M. J., and Mather, L. E.: Lidocaine and Bupivacaine Mixtures for Epidural Blockade. Anesthesiology 56: 177-183, 1982.

Schulte-Steinberg, O., Hartmuth, J., and Schutt, L.: Carbon Dioxide Salts of Lignocaine in Brachial Plexus Block. Anaesthesia 25: 191, 1970.

Tucker, G. T., Moore, D. C., Bridenbaugh, P. O., Bridenbaugh, L. D. and Thompson, G. E.: Systemic Absorption of Mepivacaine in Commonly Used Regional Block Procedures. Anesthesiology 37: 277-287, 1972.

Tucker, G. T., Boyes, R. N., Bridenbaugh, P. O., and Moore, D. C.: Binding of Anilide-type Local Anesthetics in Human Plasma. I. Relationships between Binding, Physicochemical Properties, and Anesthetic Activity. Anesthesiology 33:287-303, 1970a.

Tucker, G. T., Boyes, R. N., Bridenbaugh, P. O., et al: Binding of Anilide-type Local Anesthetics in Human Plasma. II. Implications in vivo, with Special Reference to Transplacental Distribution. Anesthesiology 33:304-314, 1970b.

Widman, B.: Plasma Concentration of Local Anaesthetic Agents in Regard to Absorption, Distribution and Elimination, with Special Reference to Bupivacaine. Br. J. Anaesth. 47:231-236, 1975.

Villa, E. A., and Marx, G. F.: Chloroprocaine - Bupivacaine Sequence for Obstetric Extradural Analgesia. Canad. Anaesth. Soc. Journ. 22 (1): 76-78, 1975.

Winnie, A. P., Tay, C-H., Patel, K. P., Ramamurathy, S., and Durrani, Z.: Pharmacokinetics of Local Anesthetics During Plexus Blocks. Anesth. & Analg... Current Researches 56: 852-861, Number 6, (Nov-Dec) 1973.

Winnie, A. P., LaVallee, D. A., Sosa, B. P. and Masud, K. Z.: Clinical Pharmacokinetics of Local Anaesthetics. Canadian Anaesthetists' Society Journal 24: 252-262, 1977.

Winnie, A. P., Durrani, Z., Masters, R. W., and Patel, K. P., Motorblock Outlosts Sensory Blocks: A Unique Characteristic of Etidocaine? Regional Anesthesia 8:44, 1983.

Surgical considerations

Aizenberg, V. L. and Moisenko, O. L.: Regional Anesthesia of the Upper Extremity in Combination with Nitrous Oxide Analgesia in Children. Khirurgiia (Moks.) 48:26, 1972.

Brandao, R. C., Lerner, S., Rangel, W. and Rodriquez, I.: Brachial Plexus Block [Spanish]. Revista Brasileira de Anestesiologia 21: 420-425 (3), 1971.

Burkhardt, V.: The Place of Brachial Plexus Analgesia in Modern Anesthetic Practice. Recent Progress in Anesthesiology and Resuscitation Excerpta Medica pp. 57-58, 1974.

Erisson, E.: Axillary Brachial Plexus Anaesthesia in Children with Citanest. Acta Anaesthesiol. Scand. 16:291, 1965.

Ferrar, M. D., Scheybani, M. and Nolte, H.: Upper Extremity Block Effectiveness and Complications. Regional Anesthesia 6: 133-134, 1981.

Harley, N., and Gjessing, J.: A Critical Assesment of Supraclavicular Brachial Plexus Block. Anaesthesia 24: 564-570, 1969.

Lanz, E., Theiss, D. and Jankovich, D.: The Extent of Blockade Following Various Techniques of Brachial Plexus Block. Anesth. & Analg. 62: 55-58, 1983.

Lombard, T. P.: The Interscalene Approach to Block of the Brachial Plexus. S. Afr. Med. J. 62: 871-873, 1982.

McClure, J. H. and Scott, D. B.: Comparison of Bupivacaine Hydrochloride and Carbonated Bupivacaine in Brachial Plexus Block by the Interscalene Technique. Br. J. Anesthesia 53: 523-526, 1981.

Niesel, H. C., Rodrigues, P. and Wilsmann, I.: Regional Anesthesia of the Upper Extremity in Children [German]. Anaesthesist. 23:178, 1974.

Rothstin, P., Aurthur G. B., Feldman, H. S., Covino, B. G.: Use of Bupivacaine for Intercostal Nerve Block in Children. Anesthesiology in press.

Schulte-Steinberg, O.: Neural Blockade for Pediatric Surgery. Chapter 21 in "Neural Blockade in Clinical Anesthesia and Management of Pain". Edited by Cousins, M. J. and Bridenbaugh, P. O., J. B. Lippincott Co., Philadelphia, pp. 503-523, 1980.

Vester-Andersen, T., Christiansen, A., Hansen, A., Sørensen, M. and Meisler, C.: Interscalene Brachial Plexus Block: Area of Analgesia, Complications and Blood Concentrations of Local Anesthetics. Acta Anaesth. Scand. 25: 81-84, 1981.

Winnie, A. P., Radonjic, R., et al: Factors Influencing Distribution of Local Anesthetic Injected into the Brachial Plexus Sheath. Anesth. & Analg. 58: 225-234, 1979.

Technical considerations

Ansbro, F. P.: A Method of Continuous Brachial Plexus Block. American Journal of Surgery 71: 716-722, 1946.

Araujo, J. B., Botelho, L. A., Filho, N. D., and Saraiva, R.: Identification of the Brachial Plexus by Electrical Stimulation. [Brasilian]. Revista Brasileira de Anestesiologia 23: 141-145, 1973.

Cruse, P. J. E., Foord, R.: A Five-Year Prospective Study of 23, 649 Surgical Wounds. Arch. Surg. 107: 206-210, 1973.

DeKrey, J. A., Schroeder, C. F., and Buechel, D. R.: Continuous Brachial Plexus Block. Anesthesiology 30: 332, 1969.

Galindo, A. and Galindo, A: Special Needle for Nerve Blocks (Regional Workshop). Regional Anesthesia 5: 12-13, 1980.

Greeenblatt, G. M. and Denson, J. S.: Needle Nerve Stimulator-Locator: Nerve Blocks With a New Instrument for Locating Nerves. Anesth. & Analg... Current Researches 41: 599-602, 1962.

Hempel, V., Van Finck, M., and Baumgartner, E.: A Longitudinal Supraclavicular Approach to the Brachial Plexus for the Insertion of Plastic Cannulas. Anesth. & Analg. 60: 352-355, 1981.

Hillman, K. M.: Brachial Plexus Block. (Correspondence) Anaesthesia 34: 73-84, 1979.

Koons, R. A.: The Use of the Block-Aid Monitor and Plastic Intravenous Cannulas for Nerve Blocks. Anesthesiology 31: 290-291, 1969.

Lanz, E., Theiss, D.: Comparison between Subclavian and Interscalene Brachial Plexus Block [German]. Regional Anaesthesie 2:57-62, 1979.

Manriquez, R. G. and Pallares, V.: Continuous Brachial Plexus Block for Prolonged Sympathectomy and Control of Pain. Anesth. & Analg. 57: 128-130, 1978.

McClain, D. A. and Finucane, B. T.: Interscalene Approach to the Brachial Plexus: Parathesiae vs. Nerve Stimulator. Regional Anesthesia 8: 39, 1983.

Montgomery, S. J., Raj, P. P., Nettles, D., Jenkins, M. T.: The Use of the Nerve Stimulator With Standard Unsheathed Needles in Nerve Blockade. Anesth. & Analg. 52: 827-831, 1973.

Perthes, G.: Conduction Anesthesia with the Help of Electrical Stimulation [German]. München Med. Wochenschr. 59: 2545-2548, (Nov 19) 1912.

Raj, P. P., Montgomery, S. J., Nettles, D., Jenkins, M. T.: Infraclavicular Brachial Plexus Block – A New Approach. Anesth. & Analg. 52: 897-904, 1973.

Raj, P. P.: Ancillary Measures to Assure Success. Regional Anesthesia 5: 9-12, 1980.

Raj, P. P., Rosenblatt, R., Montgomery, S. J.: Use of the Nerve Stimulator for Peripheral Blocks. Regional Anesthesia 5: 14-21, 1980.

Rosenblatt, R., Pepitone-Rockwell, F. and McKillop M. J.: Continuous Axillary Anesthesia for Traumatic Heand Injury. Anesthesiology 51: 565-566, 1979.

Rosenblatt, R. M. and Cress, J. C.: Modified Seldinger Technique for Continuous Interscalene Brachial Plexus Block. Regional Anesthesia 6: 82-84, 1981.

Sarnoff, S. J.: Functional Localization of Intraspinal Catheters. Anesthesiology 11: 360-366, 1950.

Selander, D., Edshage, S., and Wolff, T.: Paretheasiae or No Parethesiae? Nerve Lesions after Axillary Blocks. Acta Anaesth. Scand. 23: 27-33, 1979.

Seropian, R., and Reynolds, B. M.: Wound Infections After Preoperative Depilatory versus Razor Preparation. The American Journal of Surgery 121: 251-254, 1971.

Smith, B. L.: Forum: Efficacy of a Nerve Stimulator in Regional Analgesia; Experience in a Resident Training Programme. Anaesthesia 31: 778-782, 1976.

Theiss, D., Robbel, G., Theiss, M., Gerbershagen, H. U., Experimentel Studies to Determine the Optimal Areas of Locating Nerves Electrically [German]. Anaesthetist 26:411-417, 1977.

Winnie, A. P.: An "Immobile Needle" for Nerve Blocks. Anesthesiology 31: 577-578, 1969.

Winnie, A. P.: Brachial Plexus Block (Continuous). Anesthesiology 31 (2): (Aug) 1969 (Correspondence).

Winnie, A. P.: An Aid for Nerve Block. (Correspondence) Anaesthesia 35: 82-83, 1980.

Wright, B. D.: A New Use for the Block-Aid Monitor. Anesthesiology 30: 236-237, 1969.

Yasuda, I., Hirano, T., Ojima, T., et al: Supraclavicular Brachial Plexus Block Using a Nerve Stimulator and an Insulated Needle. Br. J. Anaesthesia 52: 409-411, 1980.

Zenz, M. and Glocker, R.: A New "Immobile Needle" for Plexus-Anesthesia [German]. Regional-Anaesthesie 4: 29-31, 1981.

V. Considerations Concerning Complications, Side Effects and Untoward Sequelae

"When there are problems with any regional technique, look for the cause first on the proximal end of the needle."

Winnie

The ideal regional anesthetic technique should fulfill the following criteria: the pertinent landmarks should be easily identifiable and provide precise localization of the nerves to be blocked to obviate the need for dangerous probing with the needle to find the nerves; the nerves should be blocked where they are contained in a closed compartment which allows a single injection of local anesthetic into the compartment, since in this situation the solution rather than the needle finds the nerves; and finally, the technique should be conceptually logical and technically simple. Traditional techniques of peripheral nerve block fall far short of this ideal, and, as a matter of fact, only spinal and peridural techniques have even approached it. However, the interfascial concept allows the perivascular techniques of brachial plexus block to come very close to spinal and peridural techniques in terms of fulfillment of these criteria. Of course, even the ideal technique can produce complications and untoward sequelae in the hands of an anesthetist who does not have a clear concept of the anatomy involved or who does not carry out the technical procedure with precision and care. Regional anesthesia is not for the casual or careless anesthetist, and perivascular anesthesia is no exception.

The appreciation of the fascial sheath investing the brachial plexus contributes as much to the *safety* of the perivascular techniques as it does to the high degree of success achieved with them. Not only does the fascia control the spread of properly injected local anesthetic agents, since the perivascular concept reduces all of these techniques to a single injection, it also reduces the likelihood of complications significantly as compared with multiple injection techniques, since each and every insertion of the needle carries with it the same risk of vascular, pulmonary, or neural damage. The purpose of this chapter is to review all of the complications possible with brachial plexus anesthesia and also to provide an understanding of the mechanism by which each of the possible complications can occur, how they can be managed if they occur, and how they can be avoided or minimized by properly performed perivascular techniques of brachial block.

Local Anesthetic Reactions

Intravascular injection

The injection of local anesthetic directly into *a vein* can be one of the most serious complications possible with any regional technique, because the rapid rise in the blood level of the agent almost invariably results in an immediate systemic reaction. While most such reactions, if handled properly, are without serious sequelae, *every systemic reaction to local anesthetic should be treated as potentially lethal.* Such a reaction is always due to an *avoidable* error in technique. Its incidence may be minimized by repeated aspiration in several quadrants *prior to injection,* but even with this precaution the needle may inadvertently be moved slightly *after* aspiration and *during* injection so that it comes to lie in a vessel. Therefore, aspiration should be carried out *repeatedly* and *intermittently* throughout the entire course of an injection, and if blood is obtained during any of these attempts to aspirate, the anesthetist should wait at least one injection-site-to-brain circulation time for the appearance of signs or symptoms before resuming the injection.

Of the perivascular techniques, the axillary is the most likely to allow an intravenous injection, as this is the only site where the major, large vein lies within the sheath. However, it is important to note that the vein or veins lie anterior and slightly inferior to the artery in the axilla. Thus, in carrying out the axillary technique of the author, the palpating finger compresses the vein and rolls it inferiorly while the needle is inserted superiorly, so that the chance of venipuncture and/or intravenous injection is greatly minimized. Obviously, the common practice of injection above and below the artery, aside from its lack of logic, only enhances the chance of an intravenous injection.

The possibility of making an inadvertent injection into the subclavian vein in carrying out the subclavian perivascular technique is rather remote, since the vein is separated from the plexus by the artery and by the anterior, scalene muscle. In order to enter this vein, the probing needle would have to be a considerable distance from the intended site of injection. Again, the chance of injection into any of the smaller veins in this area will increase in direct proportion to the number of injections utilized in carrying out a technique; so at this level the subclavian perivascular technique would seem to be the safest, both because of the constancy of its landmarks and because of the need for only a single injection.

One is much less likely to make an intravenous injection using the interscalene technique due to the paucity of veins in the area, although injection into the vertebral vein would appear to be a possibility. Strict adherence to the mandate that the needle be directed slightly caudad will avoid even the possibility of an injection into either of the vertebral vessels.

Injection into the subclavian or axillary *artery* must occur occasionally, but is apparently without sequelae, probably due to dilution and clearance of the drug in its circulation through the arm and then the lung, although it may be that such an event can not be differentiated from an intravenous injection. On the other hand, injection of local anesthetic into the vertebral artery, because of its proximity to the brain, results in the local anesthetic reaching the brain virtually undiluted and produces an immediate, violent reaction after the injection of a very small amount of local anesthetic. The author has never seen such a complication during an interscalene block, but has observed it during the performance of a stellate ganglion block, and in this case following injection of less than 1 ml of the local anesthetic, the patient grabbed the syringe, hurled it across the room, had a brief grand mal seizure, and awoke almost immediately thereafter with complete amnesia for the incident. Because this complication results from such a small amount of local anesthetic, it should not have serious sequelae.

Overdose

When a regional anesthetic technique is carried out properly but with a total dose of anesthetic that is excessive for a particular patient, as the blood level rises, systemic effects usually proceed sequentially as follows: first, premonitory symptoms such as dizziness, metallic taste, ringing in the ears, lightheadedness, and nystagmus to twitching of the fascial muscles. Then overt clonic and tonic convulsions develop, followed by central nervous system depression, in which seizure activity terminates and respiratory efforts become shallow and eventually cease, and systemic blood pressure begins to fall. Finally, progressive bradycardia leads ultimately to cardiac arrest. However, the rapid and sudden achievement of an extremely high anesthetic blood level may produce respiratory depression and cardiovascular collapse without the usual signs and symptoms of central nervous system excitation, so the sequence of events may not always be as complete as that described above.

Therefore, appropriate treatment depends on the stage to which the reaction has progressed: if the patient only has premonitory signs and symptoms, hyperventilation with oxygen to reduce the $PaCO_2$ *may* be effective in preventing further progress of the reaction by increasing the convulsant threshold. On the other hand, if convulsions have already begun, hyperventilation is still carried out, again, hoping to raise the convulsant threshold by lowering the carbondioxide tension, but also anticipating possible progression to respiratory depression. If necessary, muscle relaxants may have to be administered to allow adequate ventilatory control; and if cardiocirculatory failure is (or becomes) evident, vasopressors and positive inotropic and chronotropic agents must be utilized. For persistent and prolonged convulsions, diazepam or barbiturates may be utilized to suppress or terminate them. The author prefers diazepam, as barbiturates may superimpose their own myocardial depressant effect upon that of the local anesthetic agents. And finally, of course, if at any point the maintenance of the airway becomes a problem, endotracheal intubation should be carried out without delay.

Following a systemic reaction due to intravascular injection, when the signs and symptoms have responded to treatment, it is wise to determine the extent of anesthesia, if any, resulting from the original injection: if there is a considerable area of sensory loss, probably only a small part of the anesthetic solution was injected intravenously; whereas, if there is no anesthesia, it must be assumed that most, if not all, of the injection was intravascular.

Methemoglobinemia

In the early 1960's prilocaine was introduced into clinical practice as an agent which was as potent as lidocaine but with a markedly reduced intravenous toxicity. Presumably, the reduction in toxicity is a result of the fact that being a secondary amine (unlike all of the other amide local anesthetics), prilocaine requires no preliminary dealkylation, but undergoes immediate enzymatic hydrolysis to ortho-toluidine and N-propylalamine. While it is beyond the scope of the present work to detail the metabolism of the various local anesthetic agents, the biotransformation of prilocaine is pertinent to a discussion of its toxicity since ortho-toluidine and its aminiphenol metabolites are capable of oxidizing hemoglobin to methemoglobin. While minor degrees of methemoglobinemia occasionally follow the use of lidocaine, prilocaine is unique in its ability to reduce the blood's oxygen-carrying capacity sufficiently to cause clinically detectable cyanosis.

The ferrous porphyrin complex of hemoglobin in the red cell is continuously being oxidized to methemoglobin, a ferric complex incapable of combining with oxygen. Normally, however, the methemoglobin so formed is continuously being converted back to the ferrous state by a specific reductase, so that the non-functional complex ordinarily accounts for only 1% of a patient's total hemoglobin. Cyanosis does not become clinically detectable until at least 5–6% of a patient's hemoglobin is in the ferric state (about 0.8–1.0 grams of methemoglobin per 100 ml of blood). Furthermore, healthy individuals are not adversely affected by moderate amounts of methemoglobinemia, the dusky cyanosis being more disturbing in appearance than threatening to health. However, hypoxia can result, when a major portion of a patient's hemoglobin has been converted to the ferric state. Studies carried out by Hjelm and Holmdahl indicate that a dose of 300 mg of prilocaine will produce a methemoglobin level of 1.9%, a marginally acceptable level, while a dose of 600 mg will produce a level of 5.3%, a level capable of causing clinically appearent cyanosis. Thus by limiting the total dose of prilocaine to 600 mg, symptomatic cyanosis can generally be avoided. However, if the cyanosis due to prilocaine methemoglobinemia is sufficient to pose a threat to the patient's welfare, it can be completely reversed within 15–20 minutes with 1–2 mg/kg of methylene blue administered intravenously. It is unfortunate that this side effect of prilocaine, more distressing to the surgeon and anesthetist than to the patient, has adversely affected the acceptance of this, probably the safest of all of the amide local anesthetics.

Allergic reactions

In spite of the fact that local anesthetic agents are used extensively both in medical and dental practice, adverse reactions are uncommon occurrences. Certainly, the majority of those reactions which do occur are caused by accidental intravascular injection, by overdosage, or are a result of the patient fainting, with inadvertent intravascular injection leading to an excessive concentration of the local anesthetic in the blood, being by far the most common mechanism of the three. Obviously, then, true allergic reactions to local anesthetics are extremely rare indeed; and it has been estimated by Verril that as few as 1.0% of all reactions to local anesthetics have an immunological cause. And yet, frequently, a patient exhibiting an adverse reaction to a local anesthetic is diagnosed as "allergic" to local anesthetic and is advised not to receive local anesthetic agents in the future. Although avoidance of local anesthetic agents is often possible, such avoidance in a patient undergoing upper extremity surgery, for which brachial plexus anesthesia would be optimal, exposes the patient to an increased risk if general anesthesia is utilized solely on the basis of such an "allergic" history.

As an alternative to recommending total avoidance of local anesthetic agents in a patient with a history of an adverse reaction, Aldrete has recommended skin testing as a procedure to determine which patient with a history of an adverse reaction to a local anesthetic is truly at risk for a subsequent IgE-mediated, and thus potentially fatal, local anesthetic reaction. However, there are several facts suggesting that this approach may not accurately or safely predict true local anesthetic allergy. First of all, most low-molecular weight drugs are unable, by themselves, to elicit an allergic response. To be immunogenic, they or their metabolic or degradation products must act as haptens, combining with a protein (carrier) to form complete antigens or hapten-protein conjugates, against which the immunologic response is directed. Suitable skin testing material should thus contain the appropriate antigen or hapten-carrier conjugate for local anesthetic agents, and such is not available. Secondly, there is no reported study utilizing standard skin testing techniques which demonstrates the predictive nature of this approach. And finally, there is the potential risk of producing a severe and possibly fatal reaction when skin testing truly allergic individuals with

a drug to which they are sensitive. Intranasal and intraocular methods of in vivo screening for local anesthetic hypersensitivity have been advocated as effective alternatives to skin testing, but these in vivo methods are potentially equally hazardous, with at least one death reported from one drop of local anesthetic instilled into the conjunctival sac.

How then does one go about establishing or ruling out an allergic basis of a patient with a history of an "allergic" reaction to a local anesthetic? The most important evidence is usually provided by a detailed history: careful questioning of the patient thought to be allergic to a local anesthetic can often establish the mechanism of an adverse response. For example, the patient who describes urticaria and wheezing most likely experienced a true allergic reaction; whereas the patient who experienced a seizure after the administration of local anesthetic most probably had a systemic reaction due to inadvertent intravascular injection. Palpitations, headache, and cold, clammy skin usually indicate systemic absorption of epinephrine that was combined with the local anesthetic. And finally, fainting is more likely due to a vasovagal reaction than to anaphylaxis.

The ester local anesthetics, which have a benzioc acid ring in their structure and, thus, may produce metabolites related to para-amino-benzoic acid, are more likely to provoke an allergic reaction than amide local anesthetics, which are not metabolized to para-amino-benzoic acid. As a matter of fact, there has been only one report of a *proven* allergy to an amide local anesthetic: a patient alleged by history to be allergic to lidocaine. Interestingly enough, it was during a subsequent intradermal test with 0.2 ml of 0.5% bupiva-

225

caine that the patient developed respiratory difficulty and a measured decreased plasma concentration of complement protein C_4 and an unchanged plasma concentration of IgE antibodies, suggesting that the mechanism responsible for activating the complement system did not involve IgE antibodies.

It should be kept in mind that even a true allergic reaction following the use of a local anesthetic agent *may* be due to methylparaben or similar substances utilized as preservatives in commercial preparations of ester and amide local anesthetics, since these preservatives are structurally similar to para-amino-benzoic acid. Therefore, anaphylactic reactions may reflect prior stimulation of antibody production by the preservative and not by the local anesthetic agent itself.

Because of the lack of specific and clinically relevant information provided by skin tests, it would seem more practical to select an amide local anesthetic for administration to the patient alleged to be allergic to an ester and vice versa. Such a recommendation is based on the premise that ester local anesthetics do not manifest cross-sensitivity with amide local anesthetics. However, in making such a selection, it must be remembered to utilize a preservative-free commercial preparation of the "safe" agent, or the alternative selected may not be "safe". Incaudo and his coworkers advocate confirming the safety of the alternative selected by provocative dose testing, a carefully controlled challenge with increasing doses of the selected local anesthetic administered subcutaneously at 15 minute intervals, with careful observation for local or systemic reactions. In 50 patients with a history an "allergic reaction" to a local anesthetic, such provocative dose testing

with alternative, chemically dissimilar agents produced no adverse reactions attributable to IgE-mediated phenomena. Four of the patients experienced symptoms such as lightheadedness, drowsiness and hyperventilation without objective changes in skin or vital signs; but even in these patients, whose symptoms undoubtedly reflected patient anxiety, when the challenge was continued after an explanation to the patients, eventually tolerated 1 to 2 ml of a local anesthetic administered subcutaneously without further symptoms.

As rare as a true allergic reaction is to local anesthetics, and as successful as the use of alternative, chemically dissimilar agents is in avoiding similar reactions, because of the potentially lethal nature of an allergic reaction, it is wise to select preanesthetic medications which are capable of decreasing the incidence or severity of drug-induced allergic reactions in patients with a history suggestive of allergy. Premedicaton in these patients should logically include an H_1-receptor antagonist, such as diphenhydramine, 0.5 to 1 mg/kg orally or intramuscularly; and an H_2-receptor antagonist, such as cimetidine, 4 to 6 mg/kg orally. These drugs are effective in preventing or attenuating allergic reactions by occupying peripheral receptor sites normally responsive to histamine.

In the performance of brachial plexus block is followed within 30 minutes of the injection with a local anesthetic by urticaria, hypotension with tachycardia and bronchospasm, immediate, aggressive treatment is mandatory to minimize morbidity and prevent mortality: supplemental oxygen and intravenous epinephrine, 5µg/kg should be administered immediately. Diphenhydramine, 0.5 to 1 mg/kg, should also be administered intravenously, and crystalloid and/or colloid solutions should be infused simultaneously. In addition, corticosteroids are traditionally administered for the treatment of allergic reactions, but the theoretical basis of this treatment is not clear. While it is beyond the scope of the present discussion to delineate the mechanisms for allergic reactions and their treatment, the reader is strongly encouraged to read the extensive review of allergic reactions during anesthesia by Stoelting for a clear and precise delineation of the mechanisms involved.

Pulmonary Complications

Courtesy of Dr. S. Ramamurthy
University of Texas

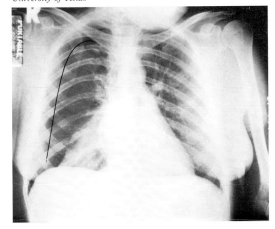

Pneumothorax

This is the most dreaded of all the complications of the supraclavicular techniques of brachial plexus block. It is virtually impossible with the currently used axillary techniques, although it was a definite possibility with some of the early techniques, such as Pitkin's, which threaded the needle all the way from the axilla to the cervical transverse processes. The incidence of pneumothorax, according to Murphy, is greatest when the classical supraclavicular approach is used; and according to Swerdlow, the risk is greater on the right, where the cupola of the lung is normally higher, and is also greater in tall, slim, long-necked patients in whom the pleura extends higher in the neck. Swerdlow also points out that there is an added risk in patients with emphysema, since puncture of an emphysematous bulla could lead to a *tension* pneumothorax. The incidence of pneumothorax following traditional supraclavicular techniques varies in the literature between 0.6 and 6%, though de Jong found an incidence of 25% when routine x-rays were taken after supraclavicular brachial block, indicating that the incidence in the literature probably only reflects those cases that became symptomatic. Moore correctly points out that with the supraclavicular technique the incidence decreases as the experience of the anesthetist increases, and certainly this is true; but the ideal technique is one where the complication rate is low *even* in the hands of the beginner. In two separate studies carried out at two different teaching institutions Sheshadri and Ramamurthy reported no pneumothoraces in a combined total of 237 subclavian perivascular brachial block, most of which were performed by residents. Compare this block with the 6.1% incidence reported by Brand and Papper in a similar large teaching institution using the more traditional technique of supraclavicular block.

Pneumothorax is *not* the result of air rushing into the pleural space through the needle that has penetrated the parietal pleura, so occlusion of the needle with a finger or syringe is not effective preventative measure. Pneumothorax, when it occurs, *is* the result of a tear in the visceral pleura and in the pulmonary parenchyma by a probing and/or improperly placed needle, and this tear in turn causes a small bronchopleural fistula with leakage of air from the lung into the intrapleural space.

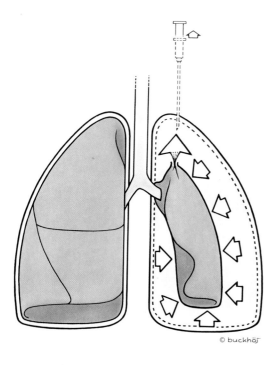

© buckhöj

Thus, because *such* tear allows only a *slow* leak, the appearance of the *objective* signs of a pneumothorax are almost always delayed for 2–6 hours, and not infrequently for as long as 12–24 hours. There are only three cases in the literature, all occurring before 1925, wherein a brachial block carried out by the technique of Kulenkampff was followed in *rapid* sequence by subcutaneous emphysema, pneumothorax and death, and in at least one of these cases there was a concomitant hemothorax (see below).

Subjective complaints of coughing, chest pain related to deep inspiration,

anxiety, and dyspnea, occurring with (or even without) subcutaneous emphysema, immediately or shortly after the performance of a supraclavicular technique should arouse suspicion. The absence of hyperresonance on percussion and decreased or absent breath sounds does not rule out the possibility that a pneumothorax is developing, for unlike the symptoms, which appear early, these signs, according to Moore, do not develop until more than 20% of the lung has collapsed. Nonetheless, whenever there is even a suspicion of pneumothorax, an x-ray should be taken immediately to establish a definitive diagnosis. Films should be taken in deep inspiration and expiration to rule out diaphragmatic paralysis due to phrenic block, a far more common cause of dyspnea occurring shortly after any supraclavicular technique (see below).

While a pneumothorax produced as described above is usually slow to develop, it must be appreciated that the application of positive pressure to the airway *after* the lung has been torn by a misguided needle can result in the precipitous development of a tension pneumothorax. This should always be born in mind when considering the use of a general anesthetic after a supraclavicular block has failed to produce anesthesia, when attempting to assist ventilation during the administration of oxygen for subjective dyspnea occurring sometime after a supraclavicular block, or even when controlling ventilation in treating a systemic local anesthetic reaction. Similarly, the use of nitrous oxide in a general anesthetic administered after a failed supraclavicular technique can cause a small pneumothorax to rapidly develop into a tension pneumothorax: Eger and Saidman have shown that due to the solubility of nitrous oxide, which is 34 times that of nitrogen, a volume of 300 ml of air in the intrapleural space can double in 10 minutes, triple in 45 minutes and quadruple in 2 hours when the inspired gas contains 68–78% nitrous oxide. Thus, nitrous oxide should be used cautiously, if at all, when a general anesthetic must be administered after a supraclavicular block has failed.

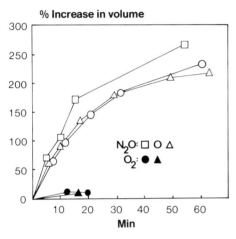

% Increase in volume

From Eger, E. J., II, and Saidman, Z. J.: Hazards of Nitrous Oxid Anesthesia in Bowel Obstruction and Pneumothorax. Anesthesiology, 26:64, 1965.
Reprinted by permission from J. B. Lippencott Company, Philadelphia.

The need for treatment of a pneumothorax depends upon the degree of collapse, and therefore, treatment should *not* be instituted until an x-ray has established the diagnosis, except for the rare development of tension pneumothorax described above, in which case insertion of a large bore needle, catheter, or chest tube is life-saving. But ordinarily the development of pneumothorax is slow, and treatment is rarely, if ever, an emergency; so panic on the part of the anesthetist or surgeon only results in needless mental and physical trauma to the patient. Usually, if the degree of collapse is less than 25%, re-expansion of the lung will occur sponta-

neously. If there is a 25–50% pneumothorax, re-expansion may or may not take place spontaneously, but in either case the patient must be followed closely with serial x-rays. Greater than 50% collapse almost invariably requires treatment, whether by needle or by catheter drainage. It would appear from the literature that more than 80% of *symptomatic* pneumothoraces require treatment. Therefore, any patient with symptomatic or roentgenographic evidence of pneumothorax should be kept at bed rest and followed closely with serial x-rays.

The insertion of a chest tube is a painful and traumatic experience for a patient, so

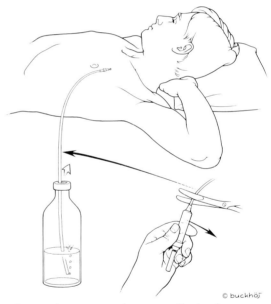

© buckhöj

the author strongly urges that whenever insertion of a chest tube is contemplated, a less traumatic alternative be tried first.

If the patient is not in respiratory distress, a skin wheal is raised with local anesthetic in the second intercostal space anteriorly in the mid-clavicular line. Then after deeper infiltration of the interspace with local anesthetic, a large-bore 16-gauge "extracath" connected to an intravenous infusion set is inserted through the chest wall *after* the proximal end of the infusion set has been placed *below* the surface of a sterile solution in a sterile container, well below the level of the patient's chest. When the system begins to bubble, the needle can be withdrawn and the intravenous infusion set connected to the plastic catheter, which is then taped in place. While the air will be evacuated more slowly with such a small-bore system than with the usual chest tube attached to underwater seal drainage, ordinarily lung re-expansion will take place fairly rapidly. When serial x-rays show the lung to be fully expanded, the system should be clamped off for several hours, and if a final x-ray shows no further air leakage, the catheter may be removed.

Obviously, if serial chest x-rays indicate that the system described is *not* effective in allowing lung re-expansion, *then* and only then should a chest tube be inserted as follows: after sterile preparation of the skin, a skin wheal is raised and deep infiltration with local anesthetic and an incision is made over the second or third intercostal space in the mid-clavicular line. The chest tube is then inserted by grasping it with a curved hemostat at the tip and bluntly pushing it through the skin incision into the pleural space.

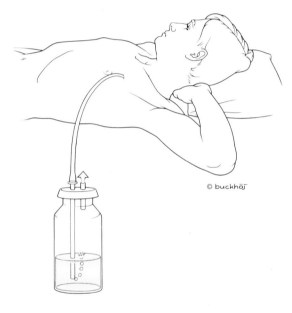

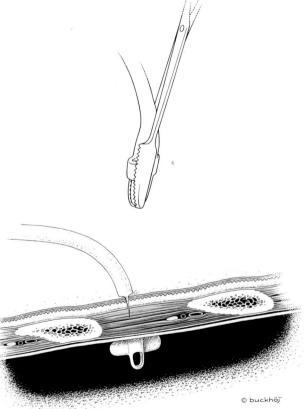

When bubbles in the water indicate good position, the tube is attached to underwater seal drainage or to an appropriate suction device, and the clamp on the catheter is removed. And finally the tube should be firmly fixed with stitches to the skin at its base to prevent accidental removal.

Obviously, this procedure is best carried out by a surgeon who is familiar with the technique. However, if the patient has developed a tension pneumothorax, insertion of a large-bore needle or extracath may be life saving, so in this situation connection to an underwater seal drainage system can be carried out sometime *after* a catheter or needle has been inserted, since the positive pressure in the chest will only allow the intrapleural air to rush *out*. Tension pneumothorax, as stated earlier, can develop when positive pressure is applied to the airway after a needle has entered the lung and represents a life threatening emergency that will not await an x-ray diagnosis. Reduced pulmonary compliance, hyperresonance, absent breath sounds and a deviated trachea, along with increasing cyanosis and decreasing blood pressure and pulse rate demand treatment: a large bore needle or extracath inserted into the chest will "hiss" as the air escapes; and if a moistened glass syringe is on the needle as it is inserted, the plunger will be pushed out by the elevated intrathoracic pressure.

In an emergency, the amputated finger of a rubber glove with the tip incised will provide an excellent flutter valve when tied over the hub of a needle or extracath until an underwater seal system can be set up. On the other hand if ventilation is being controlled, this will be unnecessary, as the positive pressure applied to the airway will re-expand the lung, but underwater seal drainage *must* be connected before discontinuing positive pressure breathing.

Pneumothorax can be prevented or at least, the incidence greatly minimized by a complete understanding of the pertinent anatomy, by the use of techniques which require a minimal number of injections, and by the use of a short needle. With those supraclavicular techniques wherein multiple injections of local anesthetic are made atop the first rib, prevention of pneumothorax depends entirely upon location of the first rib by superficial landmarks. As stated earlier, the most commonly utilized superficial landmark, the midpoint of the clavicle, lies over the first rib only 50% of the time, so it is little wonder that Adriani wrote, "when I use the supraclavicular route, I do so with a certain amount of fear and trepidation." A needle advanced medial to the first rib would certainly enter the cupola of the lung, and the need for multiple injections would increase the possibility of such "misses" proportionately. On the other hand, with the subclavian perivascular technique, the direction of the properly placed needle is parallel to the scalene muscles, and since these muscles invariably insert on the first rib, *if* the plexus is not contacted on the first insertion of the needle, the needle will "insert" on the first rib too. The fact that the plexus *is* usually encountered on the first insertion of the needle and the fact that only a single injection is required once a paresthesia has been obtained further minimizes the possibility of producing a pneumothorax with this technique. In fact, if a pneumothorax follows the performance of a subclavian perivascular technique, it is the result of a faulty technique based on incomplete knowledge of the anatomical relations described in Chapter I.

Obviously, pneumothorax is impossible with the axillary perivascular technique; and it is virtually impossible with the interscalene technique, provided that the technique is carried out at the appropriate level, which is well above the cupola of the lung. Possible, in rare cases, penetration of an emphysematous bleb on top of the cupola of the lung could occur even with a properly executed interscalene block.

Hemopneumothorax

Hemopneumothorax is an extremely rare but serious complication of brachial plexus block.

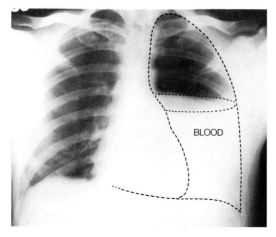

Mani: An Unusual Complication of Brachial Plexus Block and Heparin Therapy. Anesthesiology 48:213-214, 1978.
Reprinted by permission from J. B. Lippencott Company.

While it would appear that there are only two reports in the literature of unheparinized patients who developed hemopneumothorax after a brachial block, more recently Mani has reported a case which indicates that this complication, while still rare, becomes more possible if a patient is heparinized. While *spontaneous* hemopneumothorax has been reported in patients heparinized for thromboembolic disease, a hemopneumothorax occurring after a brachial block on the same side as the block can probably be attributed to the block, even if it is not detected until several days later, as in Mani's case. Obviously, other coagulopathies could enhance the likelihood of this complication in a similar manner.

The *symptoms* of hemopneumothorax may very well be difficult to differentiate from those *of* pneumothorax, though they *may* be delayed somewhat in onset; but the *physical findings* of dullness on

percussion instead of hyperresonance coupled with signs of circulatory instability, which may progress to the point of overt shock, can leave little doubt as to the diagnosis. Obviously, a chest x-ray (taken in the sitting or lateral position) will show an air fluid level. Because of the presence of air, if the patient is not heparinized, the blood may clot and needle aspiration of the pleural cavity may fail to yield blood. As a matter of fact, clotting may prevent adequate drainage even via a properly placed chest tube, and surgical drainage may be necessary. In the heparinized patient, clotting is not a problem, but with or without heparin continued or uncontrolled bleeding may also require surgical intervention. Fortunately, this is a very rare complication, but the possibility of hemopneumothorax, no matter how remote, should make one very cautious when considering regional anesthesia in the patient about to be heparinized.

When a chest tube is inserted for hemopneumothorax, it should be as large as possible (20 to 28 French), and it should be inserted in a dependent posi-

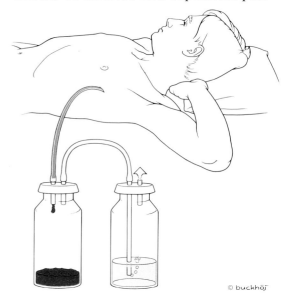

© buckhöj

tion, preferably in the eighth intercostal space in the midaxillary line. The tube is introduced with the patient in the sitting position as described for pneumothorax, but after the pleural cavity has been entered, the tube is advanced posteriorly and superiorly until at least 6 to 8 inches lie within the chest. The tube should be kept clamped during insertion, and should be connected to underwater seal drainage immediately thereafter using a multiple bottle system, the number depending on how much blood is in the chest.

Subcutaneous and mediastinal emphysema

Subcutaneous emphysema should be considered to be indicative of pneumo-

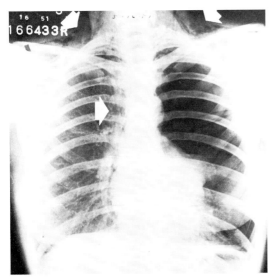

Moore D. C.: Regional Anesthesia 4.th.ed p.239, 1973.
Reprinted by permission from Charles C. Thomas, Publisher, Springfield, Illinois.

thorax when it appears following the administration of a supraclavicular brachial block.

Not infrequently there is a concomitant pneumomediastinum, which goes unrecognized unless it appears on x-ray or unless there is sufficient air in the mediastinum to produce a "mediastinal crunch" on auscultaion, a crunching sound synchronous with the heart beat (Hamman's sign). Neither of these signs are evident until the pneumothorax is clinically significant, as when a general anesthetic with nitrous oxide and/or positive pressure is administered after a failed supraclavicular brachial block. If *both* nitrous oxide and positive pressure breathing are used, in addition to the signs of rapidly developing tension pneumothorax, the subcutaneous emphysema may rapidly increase in the neck and extend into the fascial tissues ("frog-faced man"); and if there is coexistent pneumomediastinum, the increase in gas in the mediastinum may contribute to the rapidity of the cardiovascular collapse.

In the three reports in the early German literature of *rapid* death from pneumothorax referred to earlier, the pneumothorax was accompanied by massive subcutaneous emphysema and mediastinal emphysema. Yet Weil reported a patient as early as 1919 who developed mediastinal emphysema with "mediastinal crunch" but *without* evidence of pneumothorax or subcutaneous emphysema, who then went on to recover spontaneously. The interesting feature in this case was that the mediastinal crunch, a "clicking" sound synchronized with the pulse, was audible 3 to 6 feet from the bed when the patient was supine. When he sat up and leaned forward, the sound became difficult to hear, even on auscultation. This patient's only subjective symptoms were a feeling of retrosternal pressure, which developed immediately after the block was completed and persisted for 7 days, though the mediastinal

233

crunch disappeared on the fourth day.

In 1947 Dimond reported five cases of mediastinal emphysema occurring in a series of 700 supraclavicular blocks, and he noted that the characteristic findings were sudden substernal pain and the presence of the peculiar crackling or clicking sounds, synchronous with the heart beat. The electrocardiogram showed flattened and diphasic T-waves which reverted to normal as the air was reabsorbed. Only one of the five cases developed pneumothorax, and this became evident only on serial x-rays at 24 hours. Each of the patients made an uneventful recovery.

In short, subcutaneous emphysema should be assumed to indicate possible pneumothorax until proved otherwise when it develops following the performance of any technique of brachial block carried out above the clavicle. In some of these cases, the subcutaneous emphysema may indicate mediastinal emphysema, particularly if the patient complains of retrosternal pain. Hamman's sign will confirm the diagnosis of mediastinal air but will not rule out the possibility of pneumothorax, and both pneumothorax and mediastinal emphysema may fail to show up on x-ray for 12 to 24 hours. In any case, the administration of anesthesia with nitrous oxide and/or positive pressure ventilation should be avoided, if possible after a supraclavicular brachial block, *especially* if there is subcutaneous emphysema in the neck.

Diaphragmatic paralysis

Reports of diaphragmatic paralysis due to phrenic block as a result of supraclavicular brachial block appeared in the German literature shortly after the technique was introduced by Kulenkampff and have continued to appear sporadically ever

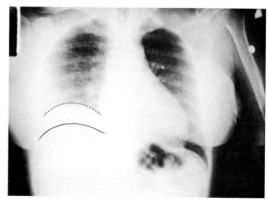

Courtesy of Dr. S. Ramamurthy
University of Texas

since. In the healthy patient with little or no respiratory disease, phrenic nerve block is usually inconsequential and asymptomatic *unless* bilateral blocks have resulted in bilateral diaphragmatic paralysis. However, in patients with severe respiratory disease paralysis of even one diaphragm may precipitate respiratory failure and result in the development of acute hypoxia. Obviously, the treatment in such cases consists of ventilatory support and the administration of oxygen. Apprehension may be considerably and may be allayed by the cautious use of small, incremental doses of diazepam administered intravenously. When the symptoms of acute respiratory distress develop shortly after the performance of a brachial block, the inexperienced anesthetist or surgeon may jump to the conclusion that the patient is developing pneumothorax. Ordinarily a phrenic block can readily be differentiated from pneumothorax by the chronology of onset: symptoms resulting from a phrenic block occur shortly after the injection of the local anesthetic, ordinarily, in the time it takes for a motor block to become established with that agent. The symptoms will persist, if untreated, only as long as the motor blockade produced with that

234

particular agent persists. As described earlier, this is quite different from the delayed onset of respiratory symptoms that can appear following pleural damage and the development of pneumothorax, and yet many inexperienced anesthetists of surgeons have panicked with the onset of respiratory distress, and have performed a needless thoracocentesis or have even inserted a chest tube unnecessarily. Though a *definitive* diagnosis of diaphragmatic paralysis can be established only by x-ray, the diagnosis should be presumed when the onset of symptoms parallels the normal onset of anesthesia, and treatment should not be delayed for roentgenographic proof of the diagnosis.

After forming from the third, fourth, and fifth cervical nerve roots, the phrenic nerve passes down the anterior surface of the anterior scalene muscle just beneath the prevertebral fascia which covers its anterior surface. Thus, the phrenic nerve is separated from the brachial plexus by the substance of the anterior scalene muscle and by its posterior fascial investment. With the subclavian perivascular and interscalene techniques, since a single injection is made behind the posterior fascia of the anterior scalene muscle, if the needle has been properly placed, it would seem unlikely that sufficient anesthetic will reach the phrenic nerve proper to produce a block. As a matter of fact, because of the *apparent* anatomical barrier to local anesthetic diffusion, the author thought that a phrenic block occuring after an interscalene or subclavian periovascular block implied faulty placement of the needle! Because diaphragmatic paralysis is asymptomatic in most patients, most reports of the incidence of phrenic block following the interscalene and/or subclavian perivascular tech-

niques of brachial block are misleading because they include only "symptomatic" phrenic blocks corroborated by x-ray. Ward, for example, reported that in his series of 33 interscalene brachial blocks, two patients (6%) developed dyspnea on deep inspiration. Both patients had radiological evidence of unilateral phrenic nerve block which disappeared when the block had worn off. Seshadri and Ramamurthy in their studies of 100 and 134 subclavian perivascular brachial blocks, respectively, reported only one patient between them who developed a symptomatic phrenic block, giving an incidence of 0.43%. The point is that it is impossible from such data to determine the true incidence of phrenic block with these techniques, for both studies examined radiographically *only* those patients who developed symptoms. However, Farrar, Scheybani and Nolte recently reported a study in which they took *routine* x-rays after performing brachial blocks using the interscalene, subclavian perivascular, and Kulenkampff techniques in 300 patients (100 in each group) and reported the incidence of phrenic block to be 36%, 36% and 38% respectively to whether the local anesthetic ascends in the sheath to block the roots of the phrenic nerve or diffuses through the anterior scalene muscle and its fascia to block the nerve itself, phrenic block is a very real possibility, to be considered pre-anesthetically, when the choice of anesthetic technique is made.

As with other pulmonary complications, it would seem logical that the incidence of phrenic block would be lower with the single-injection technique than with the more traditional multiple-injection techniques, and yet the studies of Farrar and his co-workers would seem to indicate that the incidence is the same.

The issue is rendered even more confusing by the report of Knoblanche, who demonstrated a 67% incidence of phrenic block by pleuroscopic examinations after the traditional supraclavicular brachial block technique, almost twice the incidence reported.

This is more in keeping with older radiological studies carried out following the classical supraclavicular block: for example, Hartel and Keppler and Shaw found that 80-90% of their patients showed radiologic evidence of phrenic nerve block. Dhunér found a lower incidence in his larger series, but he indicated that this may be due to the fact that the block may be so evanescent that by the time an x-ray was taken, the phrenic block had dissipated; hence he found an incidence of 28% when x-rays were taken 30-90 minutes after the block, while the incidence *appeared* to be only 15% if the x-rays were taken more than 90 minutes after the block. Obviously, postoperative films may miss many phrenic blocks, particularly if the surgery is prolonged and short-acting local anesthetic agents are utilized, and finally, the *possibility* of bilateral phrenic block should be a strong deterrent to the use of bilateral brachial block carried out above the clavicle. Obviously, phrenic nerve block and, for that matter, all of the pulmonary complications can be avoided by using the axillary perivascular technique of brachial plexus anesthesia wherever feasible.

It is significant to note that the two patients in Ward's series who developed *symptomatic* phrenic block were 18 and 34 years old and free of cardio-pulmonary disease. As were the two symptomatic patients, 39 and 42, reported by Kayerker, so it cannot be assumed, as is so often stated, that *only* those with pulmonary disease will develop respiratory embarrassment from phrenic block. On the other hand, it can and should be stated that this technique and, indeed, any technique carried out above the clavicle should be used cautiously in patients with little respiratory reserve, as indicated by Hood's report of a 38 year old woman in renal and cardiac failure who developed acute respiratory failure following a subclavian perivascular block and the phrenic block that resulted from it.

Hoarseness (Recurrent Laryngeal Nerve Block)

With the traditional multiple-injection supraclaviclar techniques of brachial plexus block, hoarseness secondary to unilateral blockade of the vagus nerve is an extremely rare occurrence for two reasons: first of all, throughout most of its course in the neck the vagus is well protected, both by the common carotid arteries and the internal jugular vein, between which it is sandwiched, and by the thick fibrous carotid sheath, which provides a tubular investment surrounding all three, artery, vein and nerve; and secondly, at the level at which the supraclavicular technique of brachial block is carried out, the vagus lies considerably medial and anterior to the course of the exploring needle. However, with those perivascular techniques carried out above the clavicle, because a single, large volume of local anesthetic is injected into or just above the subclavian perivascular portion of the interscalene space, the local anesthetic may very well track out along the subclavian artery on the right to the point where the recurrent laryngeal nerve, leaves the vagus and loops around the artery to ascend to the larynx. Of course, hoarseness *could* also result from blockade of

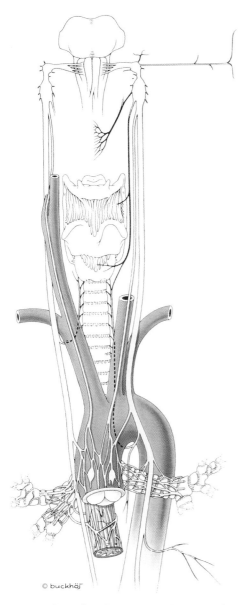

© buckhöj

the vagus itself as it travels along and/or crosses the first part of the subclavian artery just medial to the insertion of the anterior scalene muscle.

On either side since the vagus makes fairly intimate contact with the first portion of the subclavian artery on both sides, crossing the artery on the right and travelling parallel to it on the left. Howev-

er, because of the fact that hoarseness has been reported only following interscalene or subclavian perivascular blocks "carried out on the right side", it would *seem* that hoarseness represents a true recurrent laryngeal block.

Nonetheless, while the right recurrent nerve is given off as soon as the vagus has crossed the subclavian artery, and the left is not given off until the carotid has joined the aorta, after the left recurrent nerve has looped around the aorta, it ascends toward the neck, where it does travel in close contact with the first part of the subclavian artery on its posteromedial aspect; so at least theoretically, hoarseness *could* follow a perivascular brachial block on either side.

Probably the reason there is only occasional mention of this "complication" is that hoarseness is of little clinical consequence, provided it is due to paralysis of only one vocal cord. Bilateral paralysis following bilateral brachial block has never been reported, but this could result in life threatening airway obstruction due to adduction of the paralyzed cords. Like bilateral phrenic nerve block, this complication is a theoretical contraindication to bilateral perivascular brachial blocks carried out above the clavicle.

Ward reported one case of hoarseness following a right interscalene block, which in his series of 34 blocks represented an incidence of 3%. Seltzer reported a similar case following right interscalene block which was accompanied by Horner's syndrome. In Seshadri's series of 100 subclavian perivascular brachial blocks carried out at the author's own institution, the incidence of hoarseness as a side effect was 6%, while in Ramamurthy's series of 134 subclavian perivascular blocks, the incidence was only 1.5%.

Cardiovascular Complications

Hematoma formation

Puncture of the axillary or subclavian arteries during performance of a brachial block is usually harmless and without sequelae. The needle is relatively small, and the arteries, with their thick, muscular layers, quickly seal off the puncture site. As a matter of fact, puncture of the artery, whether intentional or unintentional, tells the anesthetist the exact location of his needle: with the subclavian perivascular technique, the appearance of arterial blood indicates that the needle lies slightly anterior to the plexus, and must be withdrawn and reinserted slightly more posteriorly, closer to the middle scalene muscle; and with the axillary perivascular technique, if the artery is entered, the needle is simply advanced further until the flow of blood ceases, indicating that the posterior wall of the vessel has been penetrated, at which point the contents of the syringe are expelled. In either case, as the needle is withdrawn from the vessel, firm digital pressure over the artery followed by vigorous massage will usually minimize the amount of blood that escapes.

In carrying out 134 subclavian perivascular blocks, Ramamurthy and his co-workers punctured the subclavian artery in 29 of the cases (22%), but a palpable hematoma developed in only 2 of the patients (1.4%); and in Word's series of 34 interscalene blocks, blood was aspirated in seven patients (21%), but a palpable hematoma developed in only 1 (3%). In a series of 246 axillary perivascular brachial blocks, Brand and Papper did not note the incidence of arterial or venous penetration, but they did report that 3 patients developed palpable hematomas (1.2%). The important point is that none of the patients in any of these series developed any neurological sequelae whatsoever. Moore feels that the occasional hematoma that develops following venous or arterial puncture may be a result of the vasodilator effect of the local anesthetic bathing the vessel, preventing retraction of the vessel and sealing of the puncture. Obviously, if a patient is on anticoagulants or has a coagulopathy of any type, the chance of hematoma formation is increased, and for this reason regional anesthetic procedures should be used with great caution in these patients. Usually, even if a hematoma does form, it rarely persists for more than a week or two and even more rarely results in sequelae. However, of the five patients Wooley and Vandam reported who had neurological sequelae following supraclavicular brachial block, two had developed hematomas during the block. In one of these patients tenderness and paresthesias persisted for a few days, but in the other patient paresthesias and numbness persisted for more than 9 months. In the 10 cases of neurological sequelae reported by Selander after axillary block, only 1 patient had a hematoma; but in this patient total deficits of median, ulnar and radial nerves were apparently permanent. Surgical exploration revealed a severe constrictive epineuritis, but neurolysis was without benefit. Staal, in reporting complications of axillary artery puncture for angiography pointed out that axillary artery puncture with large needles can produce hematomas which in time may cause fibrous tissue entrapment of the plexus in the axilla, but fortunately this is exceedingly rare. Nonetheless, one should heed the admonitions of Wooley and Vandam that repeated insertions of the needle increase the possibility of hematoma formation. Obviously, then, the single-injection techniques should minimize the possibility of this complication. In addition, because of the obviously increased hazard, brachial block should be avoided or used very cautiously in patients on anticoagulant therapy or with prolonged clotting time.

Vascular insufficiency

This unique, puzzling, and obviously very rare sequel to a trans-arterial axillary block was described by Merrill, who reported the case of a 49 year old patient who experienced "a decrease in sensation and a feeling of warmth in the arm immediately following the injection of 20 ml of a mixture of lidocaine 1%, tetracaine 0.05%, and epinephrine. 1:200,000, 10 ml deep to the artery and 10 ml superficial to it. About 2 to 3 minutes later the entire hand and arm blanched. Radial, ulnar, brachial, and axillary pulses were not palpable ... No hematoma or mass was palpable in the axilla". Palpable pulses reappeared spontaneously approximately 15 minutes later. The patient developed a good sensory and motor block, and when the block wore off, there were no adverse sequelae. In these differential diagnosis of the possible etiologic mechanisms, the authors include the effects of intra-arterial local anesthetics or intra-arterial epinephrine, subintimal injection into the arterial wall sufficient to cause mechanical obstruction, and severe vasospasm due to mechanical stimulation by the needle as it penetrated the two walls of the axillary artery. They favored the last mechanism, but the sequence of a subjective feeling of warmth shortly after the injection, followed by blanching of the skin and loss of the pulses after 2 to 3 minutes and then complete restoration of skin color and pulses to normal after an additional 15 minutes can be more adequately explained by the pharmacology of the injected drugs: only a few ml of epinephrine 1:200,000 are required when injected intra-arterially to cause intense vasoconstriction, following an initial feeling of warmth. Then when the motor, sensory, and sympathetic block is complete (and 15 minutes may be required when the volume injected into the axillary sheath is only 20 ml minus the volume injected intra-arterially), the resultant increase in blood flow would effectively dilute and wash out the epinephrine sequestered in the microcirculation of the skin.

An alternative explanation was suggested by Lennon and Linstromberg; they postulated that large volumes of local anesthetic injected into a noncompliant sheath might increase "intrasheath pressure" sufficiently to compromise the axillary artery and diminish distal flow. To test their hypothesis they placed a needle trans-arterially and injected 50 ml of local anesthetic in 10 ml increments, measuring intrasheath pressure prior to the block and after each 10 ml increment. They found that the intrasheath pressure did rise progressively after each sequential incremental injection, but never exceeded mean arterial pressure for periods longer than 60 seconds. In fact, the sheath proved to be sufficiently elastic that one minute after the fifth 10 ml increment, the sheath pressures ranged from 28–47 mm Hg *in patients with successful blocks*. Interestingly, in those patients in whom the needle was apparently improperly placed (as attested to by unsuccessful blocks), the pressures did *not* rise progressively after each sequential incremental injection. This difference between the elastance ($\Delta\varphi/\Delta V$) of a successful block and that of an unsuccessful one suggested to Lennon and Linstromberg the possibility of utilizing such measurements as a means of predicting success with axillary blocks. While such a test would be a bit complicated for routine use in carrying out brachial plexus anesthesia, the data obtained in their study clearly indicate that intrasheath pressure does not increase sufficiently, even after 50 ml have been injected, to produce the vascular insufficiency described by Merrill, particularly since Merrill had injected somewhat less than 20 ml. However, as indicated by Lennon and Linstromberg, their data does provide scientific evidence indicating "that a functional sheath exists" and that the elastance of the sheath is 0.8 ± 0.1 (mean $\pm$ standard error of the mean).

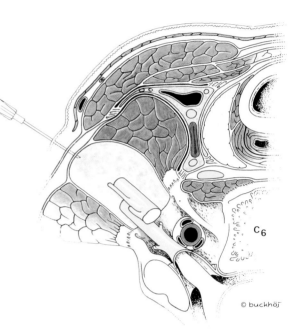

Carotid bruit

During placement of a precordial stethoscope after the administration of an interscalene brachial block, Siler reported that

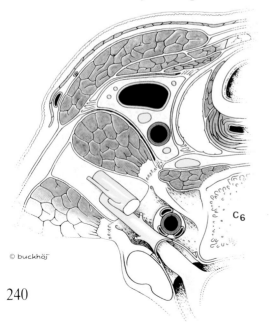

the stethoscope head slipped onto the patient's neck, at which time a carotid bruit was heard. The bruit had not been present at the time of the preoperative physical examination and it disappeared by the end of the 2½ hour surgical procedure. The development of the bruit was presumably caused by compression of the carotid artery by the distended interscalene compartment, which would cause the anterior scalene muscle to compress the carotid sheath and thus produce a narrowing of the lumen of the artery and a bruit. While this side effect was without any clinical significance in the patient reported by Siler, in an elderly patient with advanced atherosclerosis and pre-existent carotid insufficiency, such compression of the common carotid artery could be more serious.

Cardiac arrest

This complication is discussed under Neural Complications in the section on Subarachnoid Block.

240

Neural Complications

Phrenic nerve block

This complication is discussed under Pulmonary Complications.

Recurrent laryngeal nerve block

This complication is discussed under Pulmonary Complications.

Sympathetic block

The development of Horner's syndrome has been reported to occur in as many as 70–90% of all patients receiving brachial plexus block by the traditional, multiple-injection, supraclavicular techniques using 50 ml or more of anesthetic solution. Though the distance between the cervical sympathetic chain and the roots of the plexus is not great, the two are separated by the prevertebral fascia, which at the level of the block has split to invest the scalene muscles. Nonetheless with multiple injection techniques, it is not unlikely that at least one of the injections is made deep to the prevertebral fascia, resulting in sympathetic blockade and the development of Horner's syndrome. With the subclavian perivascular or interscalene techniques, where all of the solution is deposited within the sheath, while those sympathetic fibers traveling with the subclavian and vertebral arteries would, of course, be blocked, it would *appear* anatomically that blockade of the cervical sympathetic chain would be improbable, if not impossible. However, in a prospective study of 130 patients receiving a subclavian perivascular brachial block, Ramamurthy and his co-workers at the University of Texas in San Antonio found that Horner's syndrome occurred in 64% of the cases; and similarly, Seshadri at the University of Illinois found an incidence of 52% in 100 consecutive cases, also after subclavian perivascular block. Vester-Andersen in a prospective study of 100 patients developed Horner's syndome, and our experience with the interscalene technique has indicated a similar, incidence, so obviously, while the fascial investment of the plexus above the clavicle is important in the initial distribution of the local anesthetic injected within it, the fascia is certainly not "water-tight", and with time the local anesthetic diffuses through the fascial barrier to block the cervical sympathetic chain. Clearly, this side effect is virtually impossible with the axillary perivascular technique, unless excessive volumes are injected so that the solution reaches the interscalene compartment.

Because the vascular supply to the conjunctival and sclerae, the iris (which controls the size of the pupil), and Müllers superior palpebral muscle (which controls the level of the upper eyelid) are all under sympathetic control, mediated by *alpha* adrenergic receptors, Horner's syndrome can be reversed if it is upsetting to the patient by simply instilling a 0.1% ophthalmic solution of pnenylephrine in the eye.

Except in patients with headinjuries, where the inequallity in pupilsize could be misinterpreted, the development of Horner's syndrome which is usually assymptomatic is of little concern to anesthetist, though the symptoms should be explained to the patient.

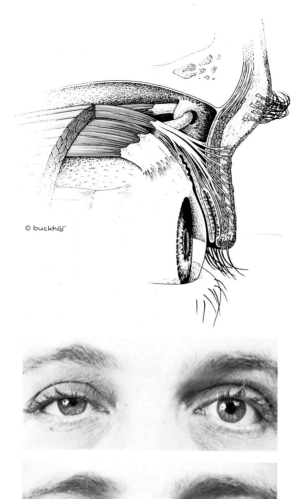

© buckhöj

Winnie, A. P., Ramamurthy, S., Durrani, Z., Radonjic, R., & Shaker, M. H.: Pharmacologic Reversal of Horner's Syndrome Following Stellate Ganglion Block. Anesthesiology 41: 615-617, 1974. Reprinted by permission from J. B. Lippencott Company.

However, while the signs and symptoms of sympathetic block are *usually* without adverse effect, Lim reported the development of severe bronchospasm shortly after the administration of an interscalene brachial block, the onset of wheezing being concomitant with the onset of Horner's syndrome. Thus, supraclavicular brachial block of any type should be used with caution (if at all) in a known, severe asthmatic.

Subarachnoid block

There are three ways that local anesthetic agents can enter the subarachnoid space during or following the performance of a brachial plexus block above the clavicle:

First, the needle may be advanced through an intervertebral foramen and the anesthetic injected directly intrathecally. Of the perivascular techniques this would appear to be possible only with the interscalene technique, and even then, *only* if the needle is *improperly* directed in a directly mesiad (horizontal) direction. Ordinarily, a needle so directed will encounter a nerve root or the vertebral artery or vein, so the anesthetist is alerted

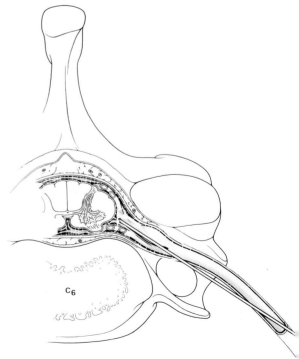

C6

to the fact that the needle has penetrated too deeply; but if these structures are missed by the advancing needle, there is nothing to prevent it from penetrating the dura and entering the subarachnoid space. On the other hand, if the needle is properly directed in a slightly caudad direction, as indicated in Chapter III, should the needle miss the roots of the plexus as it advances, it will encounter the transverse process of the next cervical vertebra below the level at which the needle was inserted.

Secondly, it occasionally happens that a dural cuff accompanies a nerve some distance distal to the intervertebral foramen through which it passes, so that a direct intrathecal injection could be made in such a situation, even if the needle has been properly placed outside of the intervertebral foramen. Postmortem studies have demonstrated that dural cuffs can extend as far as 8 cm past the interverte-

bral foramen! In such cases intrathecal injection is obviously possible, though rare, with any of the techniques carried out above the clavicle, perivascular or otherwise. Bonica described the performance of a supraclavicular brachial block in which, after eliciting parethesias and injecting part of the local anesthetic, spinal fluid was aspirated, presumably from a long dural cuff. He also reported high or total spinal anesthesia following 2 out of 3100 supraclavicular brachial blocks, an incidence 0.6%, so the occurrence with the conventional supraclavicular technique of brachial block is also rare but possible.

And thirdly, local anesthetics injected intraneurally can find their way back into the subarachnoid space: as early as 1875 Key and Retzius showed that solutions injected into peripheral nerves could later be detected in the spinal fluid and in the parenchyma of the central nervous sys-

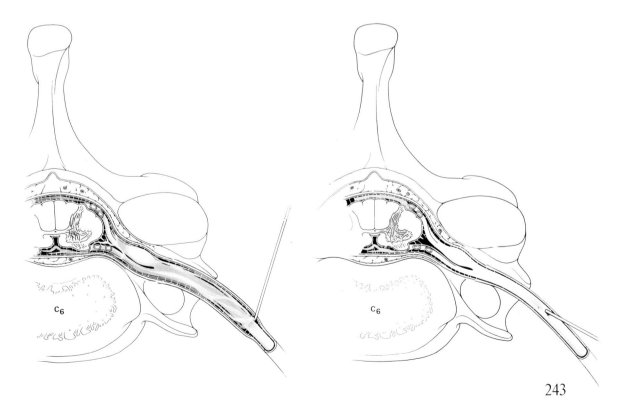

tem. More recently French, using roentgenographic studies with radiopaque dye, showed that solutions injected entirely intraneurally spread centrally, entering the parenchyma of the spinal cord and the subarachnoid space. These investigators felt that the epineurium of a peripheral nerve is simply the continuation of the pia mater and that after a subepineurial injection the perineural spaces provide a pathway for intraneurally injected local anesthetics to reach the spinal cord. Moore, using solutions colored with methylene blue, showed that when the cervical nerves of monkeys were injected intraneurally 3–4 cm from the intervertebral foramen under direct vision, the solution immediately spread centrally, reaching the parenchyma of the spinal cord in 2–5 minutes. He also noted that after 10–15 minutes the solution began to penetrate the pia mater in a sufficient concentration to tinge the spinal fluid lightly, though the spinal fluid did not become heavily stained for 35–40 minutes. Moore postulated that the delay required for penetration of the pia might explain those puzzling cases where the onset of a high spinal is delayed 30–40 minutes after the performance of a block. While Moore also felt that it is the interstices between nerve fascicles which form the avenues for retrograde diffusion of intraneurally injected local anesthetics, more recently Selander has shown that the injection must be intrafascicular (*subperineurial*) in order for the solution to spread rapidly towards the central nervous system, since *subepineurial* injections tend to simply rupture the epineurium, making further central spread impossible. This concept is supported by the work of Shanthaveerappa and Bourne, who have shown that it is the perineurium which is a direct peri-

pheral extension of the piameter, not the epineurium, which is an extension of the dura.

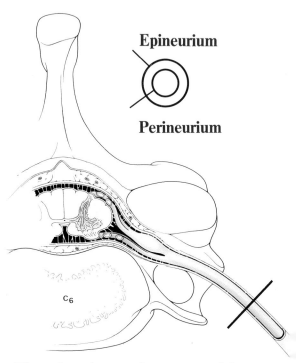

Thus, there is a continous potential space under the perineurium of peripheral nerves that extends centrally and becomes the potential subpial space next to the cord. Therefore, local anesthetic solutions injected subperineurally into a peripheral nerve can travel centripetally and rapidly reach the surface of the cord. If the onset of a high spinal following such an injection is delayed, as described by Moore, the delay represents the time required for penetration of the intact pia-arachnoid by the local anesthetic. However, as Selander has shown, intrafascicular injection into a peripheral nerve can produce pressures as high as 750 mm Hg, more than three times the pressure which French found was necessary to rupture the pia-arachnoid barrier, so *rapid* onset

244

of high or total spinal could occur by this mechanism as well.

Theoretically, then, spinal block resulting from such an intraneural injection is possible with any of the techniques of brachial plexus block, and this possibility should increase as the distance from the injection site to the spinal column decreases. Furthermore, the likelihood of such an occurrence should be greater with a technique that utilizes a single, large volume injection than with techniques which utilize multiple, smaller volume injections. In practice, however, such an occurrence is extremely unlikely, for at the beginning of an injection, even if the needle tip is intraneural, the thrust of the first few ml's of the injected solution will almost invariably push the nerve off the tip of the needle. Anyone who has *attempted* to make a deliberate intraneural injection in a cadaver realizes that to do so is almost as difficult as trying to make an injection into the substance of a wet noodle! Only if a very thin, very shortbevel needle is place *totally* intraneurally at a point where the nerve is completely fixed, could such an injection be carried out; and even then the anesthetist would be alerted to the possibility of intraneural injection because of the agonizing pain such an injection causes the patient. It would appear, again from Selander's work, that the characteristic, excruciating pain of a true intraneural injection is produced by the phenomenal pressure generated when an injection is made under the perineurium within a fascicle. Obviously, then, should an injection be accompanied by a complaint of agonizing pain in the arm, or even worse, of severe headache, the injection should be stopped immediately and the possibility of subarachnoid block anticipated.

Because of the *potential* seriousness of total spinal blockade, the rapid development of apnea, hypotension, bradycardia, and unconsciousness following the performance of a brachial block should be *assumed* to represent intrathecal injection, whatever mechanism is involved. As the complication develops, it may simulate the "depressant" phase of a systemic reaction to the local anesthetic; and though spinal block can be readily differentiated from a systemic reaction by the presence of apnea, anhidrosis, and miosis, time should not be lost in attempting to differentiate between the two complications, since the treatment is identical. And as stated earlier, if such a clinical picture develops after a delay of as much as 20–40 minutes, the diagnosis of total spinal block should not be ruled out simply on the basis of its slow onset.

Obviously, careful placement of the needle and repeated aspiration for spinal fluid prior to injection will minimize the incidence of this complication, but it is clear from the preceding discussion that failure to obtain spinal fluid on aspiration does not preclude the possibility of its occurrence. Once the diagnosis of total spinal has been made, management by a competent anesthetist is straightforward, and the complication should be without serious sequelae. On the other hand, if a total spinal is *not* recognized quickly and treatment is not instituted immediately, it may be rapidly fatal. Obviously, then, a brachial block should *never* be undertaken unless means of supporting ventilation and circulation are readily available, since ventilatory support and the administration of vasopressors promptly converts a potentially lethal complication into a harmless, though frightening, experience. There are two cases of total spinal following interscalene brachial block reported in the literature, and they illustrate the importance of rapid resuscitation to a good outcome: in the first case, reported by Ross and Scarborough, the patient developed dysphonia after only 5 ml had been injected; but because the patient could still move his upper extremities on command, the injection was continued, and by the time 30 ml had been given, the patient lost consciousness and stopped breathing. Had they discontinued the injection at the time of the early warning signs, the total spinal would have been averted. Nonetheless, the patient was intubated and ventilated, and the blood pressure was supported pharmacologically; and the patient recovered in $2\frac{1}{2}$ hours without any sequelae and without any recall of the events that followed the block. In the second case, reported by Edde and Deutsch, a 6 cm needle was utilized to perform the block, and in spite of negative aspiration for blood and CSF, shortly after the injection of 20 ml of 0.5% bupivacaine the patient lost consciousness, and the electrocardiogram showed ventricular fibrillation. The trachea was immediately intubated and the lungs ventilated with 100% oxygen; and after appropriate doses of sodium bicarbonate, epinephrine and calcium chloride, defibrillation effectively restored a normal sinus rhythm. After about $1\frac{1}{2}$ hours the patient awoke and was extubated, and again, he recovered without any neurological sequelae.

As stated in Chapter III, a needle longer than $1\frac{1}{2}$ inches is *never* necessary. The author was told of another case (not in the literature) where the use of a spinal needle to perform an interscalene block led to an intramedullary injection and total spinal anesthesia, and when the spi-nal wore off, the patient had a permanent Brown-Sequard syndrome. During the injection, the anesthetist had been forewarned by the agonizing pain produced by the injection that the needle was improperly placed, but the injection was completed with the devastating results already alluded to.

Epidural block

If a misplaced needle enters an intervertebral foramen but does *not* penetrate dura, the injection of local anesthetic will most likely result in a high epidural block rather than a spinal block.

As a matter of fact, this complication was so frequent following the paravertebral nerve block techniques developed by Kappis in the first decade of this century that it caused him to abandon his technique at all but a few levels of the vertebral column. Less obvious, however, is the fact that from work as early as that of Dog-

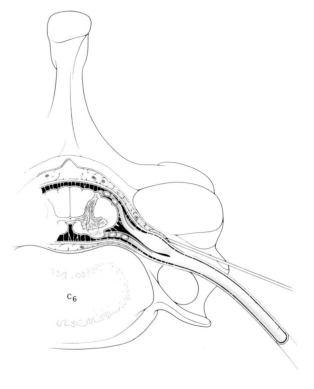

c_6

246

liotti, it would appear that under the right circumstances epidural block could result from a much more peripheral injection. Dogliotti showed that the "peridural tissue" filling the epidural space is continuous with the "perivertebral tissue" that continues towards the periphery with the segmental nerves. He demonstrated this "tissue continuity" by showing that radiopaque solutions injected into the epidural space diffuse out of the foramina and along these perineural tissues in the first 20–30 minutes post–injection, and ultimately progress as far as 10–15 cm beyond the foramina over the next few hours. Thus, it would appear that the reverse should be possible, that is, for solutions injected into these perivertebral and perineural tissues during the performance of a brachial block to diffuse centrally into the epidural space, resulting in an epidural block. On the other hand, this possibility would *seem* to be ruled out by the repeated x-rays taken by the author after the injection of radiopaque dye into the interscalene, subclavian perivascular, and axillary perivascular spaces, all of which failed to show such epidural extension; however, unlike the radiopaque dyes utilized by Dogliotti, we used water soluble dyes which are rapidly absorbed and excreted, so that after 10–15 minutes, the location of the contrast media could no longer be determined. Therefore, it is possible that the dye was absorbed before extension into the peridural space could take place. That such is *possible* was demonstrated clinically as early as 1947 when Macintosh and Mushin reported that when they placed needles in the paravertebral spaces on opposite sides of the vertebral column, fluid injected into one side came out through the needle on the opposite side, indicating the continuity between epidural and paravertebral perineural spaces. They later demonstrated the continuity of these spaces by anatomical dissections. Certainly, this not only explains the development of epidural anesthesia as a complication of brachial block, but also the occasional reports of "bilateral spread of analgesia with interscalene brachial plexus block."

Nonetheless, when high epidural block does occur following the performance of a brachial plexus block, it is characterized by a *gradual* onset of bilateral anesthesia. The extent of the resultant block, and hence the severity of the sequelae, will depend on how much of the local anesthetic injected reaches the epidural space. Both Moore and Adriani have described inadvertent high epidural block following stellate ganglion blocks, but in their cases only 10 ml of the local anesthetic solution was utilized, so the resultant block involved only the upper extremities; and their patients simply complained of the inability to move their arms until the block wore off. However, if an entire injection of 30–40 ml is made at this level into the epidural space, hypoventilation, bradycardia, and hypotension will result, though the onset will be more gradual than with a spinal block, and the patient will usually remain conscious *unless* circulatory collapse is allowed to occur. As with spinal block, support of ventilation and circulation should be undertaken at the first sign of this complication, though the administration of oxygen and atropine may be all that is required.

Obviously, of the perivascular techniques of brachial plexus block, the interscalene technique is the most likely to produce an inadvertent epidural block, and yet this complication has *only* been described with 4 patients who had undergone a brachial block using the interscalene technique. However, it is virtually impossible to enter an intervertebral foramen if the interscalene technique is carried out exactly as described (see Chapter III), for the slight caudad direction of the needle will cause it to impinge on bone before it can reach an intervertebral foramen. Only if the needle is inserted directly mesiad, i.e., in a horizontal direction, can it reach the intervertebral foramen if it is advanced far enough and that is precisely what happened in the three cases in the literature.

Nerve damage

When apparent nerve damage follows a surgical procedure carried out under brachial plexus anesthesia, as evidenced by the appearance of persistent sensory and/or motor deficit, with or without paresthesias, the etiology is extremely difficult to assess because of the multitude of factors that might be involved. Preoperative factors include pre-existing neurological disease or damage, latent or overt, while *intraoperative factors* include the spontaneous development of neurological dysfunction, nerve damage due to the surgical procedure and its accompanying trauma, damage due to the tourniquet utilized for hemostasis, and chemical damage due to the local anesthetic agent itself. Another more common and frequently overlooked cause of intraoperative nerve damage is malpositioning of an anesthetized extremity on the operating table. And finally, the most important *postoperative* cause is trauma that can occur when the anesthetized extremity is paralyzed and insensitive to pain during the subsequent recovery period, while the block is wearing off.

The best way to avoid incrimination of the anesthetic technique for "postanesthetic nerve damage" which actually existed preoperatively is to be certain that a careful neurological examination has been done *prior to* the performance of the block. Even this is not infallible as a means of exonerating the anesthetic, for in cases of severe trauma, subsequent edema, hematoma formation, or unrecognized nerve damage may result in *delayed* loss of function, which would become obvious only *after* the surgical procedure and the administration of the anesthetic. The intraoperative herniation or extrusion of a cervical disc, and to a lesser degree, trauma to nerves by bony spurs and other arthritic changes which comprise the mobility of the nerves and nerve roots when a fully paralyzed anesthetized arm is manipulated, may also cause neurological dysfunction that becomes apparent in the postoperative period. Direct intraoperative trauma to the nerves can result from the surgical procedure itself as well as from traumatic placement and pulling of retractors. Following the onset of anesthesia of the brachial plexus, especially when the subclavian perivascular and interscalene techniques have been utilized to anesthetize the entire arm and shoulder girdle, extreme care must bee taken to protect the anesthetized arm before, during, and after surgery, until the anesthesia has completely dissipated: because of the sensory block the patient will not feel or appreciate trauma to the arm; because of the proprioceptive block the patient will be unaware of the position of the arm; and because of the motor block and relaxation of the muscles of the shoulder girdle and arm, if the arm is not carefully protected, it could fall off the table, stretcher, or bed, with resultant neural and/or vascular damage, and even dislocation of the shoulder. Furthermore, if the arm is kept in hyperextension for a prolonged period of time, especially if the position is accompanied by external rotation and traction, neural damage can result in as little as 45 minutes. Usually, though not always, this latter type of damage will be apparent immediately after the anesthetic has worn off, so the importance of seeing the patient as soon as possible after dissipation of the anesthetic effects of a block cannot be emphasized enough. While recovery may not be complete for a considerable time after a block carried out with the newer protein-binding local anesthetics, a quick postanesthetic assessment of neurological function should be carried out as routinely as a preoperative one.

Tourniquet paralysis syndrome

In the early reports of complications following surgery carried out under brachial plexus anesthesia it would appear that the vast majority of cases of nerve damage were due to the common practice of using thick rubber tubing as a tourniquet, a practice subsequently shown to cause actual mechanical trauma and damage to nerves, especially those unprotected by the neighboring musculature. When the Esmarch bandage replaced rubber tubing as the tourniquet, the incidence of "tourniquet paralysis" decreased considerably, and then with the advent of the pneumatic tourniquet, which allowed the application of a *controllable* amount of pressure over a larger area, this syndrome became exceedingly rare. The reduction in the incidence of tourniquet paralysis with the improvement of tourniquet technology would seem to indicate that ischemia was

not the cause of this complication, for the degree of ischemia should be the same for any tourniquet, rubber or pneumatic. Thus, it appears more likely that mechanical pressure played the predominant, if not the only causative role in the production of the syndrome. However, even with a pneumatic tourniquet this complication is possible if the *pressure utilized* is excessively high or if the *time of application* is excessively prolonged. Therefore, good practice dictates that a tourniquet on the arm should not be inflated to pressures exceeding 350 mm Hg and should be deflated approximately every 60 minutes. Even with religious adherance to these rules, several cases of tourniquet paralysis were recently reported as the result of a faulty aneroid manometer, which registered 350 mm when in reality over 1200 mm Hg of pressure was being applied by the tourniquet! As a result, in some centers valves have been incorporated into the system by means of a T-piece between the manometer and the tourniquet, which will not allow the tourniquet pressure to exceed 350 mm Hg, regardless of the reading on the manometer.

As elucidated by Mouldaver, the tourniquet paralysis syndrome is a definitive entity with specific distinguishing signs and symptoms, which along with a characteristic response to electrical stimulation, provide four definitive diagnostic criteria: first, there is *motor dysfunction* with paralysis and hypotonia or atonia, but no appreciable atrophy: second, there is *sensory dissociation* wherein the modalities of touch, pressure, vibration, and position sense are usually absent, while temperature and pain remain intact. In fact, in most cases there is actual *hyper algesia*, which may persist even after the other modalities have returned to normal. In severe cases even the fibers subserving pain and temperature can be affected, but this is quite rare. In any case, there are no paresthetias or tingling sensations after release of the tourniquet because of damage to the fibers subserving touch; nor is there a positive Tinel's sign (production of paresthesia by tapping over a nerve). Third, *sympathetic function* is not affected, so that pilomotor and psychogalvanic reflexes are intact, and the skin color, temperature, and plethysmographic findings are all normal. And fourth, the *response to electrical stimulation* indicates a conduction block characterized by no response to stimulation of the motor nerve above the level of injury but a good response below it. Further, there is no tingling sensation on stimulation of sensory fibers distal to the site of injury, but there is a tingling sensation produced when the stimulation is proximal to the lesion.

Mouldaver concluded from these diagnostic criteria that the tourniquet paralysis syndrome is a localized form of mechanical nerve damage which affects primarily the larger A-alpha and A-beta fibers, so that the motor power, touch, pressure, vibration, and proprioception are affected rather than pain and sympathetic function, which are subserved by the smaller A-delta and C fibers. Mouldaver also pointed out that the resultant impairment required 3 or more months for complete recovery, but that recovery was the rule rather than the exception.

Positional paralysis
Perhaps the commonest cause of postoperative paralysis of the brachial plexus, and certainly the most commonly overlooked cause, is malpositioning of the extremity during surgery. As early as 1894, before any local anesthetic other than cocaine was available and before percutaneous brachial plexus block had even been described, Budingir described brachial plexus palsies that occurred at the operating table. Three years later Garrigues described the cases reported up to that time and concluded that the real exciting cause in the cases of peripheral origin is pressure exerted locally on nerves or blood vessels due to improper position of the arm on the table. As alluded to earlier, it was because of an unexplained case of brachial plexus palsy following surgery that Wright carried out his study, which showed that simple hyperabduction of the arm above the head obliterated the radial pulse at the wrist in 82–83% of those studied. Furthermore, Dhuner examined the records of 26 cases of "postanesthetic brachial plexus palsy" following surgical procedures and found that not a single one of the patients had received a brachial plexus block and that malposition of the arm explained virtually every case. And finally, the data indicate clearly that injury to the brachial plexus is far more common after general than after regional anesthesia, and that the commonest cause of such injury is improper position of the arm on the table. So it is obvious that damage to the brachial plexus can occur due to malposition during surgery, regardless of whether the surgery is carried out under brachial plexus anesthesia or general anesthesia; but if it occurs when the surgery has been carried out under brachial plexus anesthesia, it is the anesthetic that is usually incriminated.

Clausen has elucidated the mechanism by which positional injury to the brachial plexus occurs most commonly dur-

250

ing upper extremity surgery: he pointed out that anatomically the nerves are fixed proximally at the transverse processes by invaginations of the prevertebral fascia and distally in the upper arm by the axillary fascia. Thus, any structure or structures tending to increase the distance between these points of fixation of the nerves beyond normal limits will cause injury by stretching the nerves. There are four such structures, according to Clausen:

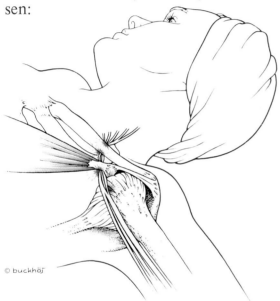

© buckhöj

The first is the arch formed by the tendinous attachment of the pectoralis minor to the coracoid process, which acts as a fulcrum in the axilla, around which the neurovascular bundle must pass; the second is the clavicle, which in extreme abduction and extension actually compresses the plexus and the subclavian vessels against the first rib and increases the tension on the nerves distal to the point of compression; the third is the prominence formed by the head of the humerus, which with the arm in external rotation,

abduction, and extension produces an axillary prominence around which the nerves and vessels must pass; and the fourth is the first rib, which interacts with the clavicle as stated above. Obviously congenital anomalies such as the presence of a cervical rib, anomalous derivation of the plexus (especially a "prefixed plexus"), hypertrophy of the scalene muscles, or presence of a scalenus minimus muscle can make the nerves even more vulnerable. It would seem obvious that with the arm externally rotated, hyperabducted, and extended, especially with the head deviated and extended to the opposite side, the plexus is stretched between the various points of fixation and compression and ischemic and/or mechanical nerve damage can result. Furthermore, if the arm is allowed to fall backward off the table while it is flaccidly paralyzed from the brachial block, the plexus may actually be avulsed at one of the points of fixation and/or compression.

If apparent positional injury has occurred, the extent and degree of paralysis should be noted immediately upon awakening. According to Clausen, sensation is less frequently affected than motor power, and in many cases, it may not be involved at all, though he did report some patients who complained of anesthesia, hypoesthesia, hyperesthesia, and even paresthesia. He stated that reflexes may or may not be present, depending on the severity of the injury, and that usually, but not invariably, tenderness appeared in the supraclavicular space 5–10 days after operation. In several of Clausen's cases Horner's syndrome was also noted, indicating damage to the lower roots of the plexus with resultant sympathetic dysfunction. While there is no specific treatment for

251

positional paralysis, fortunately the return of function is usually rapid and complete; and sensation, if impaired, returns to normal very quickly. In a few patients, full motor recovery may require several months; but according to Kwaan, there has not as yet been a single case of *permanent* injury reported in the English literature. Obviously, the best therapy for this complication is its prevention by careful positioning and protection of the extremity.

Toxic, chemical neuropathy

Another potential source of nerve damage following brachial plexus block, perhaps more theoretical than real, is chemical damage from the anesthetic solution itself. The vast majority of local anesthetic agents in clinical use today are extremely safe, provided they are utilized in the recommended concentrations and in the recommended total doses. In the experimental laboratory it is necessary to use concentrations of local anesthetics far in excess of those used clinically to produce irreversible nerve damage. Selander recently demonstrated that when bupivacaine is *topically* applied to periphral nerves (to simulate perineural injection) in concentrations as high as 2%, no significant degenerative changes occurred within the nerve. Only when a concentration of 4% was applied did adhesions, epineurial thickening, and degenerative changes occur, but in the study protocol even these changes were not statistically significant. Selander did show, however, that *intrafascicular* injection of bupivacaine, even in a concentration of 0.5%, caused *significant* axonal degeneration, the magnitude of which increased somewhat with concentration but much more with the addition of epinephrine; but he

subsequently showed that the acute effects of intrafascicular injection were due more to the trauma of injection than to the toxicity of the local anesthetic and/or epinephrine. Nonetheless, Bonica and Moore have stated repeatedly that they believe that the incidence of neuropathy *is* related to the concentration of the local anesthetic agent injected, and hence they advocate limiting the concentration of local anesthetic in brachial plexus block with lidocaine and mepivacaine, for example, to a 1% concentration. Both of these authorities base this opinion on their review of many case reports of neurological damage following brachial plexus blocks performed with lidocaine and mepivacaine, and both feel that the incidence of such damage was higher when the blocks were carried out with 1.5 or 2% concentrations than when they were carried out with a 1.0% concentration. Moore admits, however, that "whether these resulted from the agent or from trauma to the plexus was undetermined." It is puzzling to the author to note that both of these authorities in the field of regional anesthesia advocate the use of 1.5–2% concentration of these same agents in the epidural space; and yet it would appear that the nerves have no greater protection (by virtue of additional perineural investments) in the epidural space that in the periphery, so it does not seem logical that the nerves should be less resistant to the concentration related toxicity of local anesthetics in the periphery than in the epidural space. Obviously, this issue awaits objective documentation before it is settled, but in the meantime, it is fortuitous that increased concentrations of local anesthetic agents are only rarely necessary to block all of the modalities within the brachial plexus, so unless profound muscle relaxation is mandatory in the muscles of the forearm and hand, a concentration of 1% lidocaine or mepivacaine is sufficient.

Occasionally epinephrine has been incriminated as a factor in causing neural damage. It is well documented that, except in the spinal canal, the efficacy of epinephrine in prolonging anesthetic duration and decreasing systemic absorption of local anesthetics increases with increasing concentrations up to a concentration of 1:200,000, beyond which there is no further increase in efficacy, only an increase in the systemic effects of the epinephrine. Furthermore, it is equally well documented that local anesthetics with epinephrine 1:200,000 are no more neurotoxic than the same local anesthetics alone, again, provided that intraneural injection is carefully avoided. A special problem can be presented by the use of multiple dose vials of local anesthetic agents containing epinephrine: irritating copper, nickel, and zinc ions may be released by the action of local anesthetics on metal needles used to carry out nerve blocks; and while these ions are usually absorbed before they can result in neurotoxicity, since the injected solution contains epinephrine, at least theoretically, the ions may be kept in contact with the nerves long enough to cause some degree of neuritis. Therefore, it is considered bad practice to keep multiple dose vials of local anesthetics containing epinephrine for any length of time.

In short, the concentration of local anesthetics should be tailored to the needs of the particular surgical patient, and obviously, the weakest concentration required to provide the desired degree of blockade should be utilized; and even this should be reduced in the presence of peripheral neurological disease. Similarly epinephrine should be added only when necessary to increase the duration of action of a particular agent or to decrease the systemic absorption, and it should be carefully measured and added just prior to its use. The impact of epinephrine on the pharmacokinetics of the various local anesthetic agents is quite different, so epinephrine should never be utilized routinely, only when specifically indicated and when not contraindicated by systemic cardiovascular or peripheral neurological disease. If apparent chemical nerve damage should occur in spite of the above precautions, Wooley and Vandam have indicated that such damage can be differentiated from damage due to pressure (tourniquet or positional damage) in that chemical damage characteristically involves small fibers. Hence, toxic damage causes anesthesia, analgesia, hypesthesia, hypalgesia, hyperalgesia and spontaneous paresthesias and in addition, there may be disturbances in sympathetic function. These findings are in direct contrast to those produced by damage due to pressure, which, as pointed out earlier, results in dysfunction of the larger fibers, leading to losses in motor, touch, and proprioceptive function with preservation of pain and temperature and with no paresthesias.

Neural damage due to needle trauma and/or intraneural injection

In Chapter III the author has recommended strongly that paresthesias deliberately be sought in carrying out the interscalene technique and the subclavian perivascular technique of brachial plexus block, and while paresthesias are not *deliberately* sought by the author in carrying out the axillary perivascular technique, Selander has shown that paresthesias will be encountered 40% of the time. Therefore, one certainly must consider, at least, the possibility that when paresthetias are produced, the needle and/or the subsequent injection could cause mechanical damage to the nerve encountered. In an attempt to asses the role that paresthesias might play in the production of nerve lesions, Selander studied a group of 533 patients undergoing hand surgery under axillary brachial block: in 290 of the patients the brachial plexus was located by actively seeking paresthesias, and in 243 patients paresthesias were avoided and two needles were inserted into the neurovascular sheath close enough to the artery that the needles oscillated synchronously with the pulse. Postoperatively 10 patients had nerve lesions that appeared to be related to the axillary block, and in all 10 of the patients paresthesias had been produced prior to the injection of the local anesthetic, although 2 of these patients were in the group where the anesthetists had tried to avoid such paresthesias. This study, probably the only *prospective* study in the literature, would appear to set the incidence of postanesthetic neuropathy due to needle trauma at almost 2%, a figure that is significantly higher than that observed by most previous authors. Three of the 10 patients who developed evidence of neuropathy had reported that their paresthesias were enhanced during the actual injection of the local anesthetic, probably indicating that at least some of the anesthetic was injected intraneurally. In one patient the axillary block was repeated, perhaps increasing the possibility of nerve damage, because a supplementary injection into a partially blocked plexus may cause damage to an already blocked nerve, since contact with the needle will not produce the usual warning signs. Another one patient who developed a neuropathy also developed an axillary hematoma, so this may have contributed to the postanesthetic signs and symptoms, or it may even have produced the neuropathy itself, as discussed earlier. The symptoms described by the patients who developed complications in this study varied from "light paresthesias" of a few weeks' duration to serious paresthesias, aching pain, sensory disturbances, and overt paresis lasting more than a year. Of the 10 patients, 9 complained of ache, radiating pain, and axillary tenderness, and palpation of the axilla or elevation of the arm produced paresthesias. Selander stated that it was difficult to determine precisely when the symptoms actually arose, but indicated that the earliest appeared within 24 hours of the block and the latest not later than the third postoperative week. In 6 patients there were signs of paresis, most of them minor, but one patient developed complete and apparently permanent paresis. In 7 of the 10 patients the signs and symptoms disappeared spontaneously within 2–12 weeks, but in 3 patients the symptoms persisted for over one year. Two of these patients were explored surgically, and external neurolysis was performed, as there were signs of constrictive epineuritis. In one of the two, it appeared that surgery led to some improvement, but in the other there was little evidence of any benefit.

As stated earlier, this report by Selander is virtually the only prospective study in the literature, and compared to *most* of the earlier retrospective studies, the incidence of neuropathy after brachial plexus block anesthesia appears high, although in all studies, prospective and retrospective, it appears to be lower than the incidence of nerve damage following general anesthesia! It is entirely possible, of course, that in the retrospective studies, some cases of nerve damage were missed because the signs and symptoms were insufficient in magnitude or were sufficiently delayed in onset that the anesthetist was unaware of them. Thus Kulenkampff and Persky reported only one case out of 1000, de Pablo and Diez-Malloy reported 5 cases out of 3000, and Bonica reported 4 cases out of 1100; so reports like these would seem to indicate an incidence of neuropathy of 0.1–0.4%. On the other hand, in smaller studies where a deliberate, careful postanesthetic examination was carried out, the incidence was significantly higher. For example, Johnson and Greifenstein reported 6 out of 432 patients who had significant nerve damage after brachial plexus block that was "apparently related to anesthesia," and Moberg found 17 out of 300 patients who had persistant paresthesias after brachial block, indicating an incidence of 1.4–5.6%.

Whatever the incidence, it is clear that though rare, nerve damage secondary to brachial plexus block is possible, either because of damage produced by the needle itself or because of damage produced by an intraneural injection. In carefully conducted studies using electroneurography to detect signs of postinjection nerve damage, Löfström and his co-workers demonstrated the fact that rapid intraneural injection may cause mechanical nerve damage, but that the most important factor in producing residual dysfunction was the trauma produced by the insertion of a needle into the nerve, particularly if the needle was inserted repeatedly. Interestingly enough, the electroneurographic signs of damage had a delayed onset, appearing in no less than a week, reaching a peak in about 3 weeks, and showing evidence of regression about 2–3 months later. While it should be appreciated that these were only electroneurographic changes which were infrequently accompanied by symptoms, these studies do provide evidence that the chance of producing mechanical nerve damage is directly proportional to the number of paresthesias produced; so in light of these data, it would appear that the single injection perivascular techniques should reduce the incidence of neuropathy associated with previously utilized multiple injection techniques, whatever that incidence is.

Again, Selander has carried out an elegant study of the factors determining the extent of peripheral nerve injury due to the characteristics of the needles utilized in carrying out regional blocks; and these studies indicate clearly that a short-bevel (45°) needle significantly diminishes the risk of fascicular injury as compared to the more traditional, long-bevel (12°) needle. This difference, according to Selander, is propably a result of the fact that a nerve tends to slide or roll away from a short-bevel needle more than it does from a long–bevel needle, which impales it. These same studies also indicate that the magnitude of fascicular injury is considerably less when the bevel of the needle is inserted parallel to the nerve fiber axis, rather than across that axis, especially when using a long–bevel needle.

Selander's experimental demonstration of the relative superiority of the short bevel needle in minimizing nerve trauma is gratifying to the present author who has long advocated the use of a short–bevel needle for performing nerve blocks, but only because the short bevel allows a greater tactile perception of the penetration of fascial planes by the needle; but when this advantage is coupled with the advantages pointed out by Selander, it is obvious that *only* short–bevel needles should be utilized in carrying out peripheral nerve blocks. In addition, the present author has always indicated that needles longer than 1½ inches (38 mm) should *never* be used for any of the perivascular techniques of brachial plexus anesthesia, and in the only two patients known to the author (one published and one unpublished), who sustained permanent neurological damage secondary to an interscalene brachial block, a spinal needle was utilized: in one case it would appear that an intraforaminal injection was made into a motor nerve root through a horizontally placed spinal needle, and in the other case an intramedullary injection was apparently made after an earlier partial injection, also using a spinal needle. In both cases, the misplaced injection would have been much less likely, if not impossible, had the shorter needle advocated been utilized. Also in both cases, severe pain was produced by the injection, indicating an intraneural injection, yet the injection was not abandoned as should have been done. These two cases illustrate the price paid when two fundamental principles of nerve blocking are violated: the first, whenever an injection produces *severe* pain, the needle must be *presumed* to be intraneural, and the injection must be abandoned; and the second, once local anesthetic has been injected into the sheath, one should no longer attempt to produce paresthesias, since partially anesthetized nerves can be traumatized severely without the usual paresthetic warning being provoked.

Obviously, the diameter of a needle must be an important factor related to the *degree* of nerve injury produced by a needle, and yet while Kulenkampff and Persky stated as early as 1928, "to avoid injury to the cords of the plexus a very fine caliber needle is to be used," the importance of the caliber of the needle in the production of nerve injury has not been subjected to experimental evaluation. Nonetheless, most authors suggest the use of the smallest needle possible in order to minimize the degree of damage that might be produced from needle. The author and his co-workers feel that a 22–gauge needle is the best compromise in size, since it is small enough to minimize the degree of trauma that might be due to the caliber of the needle but large enough that the force of the injected solution can push the nerve which has been contacted away from the tip of the needle. We feel that with 25–gauge needles the force of the injected solution is attenuated sufficiently that the chances of an intraneural injection might be enhanced. We do use a 25–gauge needle in infants and children in an effort to minimize the pain of the needle insertion, but in this group of patients we do not attempt to produce a paresthesia.

Moore has challenged the fact that intraneural injections cause nerve damage on the basis that he and his colleagues have deliberately made intraneural injections into the brachial plexus without causing nerve damage; however, his criterion for an injection being intraneural was paresthesias and aching in the extremity during the injection of the anesthetic solution. As stated in Chapter III, the dull aching pain produced during a rapid injection into the perivascular compartment containing the brachial plexus is simply a sign of rapid perineural, rather than intraneural injection, and is caused by the sudden increase in pressure within the sheath, similar to the sensation produced by rapid injection into the caudal canal. As a matter of fact, the author has demonstrated repeatedly in cadavers that if you deliberately attempt to make such an injection into one of the nerves of the brachial plexus, as soon as pressure is applied to the syringe, the anesthetic solution pushes the nerve off the needle, particularly if a 22–gauge short–bevel needle is utilized. It would appear that the only circumstance under which this would *not* be the case is that in which the needle impales a nerve where it lies against bone, so that movement of the nerve away from the needle during the injection is impossible; and in this case severe pain occurring during the injection would warn the anesthetist of the intraneural placement of the needle.

Moore has also said that "to elicit paresthesias it is obvious that the needle must come into direct contact with the nerves and at times pierce the epineurium and enter the fasciculi, yet to date we have seen no neuritis or other nerve lesions when aqueous solutions were used." Selander has studied the effects of actual intraneural injection in animals and showed that injections *under the epineurium* produced transient, minor increases in the intraneural pressure (25–60 mm Hg) and hence caused limited spread of the injected solution (2.5–6.5 cm). On the other hand, injections made into a nerve fascicle *within the perineurium* produced very prolonged and marked increases in pressure (330–750 mm Hg) and caused a rapid spread over long distances within the fascicle (4–15 cm). In those intrafascicular injections where the injected solution reached the spinal medulla, the solution then spread superficially under the pia mater. This finding confirms the concept of Shanthaveerappa and Bourne, who stated that the perineurium is a direct peripheral extension of the pia-arachnoid, and also explains the reports of sudden, unexpected *spinal* anesthesia following nerve blocks carried out close to the spine, such as interscalene brachial plexus blocks. During subepineurial injection, Selander noted that the epineurium easily expanded and usually formed an irregular bleb around the injection site. Furthermore, the injected solution spread for much shorter distances than a similar solution injected subperineurially and frequently ruptured the epineurium. In a clinical setting if such spread and rupture occurred several centimeters proximal to the site of injection during the performance of an interscalene block, it could represent another mechanism by which unexpected *epidural* anesthesia could follow the performance of an interscalene brachial block, since the epineurium is simply a peripheral extension of the duramater. The likelihood of this possibility would even be greater in man than in Selander's rabbits, for man has a firmer epineurial sheath than rabbits. However, a much more important finding in Selander's study is the fact that the *magnitude* of the intrafascicular pressure developed during and after intrafascicular injection may exceed the capillary perfusion pressure for 10–15 minutes! Such a period of intraneural ischemia might very well render ordinarily nontoxic concentrations of local anesthetic agents toxic, particularly if the presence of epinephrine enhanced the degree and duration of the ischemia even further. And indeed, in the final phase of the study, Selander did demonstrate that the intrafascicular injection of agents which were harmless when applied topically produced significant axonal damage and that the damage increased *significantly* when epinephrine was added to the solution. Obviously, the conclusion to be drawn from these studies is that, as stated earlier, epinephrine should not be utilized for nerve blocks *routinely,* but only when specifically indicated to minimize the possibility of systemic effects of local anesthetics and when not contraindicated by cardiovascular or neurological disease. Today, with the advent of the long-acting protein-binding local anesthetics, epinephrine is virtually unnecessary to provide a longer duration of action.

As indicated in Chapter IV, Galindo has designed special needles which are teflon coated except at the tip, to allow more accurate localization of nerves when using a nerve stimulator, and which have a "pencil point" tip to minimize trauma to the nerves being blocked. Since Selander's studies seemed to indicate that the damage done to a nerve by a needle inserted into it was due to the cutting edges of the needle, Galindo felt that the pin-type would separate nerve fascicles without cutting them. And indeed, when he compared the degree of nerve damage produced by a 22-gauge pin-point needle with that produced by a 22-gauge short-bevel needle, Galindo did find that there was no damage during nerve penetration with the pin-point needle as compared with 50% damage produced by a short-bevel needle. Unfortunately, the significance of the difference is minimized by the fact that the short-bevel needle was inserted with the bevel transverse to the nerve fibers, the bevel orientation which Selander's studies indicated produced more damage. The other beneficial effect

of the pencil-point needle in reducing nerve trauma was demonstrated by the fact that Galindo could not produce an intraneural injection with his needle, due to the fact that the aperture is proximal to the point. This is in contrast to the short-bevel needle, through which deliberate intraneural injection produced a mean pressure of 755 mm Hg. Thus it would appear that the inability of the special point of this needle to cut nerve fascicles and the placement of the apperture proximal to the pin-point to prevent intraneural injection *should* reduce even further the already low incidence of nerve damage following the administration of a nerve block. Obviously, extensive clinical testing will be necessary before final judgment can be passed. Certainly, the fact that these needles are "special equipment" and not readily available may discourage their use prematurely.

While it is important that the regional anesthetist be aware of all of the factors which are capable of producing nerve damage, in order to accurately access the role of the anesthetic and surgical factors, as stated earlier one must have, at least, a cursory preoperative evaluation of neurological function. While it is impractical to expect a careful, detailed neurological examination prior to every elective surgical procedure on the upper extremity, it is possible to utilize Livingstone's method of rapid identification of neuropathies of the major peripheral nerves derived from the brachial plexus, which consists of five simple steps:

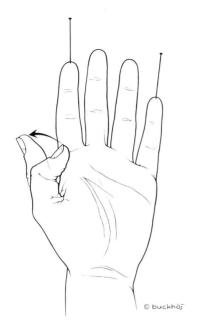

© buckhöj

(1) The *median nerve* is tested by pinprick over the palmar surface of the distal phalanx of the index finger; (2) the *ulnar nerve* is tested in a similar manner by pinprick over the palmar surface of the distal phalanx of the fifth finger; (3) *radial nerve* function is checked by extension of the distal phalanx of the thumb; (4) *musculocutaneous nerve* function can be assessed by flexion of the forearm; and (5) *axillary nerve* function can be tested by abduction of the arm. Livingstone's method is so simple and fast, it *can* be carried out routinely preoperatively. Obviously, if the patient is undergoing surgery for trauma that may already have produced nerve damage, a complete neurological examination is mandatory. But in the elective case where postoperative neurological dysfunction is not anticipated, Livingstone's test is more than adequate. Furthermore, it is only by such *routine pre* and *post*-operative testing that the *true* incidence of nerve injuries due to anesthesia can be determined.

If and when neurologic sequelae do arise after a brachial plexus block, careful evaluation of the sensory and motor function of each of the major nerves will usually indicate not only which nerve is damaged, but at what level the damage has occurred, and depending on which nerve or combination of nerves is damaged, one can tell whether the damage is at a root, trunk, cord or peripheral nerve level. As stated in Chapter I, detailed knowledge of the neuroanatomy of the upper extremity is absolutely essential to such an evaluation. For this reason the sensory and motor deficits resulting from damage to the five major derivatives of the brachial plexus are illustrated in these sections devoted to the distribution of each nerve.

Whenever neurologic dysfunction is evident in a patient who has undergone upper extremity surgery under regional anesthesia, the possibility of other causes should be carefully investigated *before* the nerve block itself is incriminated. Marinacci has emphasized the importance of performing electromyography as soon as a neurological complication becomes manifest in order to accurately assess the etiologic role (or to establish the lack of such a role) of the anesthetic and to investigate the possibility of a pre-existing lesion, concurrent disease, or concomitant trauma. Marinaci points out that the electromyogram records two specific types of muscle activity: normal activity recorded from normally innervated muscle; and denervated activity recorded from muscles that have lost their nerve supply. The change from an innervated to a denervated pattern occurs 18–21 days after the actual nerve damage. Thus, if an electromyogram performed immediately after surgery shows denervation activity, obviously this activity must have resulted from a pre-existing lesion or some other concurrent disease problem, since it takes

18–21 days from the actual damage for such activity to appear. On the other hand, if the electromyogram shows normal activity immediately postoperatively and subsequently shows denervated activity 18–21 days after surgery, the damage occurred at the time of surgery. Furthermore, by carefully noting which muscles show denervated activity, knowing the nerve supply to those muscles (Chapter I), one can determine precisely what nerves are involved. And finally, by determining nerve conduction velocities along the course of the nerves involved, and the level at which slowing occurs, the precise level of the lesion can be determined, and with this information even the various etiologic possibilities operant at the time of surgery can be differentiated from each other. For example, in a patient exhibiting an ulnar neuropathy following surgical transposition of the ulnar nerve at the elbow performed under interscalene brachial plexus block, if the electromyogram and conduction velocity studies indicate that the lesion is at the elbow, clearly the interscalene brachial block cannot be incriminated. The value of carrying out electromyographic and conduction velocity studies immediately postoperatively has been documented by Marinacci, who performed EMG's on 542 patients whose neurological complaints were considered to represent possible complications of spinal anesthesia. In only 4 of these cases could spinal anesthesia actually be incriminated, and in the remaining 538 cases, the neurological symptoms were due to other conditions, which included accidental surgical section of a nerve or nerves, trauma to a nerve or nerves by surgical retractors, positional pressure, positional stretching, infectious polyneuritis, herniated nucleus pulposus, and conversion hysteria.

One other possible complication of brachial plexus block due to needle trauma is worthy of mention, in spite of the fact that it is exceedingly rare. It is well known that reflex sympathetic dystrophy can follow even the slightest neural or even perineural trauma, so obviously the performance of a rather traumatic brachial block, especially with multiple injections, could result in a reflex sympathetic dystrophy, with progressive development of pain, vasomotor, disturbances, and even trophic changes, particularly if the block failed to produce the desired anesthesia and the accompanying sympathetic blockade. Several of the cases of neurological sequelae reported in the literature after brachial block anesthesia showed the classic signs and symptoms of "causalgia", and in several of these complete relief was provided by a stellate ganglion block. Certainly, this mechanism should be kept in mind when a patient develops a delayed postoperative onset of burning pain, especially since reflex sympathetic dystrophy responds completely to *early* definitive therapy.

In summary, patients complaining of persistant paresthesias, aching, sensory disturbances and motor weakness following brachial plexus anesthesia should be carefully investigated by neurological and electromyographic examination to determine whether the nerve block procedure played an etiologic role, It is important to realize that the symptoms need not appear immediately postoperatively and, in fact, may not become manifest until 7–14 days later. If a hematoma is evident, surgical exploration and evacuation should be seriously considered. In many cases physiotherapy may be appropriate to prevent muscle atrophy while awaiting recovery, for recovery is the rule rather than the exception. A trial of sympathetic blocks may be appropriate to remove any sympathetic mechanism and to provide optimal blood flow to the recovering nerve or nerves.

Obviously the only specific treatment of the neurological complications of brachial plexus block is prevention: careful positioning of the patient and the extremities to be blocked, the careful use of needles of the appropriate diameter, length, and bevel, the production of a single paresthesia, with careful attention to the patient's response during the injection, the use of the lowest concentration of local anesthetic required for the particular procedure and avoidance of epinephrine unless necessary to prevent systemic toxicity; and finally, careful protection of the anesthetized extremity before, during and after the surgical procedure until the extremity has completely recovered. Obviously, the single most important prophylactic measure is intimate knowledge of the anatomy and complete understanding of the anesthetic technique being utilized, and that is the ultimate goal of the present work.

Infection

Infection has not been reported as a complication of brachial plexus block by any of the various approaches. Hopefully, this is, at least in part, due to strict adherence to principles of sterile technique, although an additional explanation may be the rather potent antimicrobial activity of the local anesthetic agents themselves. That local anesthetic drugs possess antibacterial properties was first suggested in 1909 by Jonnesco. Nearly half a century later Murphey demonstrated that 0.5% tetracaine was toxic to pseudomonas, and

shortly thereafter Kleinfeld and Ellis also reported that tetracaine and cocaine inhibited the growth of Staphylococcus Albus, Pseudomonas Aeruginosa, and Candida Albicans. More recently Schmidt and Rosenkranz have demonstrated that the spectrum of the antimicrobial activity of local anesthetics is much broader than anticipated, with 22 of 23 species of gram negative bacteria studied and more than half of the 5 species of gram positive bacteria being sensitive to 2% procaine and lidocaine. Even the tubercle bacillus was inhibited by both of these agents. The mechanism of the antimicrobial activity of local anesthetics is unclear, but it has been postulated that they may interfere with protein production in the cytoplasmic membrane of these pathogenic organisms.

In any case, sterile technique must still be carefully followed in carrying out a brachial plexus block, or for that matter, any regional anesthetic technique: the skin should be prepared carefully with an appropriate antiseptic solution, and gloves should be worn in carrying out the actual procedure. However, in preparing a patient for an axillary block, the axillary hair should *not* be shaved unless the individual ordinarily shaves the axilla for reasons of personal hygiene; for it has been demonstrated that shaving the operative site prior to surgery actually increases, rather than decreases, the rate of infection (see Chapter IV for additional details).

Broken needles

Moore reported breaking a stainless steel, reusable needle while seeking paresthesias for a brachial plexus block. As rare as such an occurrence is, because most needles break at the junction of the hub and shaft, both Bonica and Moore have always advocated the use of a security bead needle, the "bead" of which prevents the anesthetist from inserting the needle all the way to that point. Thus, if a security bead needle does break at the junction of the shaft and hub, it is easily removed.

The weakness at the hub-shaft junction in reusable needles was due to the fact that the metal tip of the hub was mechanically "crimped" onto the shaft at that point. The shaft of the disposable needles advocated in Chapter IV are glued to the translucent plastic hub with epoxy over a significant distance, so weakness at this junction should not exist with these needles. However, the hub-shaft junction can be weakened dangerously if the shaft of the needle is bent and then straightened, an event that is much more likely if the needle gauge is too fine and/or the length too short. This is illustrated by the report of Snow and his co-workers who utilized a disposable 25 gauge, ⅝ths inch needle to carry out an axillary block. Because of the short shaft of the needle, it had to be inserted all the way to the hub, and upon one such insertion, the needle broke at the point where it joins the hub, and the distal part of the needle remained in the patient's axilla. Repeated efforts to retrieve the needle surgically failed, and the needle remained in place. The report does not state whether the needle had bent upon insertion, but this is one of the problems of such a fine needle, and one of the reasons why the author advocates the use of the 22 gauge, 1½ inch needle.

To prevent the breaking of needles, the following recommendations are made: with rare exceptions, no less than 22 gauge, 1½ inch needles should be utilized for brachial plexus block. The length is sufficient that the needle need never be inserted all the way to the hub and the diameter sufficient that the needle should not bend. If a needle bends, it should not be straightened and reused, but discarded and replaced with another needle. Changes of needle direction should be made only after the needle has been withdrawn to the subcutaneous tissues and finally, if bone is contacted unintentionally, the needle should be examined carefully, and if damaged, it should be replaced.

References & Bibliographpy

Accardo, N. J. and Adriani, J.: Brachial Plexus Block: A Simplified Technique Using the Axillary Route. South. Med. J. 42: 920-923, 1949.

Adriani, J., Parmley, J., Ochsner, A.: Fatalities and Complications After Attempts at Stellate Ganglion Blocks. Surgery 36: 615-619, 1952.

Adriani, J., and Evangelou, M.: Complications of Regional Anesthesia. Current Researches in Anesth. & Analg. 34: 96-101, 1955.

Adriani, J.: Comment. Anesth. & Analg. 49:182-183, 1970.

Adriani, J.: Etiology and Management of Adverse Reactions to Local Anesthetics. Int. Anesthesiol. Clin. 10:127-151, 1972.

Albert, J. and Löfström, B.: Bilateral Ulnar Nerve Blocks for the Evaluation of Local Anaesthetic Agents: II. Tests With a New Longer-Acting Agent, LAC-43, and With Tetracaine. Acta Anaesth. Scand. 9: 1-12, 1965.

Aldrete, J. A., and Johnson, D. A.: Evaluation of Intracutaneous Testing for Investigation of Allergy to Local Anesthetic Agents. Anesth. & Analg. 49: 173-183, 1970.

Barutell, C., Vidal, F., Raich, M. and Montero, A.: A Neurological Complication Following Interscalene Brachial Plexus Block. Anesthesia 35: 365-367, 1980.

Beaven, M. A.: Anaphylactoid Reactions to Anesthetic Drugs. Anesthesiology 55:3-5, 1981.

Benumof, J. L. and Semenza, J.: Total Spinal Anesthesia Following Intrathoracic Intercostal Nerve Blocks. Anesthesiology 43: 124-125, 1973.

Bonica, J. J., Moore, D. C. & Orlov, M.: Brachial Plexus Block Anesthesia. Am. J. Surg. 78: 65-79, 1949.

Bonica, J. J.: The Management of Pain, Philadelphia. Lea & Febiger, 1953, pp. 216 and 223.

Bonica, J. J.: Quoted in Chapter V: High and/or Total Spinal (Subarachnoid) Block Following Peripheral Nerve Block, pp. 48-54. In Moore, D. C.: Complications of Regional Anesthesia. Charles C. Thomas Publishers, Springfield, 1955.

Brand, L. and Papper, E. M.: A Comparison of Supraclavicular and Axillary Techniques for Brachial Plexus Blocks. Anesthesiology 22: 226-229, 1961.

Brandao, R. C., Lerner, S., Rangel, W., and Rodriquez, I.: Brachial Plexus Block [Brasilian]. Revista Brasileira de Anestesiologia 21: 420-425 (3), 1971.

Brierley, J. B., and Field, E. J.: The Fate of an Intraneural Injection as Demonstrated by the Use of Radio-Active Phosphorus. J. Neurol. Neurosurg. Psychiat. 12: 86, 1949.

Britt, B. A. and Gordon, R. A.: Peripheral Nerve Injuries Associated with Anesthesia. Can. Anaes. Soc. J. 11: 514-536, 1964.

Brown, D. T., Beamish, D., and Wildsmith, J. A. W.: Allergic Reaction to an Amide Local Anesthetic. Br. J. Anaesth. 53: 435-437, 1981.

Brunner, F.: Phrenic Nerve Paralysis after Plexus Anesthesia [German]. Zentralbl. f. Chir. 40: 1104-1106, 1913.

Budinger, K.: Paralysis after Chloroform Narcosis [German]. Arch. f. Klin. Chir. 47: 121-145, 1894.

Burkhardt, V.: The Place of Brachial Plexus Analgesia in Modern Anesthesia Practice. Recent Progress in Anesthesiology and Resuscitation. Excerpta Medica pp. 57-58, 1974.

Capelle, W.: Anesthesia of the Brachial Plexus: The Dangers and How to Avoid Them. [German]. Beitr. z. Klin. Chir. 104: 122-139, 1917.

Clausen, E. G.: Postoperative ("Anesthetic") Paralysis of the Brachial Plexus. Surg. 12: 933, 1942.

Cobcroft, M. D.: Bilateral Spread of Analgesia with Interscalene Brachial Plexus Block. Anesthesia and Intensive Care 4 (1): 73, 1976.

Covino, B. G., Vassallo, H. G.: Chapter 6, General Pharmacological and Toxicological Aspects of Local Anesthetic Agents, pp. 123-148. In Local Anesthetics: Mechanisms of Action and Clinical Use. Grune & Stratton, New York, 1976.

de Jong, R. H.: Axillary Block of the Brachial Plexus. Anesthesiology 22: 215-225, 1961.

de Jong, R. H., Heavner, J. E.: Local Anesthetic Seizure Prevention: Diazepam vs. Pentobarbitol. Anesthesiology 30: 449-457, 1972.

de Jong, R. H.: Local Anesthetics. Chapter 14. Adverse Effects, p. 254. Charles C. Thomas Publishers, Springfield, 1977.

Denlinger, J. K.: Pneumothorax. Chapter 12 in Complications in Anesthesiology by Orkin, F. K. and Cooperman, L. H. J. B. Lippencott Co., Philadelphia, 1983.

Denny-Brown, D. and Brenner, C.: Paralysis of Nerve Induced by Direct Pressure and by Tourniquet. Archives of Neurology and Psychiatry 51: 1-26, 1944.

Denny-Brown, D. and Doherty, M. M.: Effects of Transient Stretching of Peripheral Nerve. Archives of Neurology and Psychiatry 54: 116-129, 1945.

de Pablo, J. S. and Diez-Mallo, J.: Experience With Three Thousand Cases of Brachial Plexus Block: Its Dangers. Ann. Surg. 128: 956-964, 1948.

DeSwarte, R. D.: Drug Allergy. In Patterson, R., Editor: Allergic Diseases. Diagnoses and Management. Philadelphia, 1972, J. B. Lippincott Co., pp. 393-494.

Dhunér, K. G.: Nerve Injuries Following Operations: A Survey of Cases Occuring During A Six-Year Period. Anesthesiology 11: 289-293, 1950.

Dhunér K. G., Moberg, E., Onne, L.: Paresis of the Phrenic Nerve during Brachial Plexus Block Analgesia and its Importance. Acta Chirug. Scand. 109: 53-57, 1955.

Dimond, E. G., Root, B., and Delp, M. H.: Mediastinal Emphysema Secondary to Brachial Plexus Block. Bull. U. S. Army M. Dept. 7: 718-721, (Aug) 1947.

Dogliotti, A. M.: Anesthesia: Narcosis, Local, Regional, Spinal. S. B. Debour, Chicago, 1939.

Drake, C. G.: Diagnosis and Treatment of Lesions of the Brachial Plexus and Adjacent Structures. Clinical Neurosurgery, 11: 110-127, 1963.

Dudrick, S., Masland, W. and Mishkin, M.: Brachial Plexus Injury Following Axillary Artery Puncture-Further Comments on Management. Radiology 88: 271-273, 1967.

Edde, R. R. and Deutsch, S.: Cardiac Arrest after Interscalene Brachial Plexus Block. Anesth. & Analg. 56: 446-447, 1977.

Eger, E. I., II., and Saidman, L. J.: Hazards of Nitrous Oxide Anesthesia in Bowel Obstruction and Pneumothorax. Anesthesiology 26: 61-66, 1965.

Evans, J. A., Dobben, G. D. and Gay, G. R.: Peridural Effusion of Drugs Following Sympathetic Blockade. JAMA 200: 573-578, 1967.

Ewing, M. R. and Edin, M. B.: Postoperative Paralysis in the Upper Extremity. Lancet, 99-103, 1950.

Eyre, J. and Nally, F. F.: Nasal Test for Hypersensitivity. Lancet 1:264-265, 1971.

Farrar, M. D., Scheybani, M., and Nolte, H.: Upper Extremity Block Effectiveness and Complications. Regional Anesthesia 6: 133-134, 1981.

Fink, B. R.: Acute and Chronic Toxicity of Local Anaesthetics. Canad. Anaesth. Soc. J. 20: 1-16, 1973.

Flesch-Thebesius, M.: Prolonged Paralysis of the Arm following Kulenkampff's Anesthesia [German]. Zentralbl. f. Chir. 46: 652-654, (Aug 16) 1919.

French, J. D., Strain, W. H., and Jones, G. F.: Mode of Extension of Contrast Substances Injected into Peripheral Nerves. J. of Neuropath & Exp. Neurology 7: 47, 1948.

Frykholm, R.: Cervical Epidural Structure, Periradicular & Epineurial Sheaths. Acta Chir. Scandinavia 102: 10-20, 1951.

Galindo, A. and Galindo, A.: Special Needle for Nerve Blocks (Regional Workshop). Regional Anesthesia 5:12-13, 1980.

Garriques, H. J.: Anesthesia Paralysis. Am. J. M. Sc. 113: 81-89, 1897.

Ghildyal, S. K., Misra, U. S. and Misra, T. R.: Neurological Sequelae of Brachial Plexus Block (A Case Report). Unpublished – submitted to Anesth. and Analg. – 1974.

Halstead, A. E.: Anesthesia Paralysis. Surgery Gynecology and Obstetric: 201-203, 1908.

Hamilton, W. K., Sokoll, M. D.: Tourniquet Paralysis (Anesthesia Problem of the Month 5). JAMA 199: 95, 1967.

Hamelberg, W. and Jacoby, J. J.: Pneumohemothorax following Brachial Plexus Block. Anesth. & Analg. 38: 251-253,1959.

Harley, N. and Gjessing, J.: A Critical Assessment of Supraclavicular Brachial Plexus Block. Anaesthesia 24: 564-570, 1969.

Hartel, F. and Kepler, W.: Experience with Kulenkampff's Technic of Brachial Plexus Anesthesia with Special Regard to Complications During and after the Block. Arch. f. Klin. Chir. 103: 1-43, 1913.

Hering, F.: Complications of Paravertebral Anesthesia and a Death after Brachial Plexus Anesthesia [German]. Zentralbl. f. Chir.47: 827-831, (July) 1920.

Hirschler, M.: Nerve Damage from Brachial Plexus Anesthesia [German]. Zentralbl. f. Chir. 40: 766-768, (May 17) 1913.

Hjelm, M. and Holmdahl, M. H.: Methaemoglobinemia Following Lignocaine. Lancet 1:53-54, 1965.

Hoffer, M. M., Braun, R. and Hsu, T., et al: Functional Recovery and Orthopedic Management of Brachial Plexus Palsies. JAMA 246: 2467-2470, 1981.

Hood, J. and Knoblanche, G.: Respiratory Failure Following Brachial Plexus Anaesthesia. Anaesthesia and Intensive Care 7: 285-286, 1979.

Incuado, G., Schatz, M., Patterson, R., Rosenberg, M., Yamamoto, F., and Hamburger, R. N.: Administration of Local Anaesthetics to Patients with a History of Prior Adverse Reaction. J. Allergy Clin. Immunol. 61:339-345, 1978.

Jackson, L. and Keats, A. S.: Mechanism of Brachial Plexus Palsy Following Anesthesia. Anesthesiology 26: 2, 1965.

Johnson, P. S., and Greifenstein, F. E.: Brachial Plexus Block Anesthesia. J. Mich. State Med. Sc. 54: 1329-1331, 1955.

Jonnesco, T.: Remarks on General Spinal Analgesia. Brit. Med. J. 2:1396-1401, 1909.

Kappis, M.: Conduction Anesthesia of the Abdomen, Heart, Arm and Neck with Paravertebral Injections [German]. München Med. Wochenscrh. 59: 794-796, 1912.

Kayerker, U. M., and Dick, M. M.: Phrenic Nerve Paralysis Following Interscalene Brachial Plexus Block. Anesth. & Analg. 62:536-537, 1983.

Kayerker, U. M., and Dick, M. M.: Phrenic Nerve Paralysis Following Interscalene Brachial Plexus Block. Anesth. & Analg. 62: 536-537, 1983.

Key, E. A. H., Retzius, G.: Studies of the Anatomy of the Nervous System under the Conjunction [German]. Stockholm, Samson & Wallin, 1875-76.

Kiese, M.: Relationship of Drug Metabolism to Methemogloboin Formation. Ann. N. Y. Acad. Sci. 123:141-155, 1965.

Kiloh, L. G.: Brachial Plexus Lesions After Cholecystectomy. Lancet, 103-105, 1950.

Klauser, R.: Phrenic Paralysis from Brachial Plexus Block [German]. Zentralbl. f. Chir. 40: 599-600, (Apr 19) 1913.

Kleinfeld, J. and Ellis, P. P.: Effects of Topical Anesthetics on Growth of Microorganisms. Arch. Ophthal. (Chicago) 76: 712-715. 1966.

Kleinfeld, J. and Ellis, P. P.: Inhibition of Microorganisms by Topical Anesthetics. Appl. Microbiol. 15:1296-1298, 1967.

Knoblanche G. E.: The Incidence and Etiology of Phrenic Nerve Blockade associated with Supraclavicular Brachial Plexus Block. Anaesth. Intensive Care 1979: 346-9.

Kulenkampff, D. & Persky, M. A.: Brachial Plexus Anesthesia: Its Indications, Technique, and Dangers. Ann. Surg. 87: 883-891, 1928.

Kumar, A., Battit, G. E., Froese, A. B. and Long, M. C.: Bilateral Cervical and Thoracic Epidural Blockade Complicating Interscalene Brachial Plexus Block: A Report of Two Cases. Anesthesiology 35: 650-652, 1971.

Kwaan, J. H. M. and Rappaport, I.: Postoperative Brachial Plexus Palsy. Arch Surg. 101: 612-615, 1970.

Lanz, E., Theiss, D. and Jankovic, D.: The Extent of Blockade Following Various Techniques of Brachial Plexus Block. Anesth. & Analg. 62: 55-58, 1983.

Lennon, R. L. and Linstromberg, J. W.: Brachial Plexus Anesthesia and Axillary Sheath Elastance. Anesth. & Analg. 62:215-217, 1983.

Levine, B. B.: Immunochemical Mechanisms of Drug Allergy. Ann. Rev. Med. 17:23, 1966.

Lim, E. K.: Interscalene Brachial Plexus Block in the Asthmatic Patient. Correspondence, Anesthesia 34: 370, 1979.

Lincoln, J. R. and Sawyer, H. P., Jr.: Complications Related to Body Positions During Surgical Procedures. Anesthesiology 22: 800-809, 1961.

Livingston, K. E.: Simple Method of Rapid Identification of Major Peripheral Nerve Injuries. Lahey Clin. Bull. 5: 118-121, 1947.

Lombard, T. P. and Couper, J. L.: Bilateral Spread of Analgesia Following Interscalene Brachial Plexus Block. Anesthesiology 58:472-473, 1983.

Lombard, T. P.: The Interscalene Approach to Block of the Brachial Plexus. S. Afr. Med. J. 62: 871-873, 1982.

Lombard, T. P. and Couper, J. L.: Bilateral Spread of Analgesia Following Interscalene Brachial Plexus Block. Anesthesiology 58:472-473, 1983.

Lundborg, G.: Structure and Function of the Intraneural Microvessels as Related to Trauma, Oedema Formation, and Nerve Function. The Journal of Bone and Joint Surgery, 57-A: 7, 1975.

Löfström, B., Wennberg, A., and Widen, L.: Late Disturbances in Nerve Function after Block With Local Anesthetic Agents – An Electroneurographic Study. Acta Anaesth. Scandinav. 10: 111-122, 1966.

Macintosh, R. R. and Mushin, W. W.: Observations on the Epidural Space. Anaesthesia 2: 100-104, 1947.

Mani, M., Ramamurthy, N., Rao, T. L. K., Winnie, A. P., and Collins, V. J.: An Unusual Complication of Brachial Plexus Block and Heparin Therapy. In Clinical Reports, B. R. Brown, Jr. (Editor). Anesthesiology 48: 213-214, 1978.

Marinacci, A. A. and Courville, C. B.: Electromygram in Evaluation of Neurological Complications of Spinal Anesthesia. JAMA. 168: 1337-1345, 1958.

Marinacci, A. A. and Rand, C. W.: Electromygram in Peripheral Nerve Complications Following General Surgical Proceduress. Western Journal of Surgery, Obstetrics and Gynecology 67: 199, 1959.

Marinacci, A. A.: Neurological Aspects of Complications of Spinal Anesthesia. The Bulletin of the Los Angeles Neurological Society 26: 170-192, 1961.

Merril, D. G., Brodsky, J. B. and Hentz, R. V.: Vascular Insufficiency Following Auxillary Block of the Brachial Plexus. Anesth. & Analg. 60: 162-164, 1981.

Moberg, E. and Dhunér, K-G: Brachial Plexus Block Analgesia with Xylocaine. J. Bone & Joint Surg. 33A: 884-888, 1951.

Moldaver, J.: Tourniquet Paralysis Syndrome. Arch. Surg. 68: 136-144, 1954.

Moore, D. C., and Bridenbaugh, L. D.: Pneumothorax: Its Incidence Following Brachial Plexus Anesthesia. Anesthesiology 15: 475-479, 1954.

Moore, D. C., Hain, R. F., Ward, A., and Bridenbaugh, L. D., Jr.: Importance of The Perineural Spaces In Nerve Blokcing. JAMA 156: 1050-1053, 1954.

Moore, D. C.: Broken Needles or Catheters. Complications of Regional Anesthesia. Chapter 26: 242-246. Charles C. Thomas Publishers, Springfield, 1955.

Moore, D. C.: Chapter V: High and/or Total Spinal (Subarachnoid) Block Following Peripheral Nerve Block, pp. 48-54. In Complications of Regional Anesthesia. Charles C. Thomas Publishers, Springfield, 1955.

Moore, D. C.: Regional Block. Fourth Edition. Springfield, Illinois. Charles C. Thomas Publisher, 1965, pp. 50 and 256.

Moore, D. C.: Complications of Regional Anesthesia. In Regional Anesthesia: Recent Advances and Current Status. Chapter 12. Clinical Anesthesia, Volume 2. J. J. Bonica, Ed., pp. 217-251. F. A. Davis Co., Philadelphia, 1969.

Murphy, T. M.: Complications of Diagnostic and Therapeutic Nerve Blocks. Chapter 6 pp. 106-116 in Complications in Anesthesiology. Edited by Orkin, F. K. and Cooperman, L. H. J. P. Lippencott and Company, Philadelphia, 1883.

Murphy, J. T., Allen, H. F. and Mangiaracine, A. B.: Preparation, Sterilization and Preservation of Opthalmic Solutions. Experimental Studies and a Practial Method. Arch. Ophthal. (Chicago) 53: 63-78, 1955.

Nelson, H. S.: Special Problems in Drug Allergies. In Advances in Asthma and Allergies, Bedford, 1977, Fison Corp. Vol. 4, No. 1, pp. 32-35.

Netter, F. H.: The CIBA Collection of Medical Illustrations, Volume 7: Respiratory System. CIBA Pharmaceutical Products, New York, 1979.

Nicholson, M. J. and Eversole, U. H.: Nerve Injuries Incident to Anesthesia and Operation. Anesth. & Analg. 36: 19-32, 1957.

Nicholson, M. J. and McAlpine, F. S.: Neural Injuries Associated with Surgical Positions and Operations. Positioning in Anesthesia and Surgery, Chapter 10 pp. 193-224 in: Martin, J. T., W. B. Saunders Co., 1978.

Nishmura, N. and Morioka, T.: Effects of Local Anesthetic Agents on the Peripheral Vascular System. Anesth. & Analg. 4:135-339, 1965.

Pacher, W.: Severe Nerve Damage after Brachial Plexus Anesthesia [German]. Zentralbl. f. Chir. 60: 2803-2805, (Dec 2) 1933.

Petrick, E. C.: Paralysis of the Brachial Plexus Following Elective Surgical Procedures. Anesth. & Analg. 34: 119-120, 1955.

Po, B. T. and Hansen, H.: Iatrogenic Brachial Plexus Injury. Anesth. & Analg. 48: 915-922, 1969.

Raeschke, G.: Prolonged Paralysis of the Arm following Brachial Plexus Anesthesia [German]. Zentralbl. f. Chir. 51: 2236-2237, (Oct 11) 1924.

Raffan, A. W.: Postoperative Paralysis of the Brachial Plexus. British Medical Journal, 149, 1950.

264

Ramamurthy, S.: Side Effects and Complications of Subclavian Perivascular Brachial Plexus Block. Regional Anesthesia, 1983.

Richards, R. K., Smith, N. T., Katz, J.: The Effects of Interaction Between Lidocaine and Pentobarbitol on Toxity in Mice and Guinea Pig Atria. Anesthesiology 29: 493-498, 1968.

Ross, S. and Scarborough, C. D.: Total Spinal Anesthesia Following Brachial-Plexus Block. Anesthesiology 39: 458, 1973.

Sabiston, D. C., Jr.: Tauma: Management of the Acutely Injured Patient. Chapter in Textbook of Surgery (The Biological Basis of Modern Surgical Practice). 12th Ed., pp. 288-400. W. B. Saunders Co., 1981.

Schammell, S. J.: Inadvetent Epidural Anaesthesia as a Complication of Interscalene Brachial Plexus Block. Anaesth. Intens Care 7: 56-57, 1979.

Schepelmann, R.: Intra- and Post-operative Complications of Kulenkampff's Brachial Plexus Anesthesia [German]. D. Zeitschr. f. Chir. 13: 558-578, (July) 1915.

Schmidt, C. R.: Peripheral Nerve Injuries with Anesthesia: A Review and Report of Three Cases. Anesth. & Analg. 45: 748-753, 1966.

Schmidt, R. M., and Rosenkranz, H. S.: Anti-Microbial Activity of Local Anesthetics: Lidocaine and Procaine. J. Infect. Dis. 121-597, 1970.

Selander, D., Dhunér, K. G. and Lundborg, G.: Peripheral Nerve Injury Due to Injection Needles Used for Regional Anesthesia. Acta Anaesth. Scand. 21: 182-188, 1977.

Selander, D., and Sjöstrand, J.: Longitudinal Spread of Intraneurally Injected Local Anesthetics. An Experimental Study of the Initial Neural Distribution following Intraneural Injections. Acta Anaesth. Scand. 22: 622-634, 1978.

Selander, D., Edshage, S., and Wolff, T.: Parethesiae or No Parethesiae? Nerve Lesions after Axillary Blocks. Acta Anaesth. Scand. 23: 27-33, 1979.

Selander, D., Brattsand, R., Lundborg, G., Nordborg, C., and Olsson, Y.: Local Anesthetics: Importance of Mode of Application, Concentration and Adrenaline for the Appearance of Nerve Lesions. Acta Anaesth. Scand. 23: 127-136, 1979.

Seltzer, J. L.: Hoarseness and Horner's Syndrome After Interscalene Brachial Plexus Block. Anesth. & Analg. 56: 585-586, 1977.

Seshadri, K., Masters, R. W., and Winnie, A. P. Subclavian Perivascular Block. (Personal Communication), 1981.

Shantha, T. R., Evans, J. A.: The Relationship of Epidural Anesthesia to Neural Membranes and Arachnoid Villi. Anesthesiology 37: 543-557, 1972.

Shanthaveerappa, T. R. & Bourne, G. H.: The "Perineural Epithelium", A Metabolically Active, Continuous Protoplasmic Cell Barrier Surrounding Peripheral Nerve Fasciculli. J. Anat. Lond. 96: 527-537, 1962.

Shanthaveerappa, T. R. & Bourne, G. H.: The Perineural Epithelium: Nature & Significance. Nature 199: 577-579, 1963.

Shanthaveerappa, T. R. & Bourne, G. H.: Perineural Epithelium: A New Concept of Its Role in the Integrity of the Peripheral Nervous System. Science 154: 1464-1467,1966.

Shaw, W. M.: Paralysis of the Phrenic Nerve During Brachial Plexus. Anesthesia Anesthesiology 10: 627-628, 1949.

Shaw, W. M.: Prevention of Brachial Plexus Paresis. Anesthesiology 14: 206-207, 1953.

Sievers, R.: Phrenic Paralysis from Brachial Plexus Block of Kulenkampff [German]. Zentralbl. f. Chir. 40: 338-341, (Mar 8) 1913.

Siller, J. N., Lierf, P. L. and Davis, J. F.: A New Complication of Interscalene Brachial Plexus Block. Anesthesiology 38: 590-591, 1973.

Slocum, H. C., Hoeflich, E. A. and Allen, C. R.: Circulatory and Respiratory Distress from Extreme Posistions on the Operating Table. Surgery, Gynecology and Obstetrics 84: 1051-1058, 1947.

Slocum, H. C., O'Neal, K. C., and Allen, C. R.: Neurovascular Complications From Malpositions On The Operating Table. Surg. Gyne. & Obst. 86: 729, 1948.

Snow, J. C., Kripke, B. J., Sakellarides, H. and Patel, K. P.: Broken Disposable Needle During an Axillary Approach to Block the Brachial Plexus. Anesth. & Analg. 53: 89-92, 1974.

Staal, A., van Voorthuisen, A. E. and van Dijk, L. M.: Neurological Complications Following Arterial Catherisation by the Axillary Approach. Br. J. Radiol. 39: 115-116, 1966.

Stein, A. E.: Phrenic Nerve Paralysis after Local Anesthesia of the Brachial Plexus [German]. Zentralbl. f. Chir. 40: 597-598, (Apr 19) 1913.

Stoelting, R. K.: Allergic Reactions During Anesthesia. Anesth. & Analg. 62:341-356, 1983.

Sullivan, W. E., and Mortensen, O. A.: Visualization of The Movement of a Brominized Oil Along Peripheral Nerves. Anat. Rec. 59: 493-498, 1934.

Sunderland, S.: Nerves and Nerve Injuries. Churchill & Livingstone, New York, 1978.

Swerdlow, M.: Complications of Local Anesthetic Neural Blockade. Chapter 22 in Neural Blockade in Clinical Anesthesia. Edited by Cousins, M. J. and Bridenbaugh, P. O. J. P. Lippencott Co., Philadelphia, 1980, pp. 526-542.

Tatlow, W. F. T., and Oulton, J. L.: Phatom Limbs. (With Observations on Brachial Plexus Block). Canadian M. A. J. 73: 170-177, 1955.

Tsairis, P., Dyck, P. J. and Mulder, D. W.: Natural History of Brachial Plexus Neuropathy. Arch. Neurol. 27: 109-117, 1972.

Tsairis, P.: Brachial Plexus Neuropathis. Peripheral Neuropathy 1: 659-681, 1975. Edited by Peter James Dyck, P. K. Thomas and Edward H. Lambert. Saunders Co., Philadelphia.

Verrill, P. J.: Adverse Reactions to Local Anesthetic and Vasoconstrictor Drugs. Practitioner 214, 380-389, 1975.

Vester-Andersen, T., Christiansen, A., Hansen, A., Sørensen, M., and Meisler, C.: Interscalene Brachial Plexus Block: Area of Analgesia, Complications of Local Anesthetics. Acta Anaesth. Scan. 25: 81-84, 1981.

Virtue, R. W.: Brachial-Plexus Palsy Following Brachial-Plexus Blockade. N. Y. J. Med. 73: 2477-2478, 1973.

Vischer, A.: Pneumothorax with Fatal Outcome Following Trauma to the Apex of the Lung during Brachial Plexus Anesthesia [German]. Corr. bl. f. Schweiz. 48: 772-775, (June) 1918.

Wagman, I. H., de Jong, R. H., Prince, D. A.: Effect of Carbon Dioxide on the Cortical Seizure Threshold to Lidocaine. Exp. Neurol. 17: 221-232, 1967.

Wagman, I. H., de Jong, R. H., Prince, D. A.: Effects of Lidocaine on the Central Nervous System. Anesthesiology 28: 155-172, 1967.

Webster, J. C.: The Irreducible Minimum. Surgery, Gynecology and Obstetrics, 200-201, 1908.

Weil, S.: Mediastinal Emphysema with "Mediastinal Crunch" after Plexus Anesthesia [German]. Zentralbl. f. Chir.: 890-891, 1919.

Winnie, A. P.: Letter to the Editor: Ward, M. E.: Interscalene Brachial Block. Anesth. & Analg. 51: 570-672, 1972.

Wishart, H. Y.: Pneumothorax Complicating Brachial Plexus Block Anesthesia. Brit. J. Anaesth. 26: 120-123, 1954.

Wood-Smith, F. G.: Post-operative Brachial Plexus Paralysis. British Medical Journal, 1115-1116, 1952.

Woolley, E. J. and Vandam, L. D.: Neurological Sequelac of Brachial Plexus Nerve Block. Ann. Surg. 149: 53-60, 1959.

Wright, I. S.: The Neurovascular Syndrome Produced by Hyperabduction of the Arms. American Heart Journal 28: 1-19, 1945.

Åkerman, B., Åström, A., Ross, S., and Telc, A.: Studies on the Absorbtion, Distribution and Metabolism of Labelled Prilocaine and Lidocaine in Some Animal Species. Act. Pharmacol, Toxicol. 24:389-403, 1966.

Index